Y0-DLB-762

Treatment planning
A PRAGMATIC APPROACH

Treatment planning
A PRAGMATIC APPROACH

Edited by

NORMAN K. WOOD, D.D.S., M.S., Ph.D.
Professor and Chairman,
Department of Oral Diagnosis,
Loyola University School of Dentistry,
Maywood, Illinois

with 219 illustrations

THE C. V. MOSBY COMPANY
Saint Louis 1978

Copyright © 1978 by The C. V. Mosby Company

All rights reserved. No part of this book may be reproduced in any manner without written permission of the publisher.

Printed in the United States of America

The C. V. Mosby Company
11830 Westline Industrial Drive, St. Louis, Missouri 63141

Library of Congress Cataloging in Publication Data

Main entry under title:

Treatment planning.

   Bibliography: p.
   Includes index.
   1. Therapeutics, Dental.   I. Wood, Norman K., 1935-   [DNLM: 1. Mouth diseases—Therapy. 2. Tooth diseases—Therapy.   WU166 T784]
RK318.T73   617.7′06   78-18375
ISBN 0-8016-5615-X

C/CB/B 9 8 7 6 5 4 3 2 1

Contributors

Richard Adelson, D.D.S.

Associate Professor of Dental Medicine,
State University of New York at Stony
Brook School of Dental Medicine,
Stony Brook, New York;
Coordinator of Medical and Dental
Education, Veterans Administration,
Northeast Regional Medical Education
Center, Northport, New York

Milton Arnold, B.S., M.A., D.D.S.

Clinical Associate Professor,
Department of Oral Diagnosis;
Lecturer, Department of Preventive Dentistry;
Lecturer, Continuing Education,
New York University Dental Center,
New York, New York

Bill R. Baker, B.S., D.D.S., M.S.D.

Professor of Diagnosis and Roentgenology and
Professor of Pathology, The University
of Texas Health Science Center at
San Antonio Dental School,
San Antonio, Texas

Ronald A. Barrett, D.D.S., M.S.

Associate Professor of Oral Medicine,
Department of Oral Diagnosis/Oral
Medicine/Radiology,
Louisiana State University
School of Dentistry,
New Orleans, Louisiana

Malcolm E. Boone II, B.S., D.D.S., M.S.

Division of Oral Diagnosis/Oral Medicine,
University of Colorado
School of Dentistry,
Denver, Colorado

Charles H. Boozer, B.S., D.D.S., M.A.

Professor and Chairman, Department
of Oral Diagnosis/Medicine/Radiology,
Louisiana State University
School of Dentistry,
New Orleans, Louisiana

Glenn T. Clark, D.D.S., M.S.

Assistant Professor and Co-Director,
Temporomandibular Joint and Facial Pain Clinic,
Section of Gnathology and Occlusion,
University of California
School of Dentistry,
Los Angeles, California

Richard P. Cohan, A.B., D.D.S., M.S.

Associate Professor of Oral Diagnosis and
Radiology, University of the Pacific
School of Dentistry,
San Francisco, California

David M. Dickey, D.D.S., M.S.D.

Associate Professor and Chairman,
Clinical Oral Diagnosis/Oral Medicine,
Indiana University
School of Dentistry,
Indianapolis, Indiana

Contributors

Daniel G. Durchslag, D.D.S.
Assistant Professor, Department of Oral Diagnosis; Director, Emergency Clinic; Assistant Professor, TMJ Perioral Pain Clinic, University of Southern California School of Dentistry, Los Angeles, California

John C. Ebinger, D.D.S.
Department of Oral Diagnosis, University of Washington School of Dentistry, Seattle, Washington

Ellen Eisenberg, D.M.D.
Assistant Professor of Oral Diagnosis, University of Connecticut School of Dental Medicine, Farmington, Connecticut; formerly Assistant Professor of Oral Medicine/Oral Pathology and Oral Diagnosis/Radiology, Harvard School of Dental Medicine, Boston, Massachusetts

Donald A. Falace, D.M.D.
Assistant Professor of Oral Diagnosis/Oral Medicine, University of Kentucky College of Dentistry, Lexington, Kentucky

Randy L. Gates, D.D.S.
Assistant Professor, Department of Oral Diagnosis, University of Southern California School of Dentistry, Los Angeles, California

Ronald E. Gier, D.M.D., M.S.D.
Professor and Chairman, Department of Oral Diagnosis, University of Missouri at Kansas City School of Dentistry, Kansas City, Missouri

Sol Goldman, D.D.S.
Assistant Professor, Department of Oral Diagnosis, Loyola University School of Dentistry, Maywood, Illinois

James W. McGuiness, D.D.S., M.Ed.
Associate Professor, Department of Oral Diagnosis/Medicine/Radiology, Louisiana State University School of Dentistry, New Orleans, Louisiana

Charles Olivieri Munroe, B.Ch.D., M.D., F.D.S., R.C.S.
Professor and Chairman, Department of Oral Medicine and Pathology, University of Toronto; Dentist-in-Chief, Faculty of Dentistry, Mount Sinai Hospital, Toronto, Ontario, Canada

C. Daniel Overholser, Jr., B.S., D.D.S., M.S.D.
Associate Professor and Chairman, Department of Oral Diagnosis, Baltimore College of Dental Surgery, Dental School, University of Maryland at Baltimore, Baltimore, Maryland

Roger G. Sanger, D.D.S., M.S.Ed.
Associate Professor and Chairman, Department of Diagnostic and Developmental Dentistry; Chairman, Division of Oral Diagnosis/Oral Medicine; Director, Hospital Relations, University of Colorado School of Dentistry, Denver, Colorado

Earl E. Sommers, D.D.S., M.S.D.
Department of Oral Diagnosis, University of Washington School of Dentistry, Seattle, Washington

Norman K. Wood, D.D.S., M.S., Ph.D.
Professor and Chairman, Department of Oral Diagnosis, Loyola University School of Dentistry, Maywood, Illinois

To my wife
Carole
and my daughters
Wendy, Sallye, and Amy

Preface

This introductory book presents an overview or philosophy of dental treatment planning for the adult patient. Although segmented aspects of treatment planning are taught extensively within the various dental school clinical disciplines, frequently such information is not integrated for the student. This problem is compounded by the dearth of general texts and general courses in treatment planning. Of course, students gain some experience in this area as they develop preliminary treatment plans and consult with faculty members in efforts to finalize treatment plans for patients. Also, treatment planning boards and clinical conferences have been initiated for the purpose of integrating information in regard to treatment planning.

Actually the basic defect is not uncommon to dental and medical education. Large segments of time, in some instances, have been devoted to teaching minute detail in one area without first ensuring that the student commands a satisfactory overview of the general subject. This often happens in treatment planning; as a result, the graduating dentist may fail to possess a well-rounded philosophy, but frequently is biased in some direction or another.

In an effort to circumvent this shortcoming, we have chosen not to devote chapters to individual clinical disciplines but have attempted to present an integrated approach to treatment planning throughout.

As one contemplates writing a textbook many decisions have to be made concerning the inclusion and exclusion of certain material or whole sections of information. Frequently in textbooks, peripheral material is included in such a manner that the finished product is an inadequate précis of the discipline. We have taken the stand that it is wiser to eliminate certain material that is covered more adequately in other treatises or indeed may be the subject of complete books. In this vein we have decided not to devote entire chapters to examination of the patient, soft tissue and bony pathology, individual clinical specialties, specific details of treatment, and considerations of the juvenile patient.

Certainly it is obvious that the complete and accurate examination of the patient is necessary before treatment planning is to be initiated; however, many excellent texts are devoted almost entirely to this subject, so it seems undesirable to include material that will be necessarily incomplete and abbreviated. However, eight steps in treatment planning are presented in Chapter 1, and throughout the book the student is reminded of the importance of considering modifications in treatment and treatment planning in light of all the data compiled from *all* phases of the examination. Cases are included to illustrate particular situations.

Likewise, concerning soft tissue and bony lesions, whole textbooks are available that deal with their diagnosis and treatment. Hence these will not be covered in this volume.

As with any textbook, the editor is indebted to a vast number of individuals for making the publication a reality. This is particularly true in this case because knowledge of treatment planning is gained little by little over the years from teachers, colleagues, students, and, of course, patients.

Specifically, it is my duty and very great pleasure to express my formal gratitude to the contributors of chapters to this volume. All proved to be extremely cooperative and expended much time and effort to ensure that their material reflected the main philosophy of the book and dovetailed with details in related chapters.

It is my particular pleasure to extend my grateful thanks to Mr. James Cockerill of the Department of Dental Photography of Loyola University School of Dentistry. Mr. Cockerill undertook the arduous task of printing most of the photographs for the book. Jim's cooperation, expertise, and attention to detail was a refreshing experience indeed.

Plaudits also are due Mrs. Sheila Wilhelmus who so diligently and painstakingly typed the numerous rough drafts and also the final manuscript. Much to her credit was her ability to understand and overlook my crankiness during certain periods of stress.

My wife, Carole Wood, deserves a kind word for her understanding and patience during these months of labor. More materially, Carole contributed several line drawings and also completed some typing of the manuscript in emergency situations.

I gratefully thank Dr. Raffaele Suriano, Dean of Loyola University School of Dentistry, for his quiet support and for easing our task in many ways.

Norman K. Wood

Contents

PART I   AN OVERVIEW

1 Introduction, 3
Norman K. Wood

2 Pragmatic versus idealistic treatment planning, 9
Norman K. Wood

3 The general dentist: coordinator of the team, 12
Bill R. Baker

PART II   MODIFYING FACTORS IN TREATMENT PLANNING

4 Dental and oral findings, 19
Glenn T. Clark
Norman K. Wood

5 Medical considerations: renal, endocrine, infectious, bone, joint, and neurologic diseases, 43
Donald A. Falace

6 Medical considerations: cardiovascular, respiratory, gastrointestinal, and hematologic systems, xerostomia, and irradiation, 81
Ellen Eisenberg

7 Behavioral considerations, 131
Richard Adelson

8 Preventive and prognostic considerations, 151
Milton Arnold

9 Additional considerations, 171
   David M. Dickey

PART III SEQUENCING, CLASSIFICATION, CASE ANALYSIS, AND CASE TREATMENT PLANNING

10 Sequence of treatment and flexibility, 179
   Earl E. Sommers
   John C. Ebinger

11 The simple case, 192
   Norman K. Wood
   Sol Goldman

12 The interdisciplinary tooth replacement case, 200
   Charles H. Boozer
   Ronald A. Barrett
   James W. McGuiness
   Norman K. Wood

13 The difficult case with alternative approaches, 215
   C. Daniel Overholser, Jr.

14 The transitional case, 235
   Richard P. Cohan
   Norman K. Wood

PART IV MISCELLANEOUS

15 Innovative approaches, 263
   Ronald E. Gier

16 Case presentation, 282
   John C. Ebinger
   Earl E. Sommers

17 Maintenance, 296
   Randy L. Gates
   Daniel G. Durchslag

18 Pitfalls in treatment planning and patient management, 305
   Charles Olivieri Munroe

PART V RECORDS

19 Problem-oriented dental record system—an alternative, 323
Roger G. Sanger
Malcolm E. Boone II

20 Problem-oriented record system—case example, 334
Malcolm E. Boone II
Roger G. Sanger

PART I

An overview

1

Introduction

Norman K. Wood

Just as success generally brings happiness to individuals, successful treatment of dental disorders brings satisfaction to dentists and their patients.

In order to achieve success consistently in dentistry, it is essential that the *best* possible treatment plan be developed and implemented for *each* of our patients in dental practice. This cannot be accomplished by quickly "eyeballing" a case and then rushing ahead with treatment of some kind. Rather, it is necessary to *systematically* "work up" each patient completely and to develop a suitable treatment plan before any irreversible work is attempted.

Treatment planning is a practical *science* requiring the clinician to follow logical scientific steps. However, it is also an *art*, as much experience is needed to become proficient and successful in treatment planning.

Treatment planning may be considered as an exercise in problem solving and may be conveniently divided into eight steps:

1. Initial classification of patient
2. Collection of data (examination of patient)
3. Analysis and synthesis of data (establishing the diagnosis)
4. Development of a treatment plan
5. Case presentation and adoption of a treatment plan
6. Implementation of the treatment plan
7. Monitoring
8. Record keeping

INITIAL CLASSIFICATION OF PATIENT

After the usual pleasantries are exchanged, it is essential that the patient's chief complaint or reason for coming be established. If necessary, ask the patient, "Why are you here to see me?" This information will enable you to immediately categorize the patient into one of the following classifications:

1. A patient presenting for emergency treatment only
2. A new patient desiring complete oral care
3. A combination of both of the above
4. A recall patient desiring a periodic examination and care

Obviously the order as well as the number of steps you follow in the workup will vary, primarily depending on the patient classification. Thus it is essential that the classification be established at the onset.

For example, a tourist suffering from a toothache while spending a day or two in your locality comes to you for relief of pain and interim treatment. In such an instance it is quite improper to put the patient through the time and expense of a complete workup including full-mouth roentgenograms. An abbreviated medical history, ensuring that there are no systemic conditions that would contraindicate your emergency treatment, is sufficient. Usually just a roentgenogram of the troublesome tooth is all that is required unless an extraction seems necessary, and then the desirability of such treatment must be weighed in light of the condition of the other teeth and periodontium.

Likewise a regular patient returning for a 6-month periodic maintenance examination does not require the retaking of the complete medical history because this is already recorded in his chart. Rather, a simple question or two bringing the history up-to-date is all that is required; for example, "Mrs. White, has your medical status changed in any way since you last visited us? Have you had any recent illnesses or hospitalizations? Have your medications been modified in any way? Do you have any oral problems that you are aware of?"

On the other hand, a new patient who presents for complete oral care is an entirely different proposition, and in such an instance a complete orderly workup with the maintenance of complete records is mandatory!

COLLECTION OF DATA (EXAMINATION OF PATIENT)

Although all eight steps are important in treatment planning, patient examination is a basic and most important step. It is impossible to consistently diagnose correctly or, in turn, to develop the correct treatment plan if the examination is faulty or incomplete. Hence a haphazard approach is to be condemned, while a systematic stepwise approach is to be considered mandatory. To illustrate the importance of this philosophy, imagine the problems a dentist may unnecessarily encounter if he fails to complete an adequate, orderly history for each patient. Such a dentist may well find himself in the untenable situation of having a patient inform the dentist *after* an extraction that he has rheumatic heart disease. If the dentist had known this fact beforehand, he could have minimized the chance of the patient developing subacute bacterial endocarditis by providing preoperative prophylactic antibiotic coverage. Or imagine the chagrin of the dentist that quickly extracts a painful carious mandibular secondary molar and later, after he has reviewed the case in more detail, wishes that he had conserved the tooth as a posterior abutment for a bridge or partial denture.

I use the following sequence of patient examination.
1. Cursory examination of oral cavity
2. Patient history
    a. Chief complaint
    b. History of present illness
    c. Medical history
        (1) Review of systems
        (2) Social, occupational, and family history
        (3) Dental history

3. Attitudinal evaluation
4. Physical examination
   a. General survey of patient
   b. Detailed examination of neck, face, and temporomandibular joints
   c. Intraoral examination
      (1) Detailed examination of all soft tissues of oral cavity and oropharynx as well as jawbones
      (2) Detailed examination of periodontium and dentition
      (3) Roentgenographic examination
5. Laboratory examination
6. Special tests
   a. Vitality
   b. Cytology
   c. Biopsy
   d. Mounted casts

ANALYSIS AND SYNTHESIS OF DATA (ESTABLISHING THE DIAGNOSIS)

When all the data (findings) become available from the examination of the patient, the clinician needs to find a quiet corner and evaluate all aspects of the case thoroughly. Facts obtained from all the modalities of the examination are integrated as the complete patient is considered. Facts that modify the case and frequently modify each other are carefully weighed. The process results in establishing the diagnosis.

In clinical oral pathology, establishing a diagnosis usually involves the following stepwise process: compiling a list of all the possible diagnoses, completing a differential diagnosis, forming a working diagnosis, and concluding with a final diagnosis, which may be rendered by microscopic study of the tissue specimen. However, in the routine dental case the intermediate steps are usually unnecessary because the common dental diseases, such as caries, gingivitis, acute necrotizing ulcerative ginivitis, periodontitis, malocclusion, and malpositions, are generally easily recognized and not readily confused with other entities.

There is another dissimilarity to the diagnosis of oral lesions. Usually there is just one entity for which it is necessary to establish a diagnosis, for example, a smooth polypoid mass on the buccal mucosa that proves to be a fibroma. In the diagnosis of the complete oral cavity, however, several diverse conditions have to be diagnosed separately.

Hence a final diagnosis for a given instance might look like this: Mrs. White has moderate caries (five lesions) with a generalized mild gingivitis. There is moderate periodontitis in the mandibular incisor region, and a class 1 occlusion is present throughout. Thus when one considers the entire dental case, the process of differential diagnosis is seldom needed.

On the other hand, questions frequently arise concerning the diagnosis of conditions involving single teeth that require a differential diagnosis. For instance, the painful tooth demands a consideration of all the processes that might be the cause. Likewise a complex workup of a patient suffering from facial pain will necessitate the development of a differential diagnosis as well as all the other intermediate steps.

DEVELOPMENT OF A TREATMENT PLAN

After the diagnosis has been established the clinician is ready to commence developing a treatment plan. Because the greater part of this book is devoted to this aspect, it will not be detailed here. Suffice it to say that the dental findings are of paramount importance in deciding what treatment is indicated. However, there are many other important factors that modify the conclusions and, if left unconsidered, may well precipitate failure of the case. Indeed, the dental clinician must go far beyond the oral findings and weigh many other factors before he can judge what is best for the patient as a whole.

CASE PRESENTATION AND ADOPTION OF A TREATMENT PLAN

After the clinician decides on the best possible treatment plan for the individual patient, the next step is to present the chosen approach to the patient. Case presentation is a very important aspect in the quest for success in dental practice, and a detailed account will be found in Chapter 16.

The dentist must become skilled in the art of case presentation so that the general, technical, prognostic, and financial aspects of the case may be conveyed to the patient in a simple, logical, and understandable manner. On the basis of this conversation the patient will decide if the plan is acceptable or not. If the plan is unacceptable to the patient, compromises or alternate ways of treatment may be worked out at the discretion of the dentist. In some instances the dentist may advise the patient to obtain an opinion from another dentist or indeed to switch to another dentist entirely. In addition, the patient may be expected to exercise the prerogative of initiating these latter two options himself. At any rate, it is essential that the patient fully agree that the treatment plan presented is the best for him at that time and that he can afford it. If such is not the case and the dentist forces the treatment plan on the patient without the patient being entirely satisfied about it, the stage is set for trouble at a later date. This is particularly true when the patient experiences trouble soon after treatment has been completed. If the patient has been entertaining doubts concerning the efficacy of the treatment plan all along, he will tend to be much more critical at this time and perhaps even hostile. On the other hand, if the patient has been in complete agreement with the treatment plan, he will be more understanding and will more readily accept the current problem and the extra expense the readjustment requires. In this context, establishing and maintaining goodwill with each patient is one of the most important secrets of successful dental practice.

In addition to the above functions, the case presentation phase permits the finalization of the treatment plan. This occurs when the dentist and the patient agree to a mutually acceptable plan. It is true that prior to the case presentation stage the dentist will have designed a treatment plan that he thinks is optimum for the patient, but this cannot be considered the final treatment plan until the patient approves it, that is, gives his consent.

Furthermore, this final treatment plan should not be considered sacred. As is discussed elsewhere in this book, a degree of flexibility must be built into the final treatment plan in case certain developments force a modification in treatment at a later date; for example, perhaps the dentist finds that a certain pivotal tooth cannot be maintained and that a partial denture would now be indicated instead of the anticipated fixed bridge.

IMPLEMENTATION OF THE TREATMENT PLAN

A lengthy consideration of treatment is entirely beyond the scope of this book. Detailed discussions concerning treatment may be found in any of the many books dealing with the various clinical disciplines. Hopefully, rendering the actual treatment and its sequence will successfully follow the previously conceived plan of approach.

MONITORING

Evaluation of treatment that we render to patients who are maintained on regular recall systems is a marvelous educational experience. Practically speaking, this is one modality that separates a successful treatment planner from a recent graduate. The old cliché that *there is no substitute for experience* is particularly applicable here. The student graduating from dental school or the dental specialist completing a formal training program has had an opportunity to follow his cases for only about 18 months at the maximum or often only 6 months at the minimum. Whether treatment or a treatment plan is successful cannot be determined in 6 months or 18 months—unless the case had failed already! Most complex cases must be followed for at least 5 years and optimally for 10, 15, or 20 years in order to determine if the treatment has been successful. This is a terribly important concept for the dental and graduate trainee to grasp. The fact is that trainees may easily receive a false impression when their complex, difficult cases appear to do well. Some of these cases develop serious problems or fail completely shortly after the students graduate, but unfortunately the fledgling dentist seldom learns about this and hence misses an excellent learning experience. Nowhere is this factor more applicable than in the field of periodontics. Frequently the overzealous trainee attempts to save almost all teeth that are periodontally involved. The seasoned periodontist through experience has a much more realistic approach. As a result, in the treatment planning stage he can much more precisely identify the teeth that he knows he cannot reasonably expect to save for a significant time, condemn them, and then concentrate his efforts on maintaining the teeth that have a more favorable prognosis. As a result, his failure rate is reduced and he is providing a better professional service for his patients.

RECORD KEEPING

Record keeping is not usually discussed in conjunction with treatment planning. Nevertheless the maintenance of records is now such an important aspect of clinical practice that we feel constrained to introduce it here.

Careful patient record keeping implies that an adequate record folder or chart be adopted and used for each patient. Many different types are commercially available, some of which may suit the need of individual practitioners. If not, individual dentists may wish to design one to meet their particular stipulations.

An acceptable patient folder should contain at least the following sections:
1. Secretarial information
2. Consent form
3. Physician's report (if indicated)
4. Medical and dental history

An overview

  5. Clinical examination
     a. Head, neck, and oral cavity
     b. Dental
  6. Treatment planning
  7. Progress report

Notations in the chart must be carefully entered and documented. Although the completion of all sections is important, it is particularly necessary to record all the details of treatment rendered, including a notation concerning prescriptions written or drugs administered. Deviations from the original treatment plan should be noted along with the reasons for change. (Equally important, the patient must be informed and consent to the change). Conscientious record keeping benefits both the patient and the operator and is of paramount importance in the event of litigation.

2

Pragmatic versus idealistic treatment planning

Norman K. Wood

CONSIDERATIONS OF QUALITY IN DENTISTRY

It is impossible to make a simple evaluation of the quality of American dentistry. This is partly due to the fact that the quality of dental services provided describes a wide spectrum ranging from poor, through mediocre, to excellent. An excellent service implies that the dentist performs a technically excellent piece of work and that this work was correctly indicated for that particular patient. In addition to the technical quality of the actual work performed, the question of the suitability of the particular treatment plan also is introduced.

It is interesting to speculate that a clinician who does technically excellent work may be a poor treatment planner. Conversely, the clinician who does technically poor work may be doing an excellent job of treatment planning. It follows then that a quality professional service is performed when a technically excellent piece of work is delivered, providing that such treatment is the most suitable for that particular patient, *all factors being considered*.

PHILOSOPHIES IN TREATMENT PLANNING

In most, if not all, dental schools, treatment plans are developed carefully and systematically. However, there is a tendency to slip into one of two possible deficiencies after graduation: (1) complete elimination of the treatment planning step or (2) idealistic treatment planning.

Elimination of treatment planning

Some dentists seldom or never take the time to develop treatment plans but, after quickly "eyeballing" a case, institute treatment in a spasmodic manner, giving little heed to the overall end result. Tight scheduling and shortage of chair time are usually the excuses given for eliminating this important step. Often such practitioners do not have enough time to do a complete examination of the patient either! The dentist that practices in such a manner may be likened to an architect or building contractor starting construction without first drawing up a complete set of blueprints and plans. The difference is that the dentist's blunders are not as obvious or as public as are those of the contractor. Suffice it to say that the dentist working without a definite plan of approach will continually have to redo work and will experience many failures, particularly with complex cases.

Idealistic treatment planning

The *idealistic* treatment planner holds *one* concept of treatment as ideal for *all* patients, regardless of the patient's individual needs. In contrast, the *knowledgeable* treatment planner pragmatically tailors an ideal treatment plan to meet the needs of the individual as a total person.

The dentist that rigidly practices idealistic dentistry is just as unsavory a character as his haphazard counterpart discussed above. Such a dentist frequently develops treatment plans that are based on some high ideals he feels he has to live up to, and nothing can prevent him from instituting his idealistic treatment plan even if it is completely contraindicated for a particular patient. These clinicians practice by dogma rather than by analyzing the findings in each case. Such stereotyped individuals are unable to comprehend "gray areas" but think only in the contrasting world of "black and white." To them a bridge is *always* better than a partial denture, and a cast restoration is *always* preferable to an amalgam regardless of the individual circumstance. Many of us have had the opportunity to examine their work after dissatisfied patients have abandoned them in search of a more understanding and flexible dentist. We have found crowns and bridges failing not because of faulty design or fabrication but because their placement was contraindicated in the first place, perhaps because of advanced periodontal disease or too long a span between supporting teeth.

Other practitioners feel that extracting a tooth is an admission of failure and go to ridiculous lengths to conserve a tooth that has an extremely poor prognosis and that really should have been condemned immediately. (In partial defense of this type of individual, however, I would estimate that for every practitioner of this type there are probably ten who are the other extreme, that is, condemn teeth too readily.) There is a time to condemn teeth in the best interests of the patient, ideologic or emotional beliefs aside. The converse is just as true for conserving teeth. It is important to stress that indications for either may vary from patient to patient. Conscientiously evaluated experience provides the seasoned practitioner the knowledge to make the right decisions.

It is commonplace for idealistic practitioners to become irate when the patient refuses to accept the complicated, expensive plan, and they may even order the patient to leave the office, saying, "I know what is best for you, and if you won't accept my approach, go somewhere else!"

Some of these individuals suffer from the "tooth-gum" syndrome; that is, they divorce the dental apparatus from the remainder of the patient, consider only local factors, and fail to recognize or ignore many other factors that should influence the treatment plan.

In addition, some practitioners approach each patient and the development of the treatment plan in a stereotyped manner. The patient is processed through rigid steps where the sequence of treatment never changes regardless of the findings in individual patients. These practitioners are fond of stating that "everyone deserves a chance to retain their teeth" and process *all* their patients through their extensive preventive periodontal program. The fact that the patient may have 12 children, be in financial difficulty, demonstrates +6 mobility in all remaining teeth, and has informed the dentist that he has come for the purpose of obtaining full upper and lower dentures does not deter the dentist from his preventive idealism. In fairness to this type of individual, his contemporaries who are rendering the population edentulous as rapidly as they enter the office are equally odious. Consider this point for a moment: if the practice of dentistry and the designing of treatment plans can be successfully completed by processing all patients in a rigid, uniform manner, than dental auxiliaries can do it. On the other hand, if all the data collected from each patient must be individually analzyed and synthesized in preparing a suitable treatment plan for a given patient, then dentists have to be the ones to do it.

PRAGMATIC TREATMENT PLANNING

The following guidelines are helpful in determining whether a particular treatment plan is correct for an individual patient.

1. Is such treatment indicated for this disease?
2. Is such treatment indicated for this patient?
3. Does the patient desire and accept this treatment?

Dr. Gordon Cheney, writing in *Dental Clinics of North America* (April 1977), states that, traditionally, dentists think the following formula is correct:

$$\text{Clinical skill} + \text{Knowledge} = \text{Successful care}$$

Dr. Cheney goes on to say that this formula frequently results in unsuccessful care. He suggests that the following formula is much more applicable:

$$\text{Clinical skill} + \text{Knowledge} \times \text{Quality of physician-patient relationship} + \text{Patient's personality and motivation} = \text{Success or failure}$$

The principles of pragmatic treatment planning are discussed in part two of this book. In this section the dental practitioner is urged to go far beyond the dental and oral findings and to evaluate all the factors when tailoring a treatment plan for the needs of the individual patient.

3

The general dentist: coordinator of the team

Bill R. Baker

In the era when the patient's total dental care was rendered by one dentist practicing alone with the aid of an assistant, coordination of diagnosis, treatment planning, and treatment rendered could be accomplished by one individual. This situation changed first with the advent of institutional dentistry and later with group practice and numerous specialties. Military dentistry was one of the areas first to feel the pinch of fragmentation of patient care. This fragmentation was the result of having diagnoses and tentative treatment plans rendered by one dentist and having the patient routed through various specialties for therapy. Even with everyone cooperating and working diligently to deliver good dental care, the patient often ended therapy with a result that was less than ideal. The problem was that the patient had no one who was managing the case; therefore the goals of treatment varied during the progress of the case.

The following case illustrates another problem seen in patients who do not have a case manager. It is not an indictment of one group because each person who treated the problem did what he or she thought was best for the problem. Unfortunately the dentists were seen in the wrong order, resulting in poor case management.

The patient is a widowed 35-year-old nurse with a 12-year-old son. She works in a federal hospital in which she is not eligible for treatment. Early last year she developed a toothache while on duty. The endodontist at the hospital was kind enough to relieve her pain by extirpating the pulp, placing a medicated dressing in the chamber, resealing the tooth with a temporary restoration, and advising her to have the tooth treated by a private dentist. She went directly to a private endodontist who treated the tooth successfully. On examination, he discovered three other teeth for which endodontic care was desirable and proceeded, with the patient's consent, to successfully treat them as well. By this time the patient had a considerable sum of money invested in endodontic therapy, but had neither a comprehensive diagnosis nor treatment plan. The endodontist referred her to a general dentist to complete the treatment. Because of the completed endodontic therapy, a number of alternative treatment plants had been eliminated by the time the general dentist saw her. The patient had rather extensive caries, extensive periodontitis, and required the replacement of several teeth. Because of the patient's financial status, much of this treatment was not possible. This case is in the progress of solution (to the embarrassment of all concerned) by sacrificing one of the treated teeth and compromising the rest of the care. So much better if the case had been temporized, diagnosed, planned with consideration of all factors, and the health care delivery performed under the management of one person who had a comprehensive goal in mind.

THE CASE MANAGER

In the present state of the art of dental care the one person best qualified to consider all the factors in treatment planning is the general dentist. The general dentist usually has the initial contact with the patient and has the responsibility for recall and follow-up care for all the patient's dental problems through the years. The general dentist should begin care with data gathering, which includes not only the current condition of the patient but also his medical, dental, social, occupational, and family history. These have great modifying influences on the treatment plan. Rarely does a dental patient have a "diagnosis." More often he is a person with multiple "diagnoses" who has a number of modifying factors to be considered in his treatment plan. Even though the generalist may not be expert in the fine diagnosis of a specific malady, he does have the overall view of the diagnosis of the patient. It may be necessary to request the service of a specialist in helping to refine the diagnosis. At this stage of case development, information should be made in the form of a *consultation* and not as a *referral* for treatment. It is good, responsible dentistry to seek help in the diagnosis and prognosis of specific problems from the specialist, but it is not good dentistry to have specialty therapy performed in the wrong sequence, especially before a treatment plan is complete. During this data-collection phase, consultation may be with medical specialists as well as with dental specialists. It is equally true that the consultations with the medical specialists are true consultations that connote a pooling of the knowledge of the physician and the dentist. Medical consultations require two-way communication between the dentist and the medical consultant. In the medical consultation a letter should be written to the consultant outlining the findings of the dentist and the suspected medical problem and requesting information about the status of the patient's health. The consultant is expected to be an expert in his field but cannot and should not be expected to give precise limits or guidelines for the dentist's treatment.

PLANNING PHASE

Ideally the treatment plan developed by the group would follow this scenario: The general dentist would have gathered all information, made appropriate diagnostic tests, have the patient available, and call the needed dental specialists together. Each specialist would then help refine the diagnosis and make recommendations for treatment in his or her particular discipline.

14 An overview

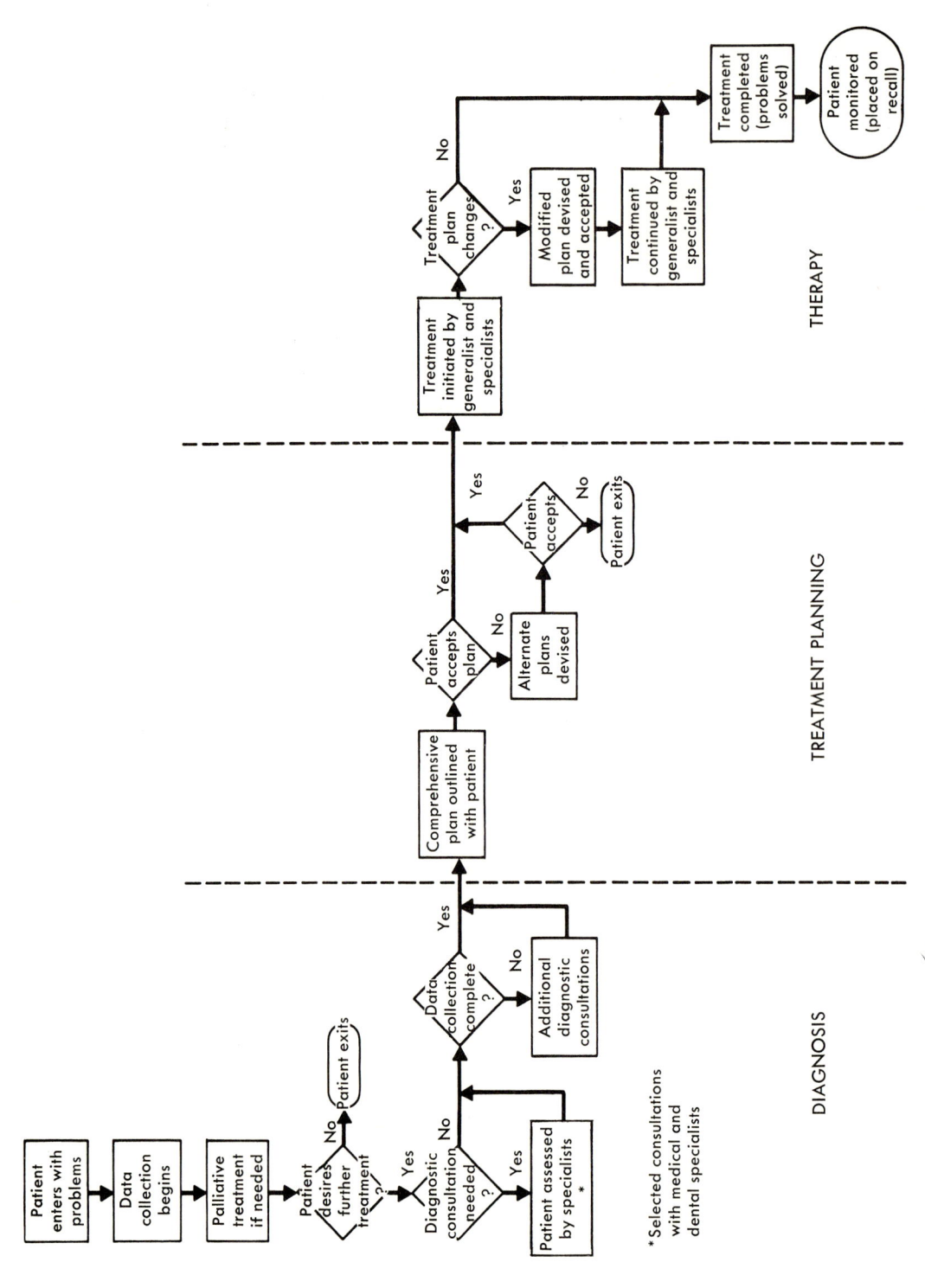

Fig. 3-1. Role of the generalist in diagnosis, planning, and therapy.

These recommendations would be synthesized, and a sequenced treatment plan would be agreed upon by the group.

In practice this is a cumbersome and inefficient way to accomplish diagnosis and treatment planning. Furthermore, it is generally necessary for the specialist to see the patient individually in his or her own office. Consultations for diagnosis and treatment planning are best made on paper. To give the specialists as much help as possible, a tentative treatment plan should be outlined. The type information needed from the individual specialist varies with the speciality. The prosthodontist should be queried concerning the selection of the desired abutment teeth and suggestions for their restoration. The periodontist should be queried primary concerning the periodontal prognosis of the teeth in question after adequate therapy and for an opinion as to their suitability as abutments. Consultation with endodontists is most often diagnostic or prognostic in nature. When the general dentist performs the major portion of therapy, only a few consultations are necessary, but several may be indicated in a complex case. The generalist should determine the order of these consultations and compile the information for the next consultant. After the round of consultations is complete, all data are analyzed and synthesized. The treatment plan is then decided on. Any significant deviation from a suggestion by one of the specialists who will be delivering part of the treatment can usually be clarified by telephone. After presenting the plan to the patient, the dentist is ready to begin treatment.

TREATMENT DELIVERY

The sequence of the treatment may or may not require the initial phases to be accomplished by the generalist. Often the first treatment will be performed by a periodontist. In whatever order specialists are seen through the progress of the case, it is desirable that the patient return to the generalist for continuing evaluation as each phase is completed. This ensures proper continuity and reassures the patient that his best interests are being kept in mind and that he is not simply being shuffled from one stranger to another to accomplish a piecemeal project. More importantly, it allows for the fact that even the best treatment plans must be flexible and dynamic. The more complex the case, the more apt is the treatment plan to require modification during therapy because of unforeseen developments. Unless these developments are reviewed and weighed by the case manager, the goal of the treatment may be lost along the way.

Follow-up treatment may be confusing to the patient. It may be reasonable that one or more of the specialists will desire follow-up in addition to the recalls of the general dentist. The necessity for follow-up care should be explained to the patient in such a manner that he understands that it is important and helps assure a good prognosis.

The general dentist must accept his responsibility as the case manager. This is best done by thinking of the specialists as consultants and therapists rather than individuals to whom complex cases be referred to avoid responsibility. The generalist, the specialist, the profession, and the patient's health profit from this integration and coordination of care. Fig. 3-1 illustrates the role of the general dentist as coordinator of the team and pinpoints specialist interaction.

PART II

Modifying factors in treatment planning

4

Dental and oral findings

Glenn T. Clark
Norman K. Wood

Unquestionably, findings obtained from the clinical and roentgenographic examination of the oral cavity, jaws, and neck play a major role in treatment planning. However, there are many other important factors to consider. These additional considerations are discussed in the next four chapters as well as elsewhere throughout this book.

This chapter deals with the manner in which *oral findings* influence treatment planning decisions. We have taken a somewhat "artificial" approach which supposes that the dental and oral findings are separate from other patient factors. This approach is necessary for the preclinical or new clinical student to gain an overview of the subject before beginning a detailed discourse. The remainder of the book is devoted to the many other considerations that are interwoven with the oral findings in deciding on a plan of treatment.

MAJOR CATEGORIES OF ORAL FINDINGS

After a complete examination of the oral cavity, face, and neck has been done, the oral findings may be categorized as follows:
1. Soft tissue and bony pathology
2. Salivary abnormalities
3. Patient hygiene
4. Pathology of the periodontium
5. Pathology of the teeth
6. Conditions of the edentulous ridges
7. Occlusal considerations
8. Conditions of the temporomandibular joint and the muscles of mastication

Soft tissue and bony pathology

The diagnosis or management of soft tissue or bony lesions of the orofacial region must be one of the first things the dentist accomplishes. This is so for at

20 *Modifying factors in treatment planning*

least three reasons: (1) the lesion may signal the presence of a serious systemic disease that could significantly influence treatment success; on the other hand, the implementation of the dental treatment may seriously compromise the systemic disease; (2) the lesion may be of an infectious and communicable nature, and the dentist will need to take steps to protect himself as well as his other patients or employees; and (3) the oral lesion may be malignant in nature; hence early diagnosis and treatment is the only hope of a cure. In addition, if the lesion proves to be malignant, the proposed dental treatment plan will usually be radically altered (Fig. 4-1).

Salivary abnormalities

The effects of abnormal salivary function in relation to treatment planning are discussed in detail in Chapter 6 and will not be covered here.

Patient hygiene

The present level of patient home care can usually be quickly determined during the oral examination. In addition, following a professional home care instructional program, an assessment of the patient's ability and desire to sustain satisfactory oral hygiene should be made. As a general rule, an extensive and expensive oral rehabilitation should not be initiated if the patient fails to demonstrate a sustained satisfactory level of oral hygiene. Of central impor-

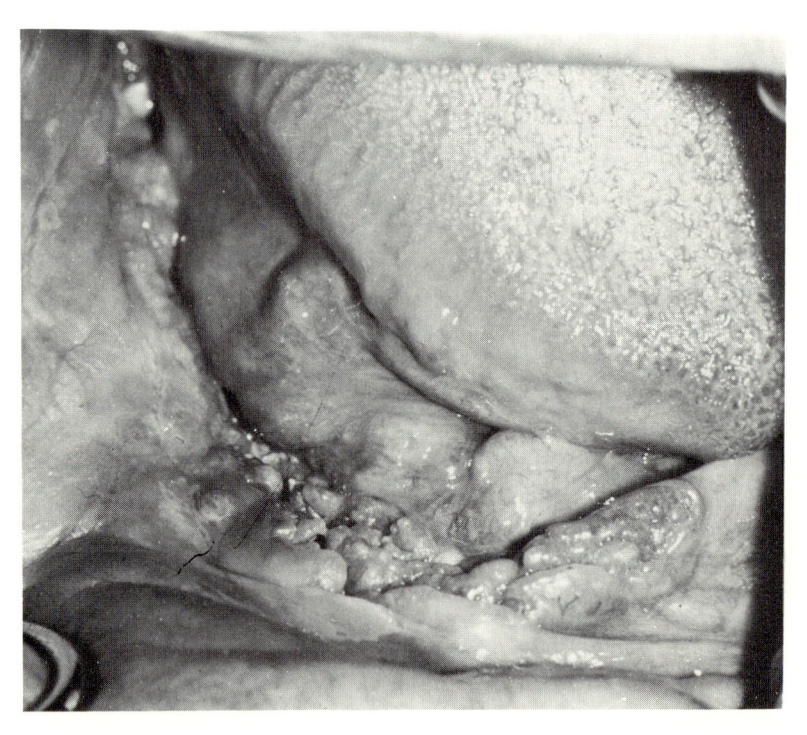

Fig. 4-1. Intraoral ulcerative lesion that was discovered during oral examination. Final diagnosis proved to be squamous cell carcinoma. Such a finding radically influences dental treatment plan.

tance here is the attitude of patients toward their teeth. The patient must care enough about saving them to justify undertaking treatment. The dentist cannot impose therapy on an uninterested patient and expect any degree of lasting success, since patient home care is an essential ingredient for maintenance of dental and periodontal health. An attitude of unconcern about the dentition may be culturally derived, since many societies place little emphasis on retention of the natural teeth. Indeed, developing proper attitudes toward hygiene may be the most important phase of a treatment plan, and failure to do so will affect all subsequent aspects of treatment.

Pathology of the periodontium

Accurate diagnosis of periodontal conditions must precede all attempts at treatment planning. It is necessary for the clinician to classify each patient according to severity, distribution, and rate of periodontal destruction. Periodontal disease may be classified as slight, moderate, or severe. Distribution may be by a local solitary lesion, several localized lesions (juvenile periodontitis), or generalized periodontitis. The rate of periodontal destruction varies considerably between patients and even at different times in the same patient. If the rate of periodontal breakdown is severe and continuous, then the prognosis is obviously not favorable. However, periodontal disease that has remained static over a number of years has a more favorable prognosis. As a general rule, the older the patient is when he develops periodontal disease the better the prognosis. If an adolescent or adult who is ordinarily more resistant develops a moderate or advanced case of periodontal disease, then this might indicate that he seriously lacks normal resistance (Fig. 4-2, A). In contrast, if a patient does not develop periodontal disease until later in life, it must be assumed his general resistance is better or the disease process itself is of a lower order.

ETIOLOGIES

Having diagnosed the periodontal conditions present, the next step is to determine the etiology or etiologies, for one cannot expect periodontal treatment to be successful until the etiologic factors are identified and minimized. The vast majority of periodontal disease in middle- and older-aged individuals is primarily caused by plaque and hard deposits on the teeth, which in turn are due to neglect of proper oral hygiene. It is known that gross dietary deficiencies will adversely affect periodontal disease; however, it is currently not clear whether minor nutritional deficiencies have deleterious effects. Other important factors may be traumatic occlusion, harmful habits such as smoking and bruxism, developmental deficiencies, and systemic disease such as poorly controlled diabetes. Concerning juvenile periodontitis, it is important for the fledgling clinician to be aware that much remains unknown about the etiologic factors; thus prognosis must always be guarded and the patient warned that the outcome of treatment is questionable.

TREATMENT

Several important questions need to be asked before definitive treatment is decided on: (1) In advanced cases should some or all of the teeth be re-

22 *Modifying factors in treatment planning*

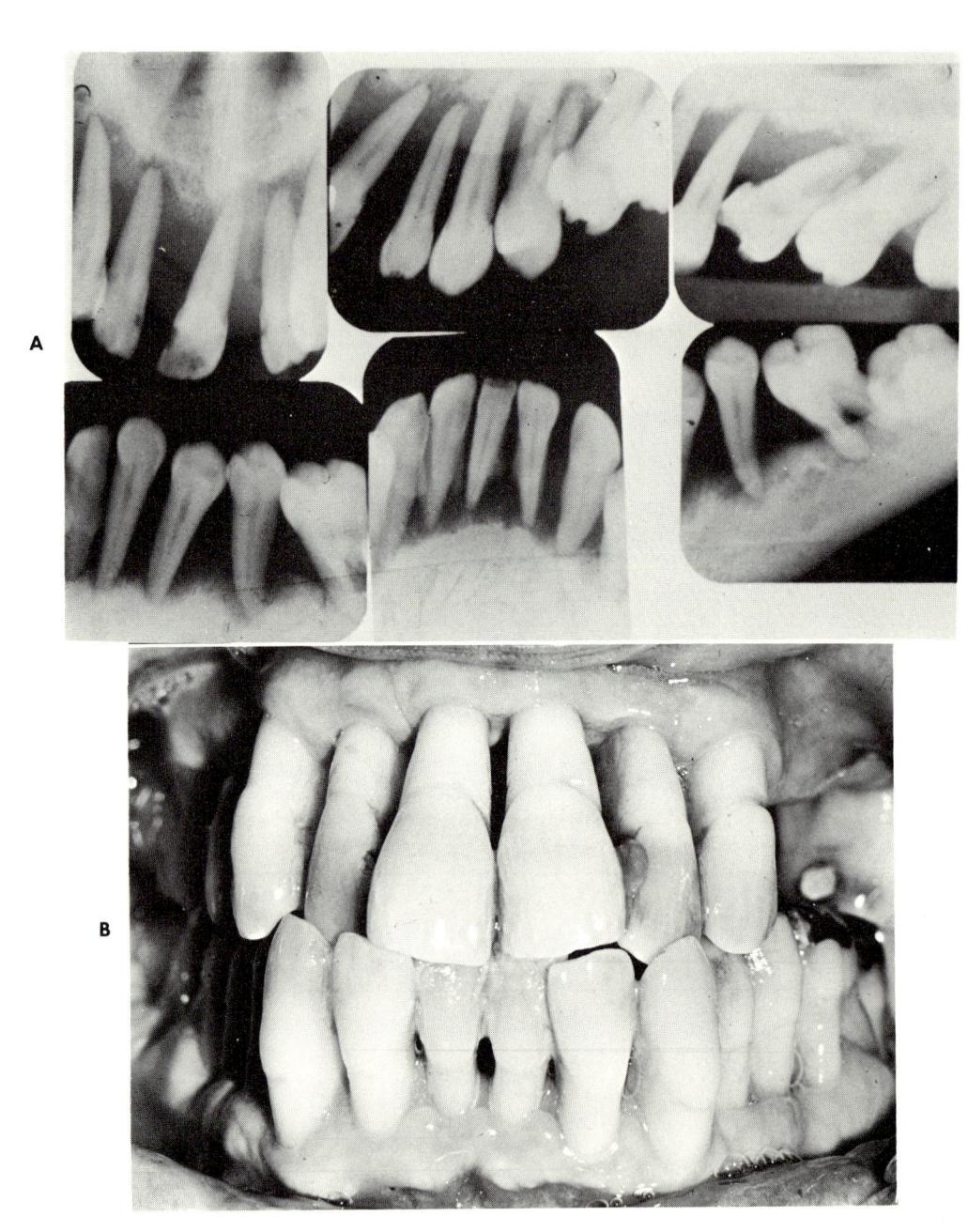

Fig. 4-2. **A,** Severely advanced periodontal bone loss in an otherwise apparently healthy 21-year-old woman. **B,** Clinical view of another patient after extensive gingivectomy. This particular patient did not mind poor aesthetics, but other patients would be very unhappy with the unsightly appearance.

moved? (2) Will you be able to obtain satisfactory oral hygiene? (This introduces the concept of sequencing of treatment. Extensive treatment should not be undertaken until the patient has proved that he or she will maintain a satisfactory level of oral hygiene.) (3) If success of the periodontal treatment depends on extensive reconstruction and splinting, does the position of the teeth allow this type of work? And can the patient afford it?

Once the clinician decides to retain some or all of the teeth, periodontal therapy should be directed toward elimination of the particular etiologic factors in each case. Hand in hand with this approach goes the attempt to eliminate the existing periodontal defects in such a way that the patient is able to reach and clean these areas satisfactorily at home. Also, do not forget the importance of aesthetic considerations in periodontal disease, such as those illustrated in Fig. 4-2, B.

Pathology of the teeth

The clinical and roentgenographic examinations will reveal the presence of pulpal and pulpoperiapical disease, the number of carious lesions, the numbers and types of restorations, and dental defects such as hypoplasia or unsightly staining (Fig. 4-3). Primary to all treatment considerations of the teeth is the amount of carious destruction evident, the rate at which the carious activity is progressing, and the age of the patient. The rate of the carious process will strongly influence the type of restoration and the type of material to be used. In some cases, advanced destruction of the teeth by caries can involve a majority of the teeth (Fig. 4-4). The treatment of choice in this situation may be extractions and complete denture construction. In general, pre-

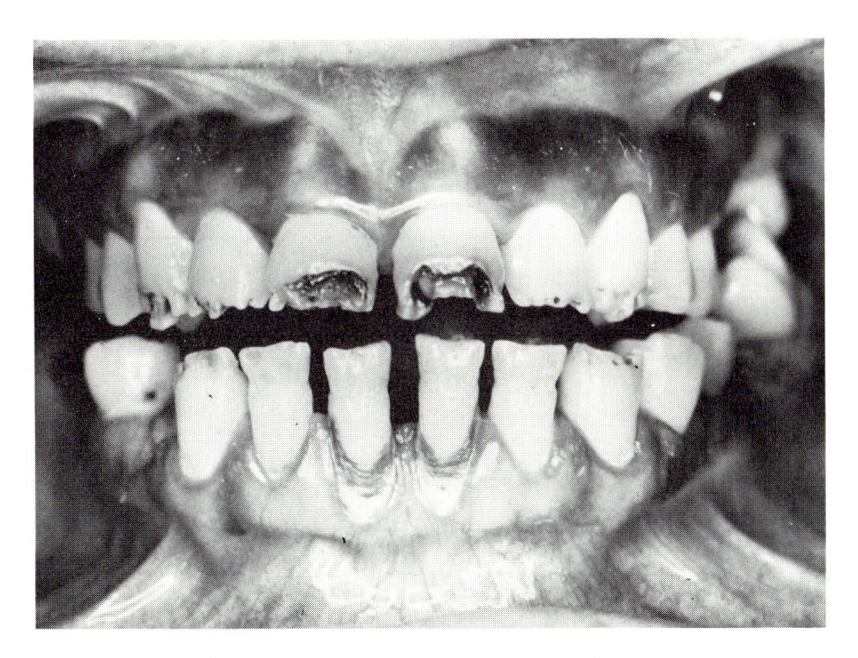

Fig. 4-3. Hypoplasia of all 12 anterior teeth probably is related to prolonged systemic insult during infancy. Note advanced carious involvement of hyperplastic areas on two maxillary central incisors.

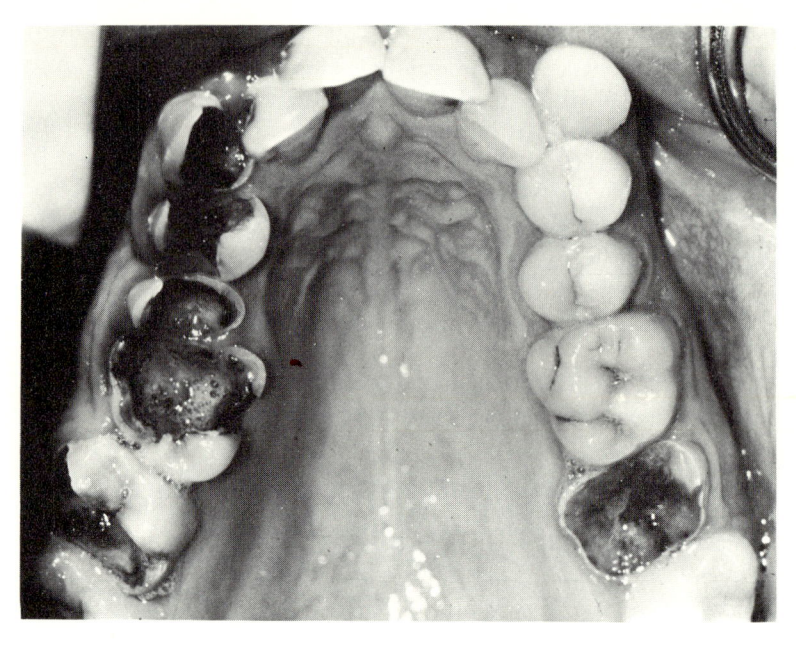

Fig. 4-4. Gross caries in maxillary teeth of 19-year-old man. Mandibular teeth were similarly involved.

vention of loss of teeth in young individuals is extremely important for maintaining future health of dental structures.

One of the most difficult problems facing the dental practitioner is that of incipient or arrested decay. Should such lesions be filled or just kept under surveillance? Some dentists fill every "explorer catch," while others wait until they are certain that the caries has reached the dentin. Patients who visit these two types of dentists successively may become very confused and may even charge the dentist with incompetence for missing cavities or for dishonesty in finding cavities that the former dentist said were not there. It is helpful to remember that a considerable number of these "explorer catches" and shallow radiolucencies restricted to the enamel surface are arrested and will never require restorations. *As a general rule*, if incipient cavities are observed in adults who have a low caries rate, they should be examined periodically instead of filled. If it appears that the patient will not keep periodic reexamination appointments (for whatever reason), then it would be advisable to restore the questionable areas. If the patient is an adolescent or adult with a high caries rate, without question, incipient areas should be restored. More details concerning the choice of restorative material are considered under "Treatment Planning for Individual Teeth."

Conditions of the edentulous ridges

Oral findings that relate to a poor prognosis for prospective denture patients prompt the dentist to make greater than ordinary attempts to conserve some of the remaining dentition. The following findings fall into this category: small or nonexistent ridge areas, knife-shaped ridges, flabby ridges, ridges in cross-bite, severe class 2 or class 3 cases, nonrepaired cleft palates, significant surgical defects in the palate or on ridges, and xerostomia. In many of these situations it is worthwhile to conserve at least a few teeth so that the patient can wear a partial denture rather than a full denture. In cases where none of the teeth can be retained and the degree of difficulty is severe, it may be wise for the general dentist to refer the patient to a denture specialist. In some instances, surgical procedures may be indicated in order to provide more satisfactory anatomy prior to denture construction.

Occlusal considerations

Decisions about treatment planning based only on skeletal classifications of occlusion will not be discussed here. Any occlusion may be anatomically and aesthetically acceptable but functionally injurious. On the other hand, not all malocclusions are injurious to the oral tissues. Occlusions should be classified and treated directly according to the functional biologic requirements and not according to any arbitrary "normal" classification of occlusion.

In biologic systems the word "normal" is used to indicate a status compatible with health and comfort. Adaptive mechanisms and the minimal demands of masticatory function in modern civilization allow health and functional comfort to be maintained with a wide range of anatomic variance. In fact, no occlusion can be considered more ideal than that existing in a mouth free of disease and dysfunction.

A uniform definition of occlusal interferences is difficult. In fact, the whole idea that cusps act as interferences is currently a controversial subject in dentistry. At present, occlusal contacts that we label as "interferences" may be divided into *supracontacts* (those contacts removed before restorative work) and *dysfunctional contacts* (those that are considered harmful and that should be removed to restore or maintain health). Harmful or dysfunctional tooth contacts can be defined as those tooth relationships that help produce abnormal jaw function. This may include an unstable maxillomandibular relationship in retruded contact position, a lack of anterior and canine segment guidance, or an unstable intercuspal position. The great majority of tooth contacts are not harmful, even if they do not fit into the "normal form." Throughout your dental career you will encounter people who have very atypical occlusal relationships, yet apparently function quite adequately. It would not be logical to tell that type of patient that he needs to have his occlusion normalized (at great expense). Decisions about treatment planning are complex enough without considering drastic morphologic modifications in the occlusal scheme when unnecessary.

Conditions of the temporomandibular joint and the muscles of mastication

It is important for the student to always remember that there are *two distinct* areas to be evaluated: (1) the temporomandibular joint and (2) the muscles of mastication.

First, an analysis for any disturbances of the joint itself is in order. The majority of intracapsular temporomandibular joint problems are caused by direct or prolonged trauma and result in a deviation in form or arthrosis of the condyle, disc, and articular surface (Fig. 4-5). The muscles of mastication are especially subject to a painful condition called the myofascial pain syndrome. This syndrome results in inflamed muscles following prolonged

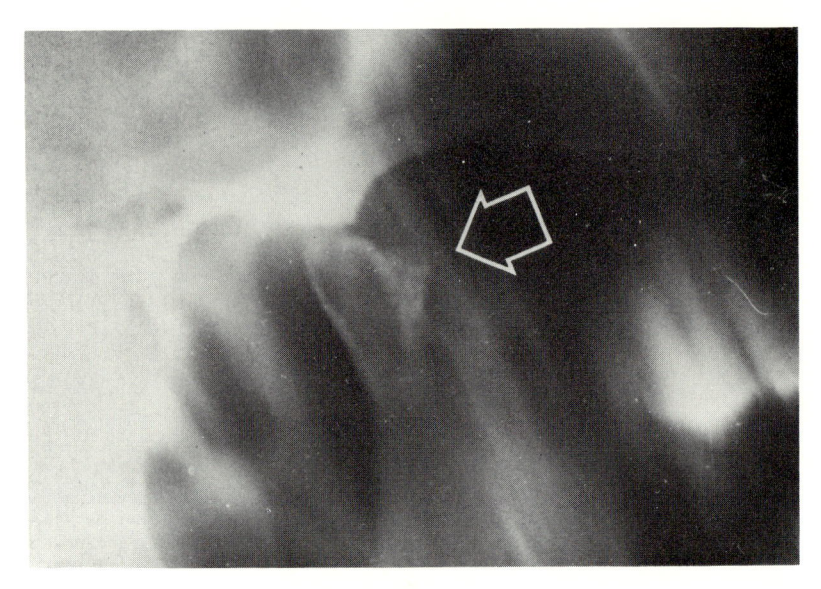

Fig. 4-5. Laminagram of temporomandibular joint showing changes typical of degenerative joint disease (osteoarthritis). Note bony spur (*arrow*) on anterior surface of condyle. This roentgenogram was taken with patient's mouth wide open.

neuromuscular tension, bruxism, or direct physical trauma to the muscles of mastication. Although this probably has a multifactoral cause, basically it is thought to be highly associated with a musculoskeletal stress response specific to the jaws.

Disturbances in the normal action of the mandibular muscles and the temporomandibular joints are a common, but poorly understood clinical problem. This lack of understanding need not be, since there are numerous signs and symptoms of abnormal jaw function. These findings can be combined with roentgenographic, psychologic, and electromyographic evaluations to provide a definitive diagnosis. The clinical examination of a patient must accurately assess the source and the characteristics of the pain and the extent of abnormal jaw function. A thorough understanding of normal function and the degrees of abnormal jaw function is necessary to estimate how much it will affect the treatment plan. Unfortunately the differentiation between healthy and unhealthy status is not clear-cut, since normal function varies widely from patient to patient. The dentist who becomes sensitive to the signs of masticatory dysfunction will avoid major mishaps in treatment planning. So often, dental examinations are limited to the teeth and the periodontium, and the muscles and joints are overlooked. If subliminal signs and symptoms of abnormal jaw function are recognized prior to treatment, one may predict the difficulty of the task ahead of time and avoid medical-legal complications. A discussion of the diagnosis, cause, and treatment of temporomandibular joint or myofascial pain is beyond the scope of this book. Obviously the management of these complex problems is much beyond the scope of the usual student practitioner.

CASE TREATMENT PLANNING

The reader is again advised that treatment planning on the basis of oral findings only, is an artificial situation. However, the fledgling student must know what options are available to him when he faces certain oral situations. The ultimate objective of such a treatment plan is the maintenance of the patient's general health, the elimination of dental disease, and the restoration of remaining dental structures to an aesthetically acceptable and functionally comfortable state.

To repeat, there are many factors that affect the final treatment plan. The dentist must always select the treatment alternatives after considering all soft tissue and bony pathology, salivary abnormalities, the level of oral hygiene, the amount of periodontal and carious disease activity, the condition of the ridges, the occlusion, and any indications of abnormal temporomandibular joint or masticatory muscle function. There are also many other considerations that may become of major importance in certain cases such as appearance, finances, treatment expectations, parafunctional habits, and patient health, to name only a few.

Case classification

It is particularly important to realize that it is not possible to develop a treatment plan for individual teeth without considering the findings of the whole case. It is also important to understand that the correct treatment for the same tooth may vary radically, depending on the overall treatment plan. It is therefore extremely useful for the clinician to make a general survey of the oral findings and to classify the case under one of the following headings prior to devoting time to treatment planning for individual teeth: (1) the simple case, (2) the tooth replacement case, (3) the difficult case, and (4) the transitional case. Such a classification, made at an early stage, benefits the clinician because certain considerations are common to cases within each of the categories. Also, early classification will prevent wasting a great deal of time over decisions on the treatment of individual teeth where an overall survey may clearly indicate extraction. Classifications of this nature should not be considered final because findings obtained later in the patient workup may dictate a reclassification of the case. Nevertheless, preliminary case classification is very useful to the clinician.

THE SIMPLE CASE

Although some will argue that there is no such entity as a "simple" case, for our purposes here we will utilize this term. If a patient requires only a prophylaxis, some moderate therapeutic root planing, a few conservative amalgams, or gold or composite restorations, then such would qualify as a simple case. Perhaps it would still qualify if a three-unit bridge was indicated under optimum conditions. Obviously, severe medical problems or financial limitations could complicate the case and cause a modification of its classification.

THE TOOTH REPLACEMENT CASE

Early in the workup of a patient it is very helpful to determine whether the patient is going to require replacement of teeth, as this will directly influence the approach to the complete case. Obviously, if several teeth are missing, they usually should be replaced. Exceptions might be made in the case of missing second and third molars if the remaining teeth are present and in good health. Occasionally clinicians will choose *not* to replace teeth even in some patients who have lost all their molars and are occluding on the anterior teeth and the premolars.

Treatment for a patient who has retained a full complement of teeth with healthy periodontal tissues is frequently quite straightforward. On the other hand, if this same patient has gross caries in many teeth or advanced periodontal disease, it may represent a difficult case for which to develop a treatment plan.

The important point is that as soon as the case appears to need a tooth or teeth replaced, the general considerations of and approach to the case change markedly. In particular, if you are going to spend the time and expense of replacing one or two teeth, then it becomes incumbent on the part of the dentist to determine much more precisely the prognosis of each of the remaining teeth. As a case in point, if a patient presents with a full complement of teeth (28) and has advanced generalized periodontal disease, you may decide to attempt to maintain all the teeth for as long a time as possible. (This approach is quite satisfactory as long as the patient fully understands all the connotations.) However, when one tooth is lost, then agonizing decisions must be made. If we go to the trouble of constructing a fixed bridge, are the remaining teeth going to be retained long enough to justify this expenditure? If we decide on a partial denture, should some additional teeth with relatively poor prognoses be extracted at this time and included in the partial denture design before it is constructed? Considering such circumstances, it becomes obvious that treatment cannot be planned for individual teeth without considering the condition of the rest of the dentition and that early case classification is very helpful.

Conventionally, teeth may be replaced in four ways: (1) the fixed bridge, (2) the removable partial denture, (3) the full denture, and (4) orthodontic treatment.

Fixed bridge. When it becomes necessary to replace some missing teeth, one of the first decisions must be whether to use a fixed bridge or a removable partial denture. Based on oral findings, a fixed bridge may be indicated if there are healthy abutment teeth on each end of a short edentulous span. The position and occlusion of the abutment teeth must be satisfactory, as should be the home care. In exceptional instances, cantilever bridges may be placed; that is, abutment teeth are present at only one end of the edentulous span. A specific instance may be when the two mandibular premolars are to be crowned, splinted together, and a *small* pontic cantilevered to the distal end. Such an approach prevents the remaining unopposed maxillary first molar from extruding and at the same time circumvents the need for a removable partial denture.

When the proper condition exists, fixed tooth replacement is an excellent method to restore teeth that have been lost. However, there are some problems encountered in fixed-bridge construction. The following are common causes for failure:

1. Poor periodontal health of the abutment teeth. It has been demonstrated recently that long-span bridges can be maintained on teeth with reduced periodontal support as long as they remain free of plaque. A tooth that has plaque and resulting periodontal inflammation will not withstand the

extra stress of fixed bridgework. Unfortunately, fixed splints and bridges render proper home care much more difficult.

2. Lack of adequate retention. Teeth with short or cone-shaped roots generally prove to be less than satisfactory abutments because they will not support the forces of normal mastication. Clinical crowns may be so short or so fragile that adequate retention is unattainable. This can be corrected in some cases through the use of posts and cores or even osseous surgery to gain clinical crown length. It is essential that maximum retention and stability be incorporated into the design of the abutment.

3. Periodontal support. The amount of periodontal osseous support is also an important consideration. The root may be of generous size, but recession may have decreased the length of root remaining in bone to such a degree that the present crown-to-root ratio is unacceptable (Fig. 4-6). In some instances this ratio may be reduced to acceptable levels by gross reduction of the length of the clinical crown.

4. Excessive occlusal forces. If excessive or unfavorable occlusal forces are present, they may cause tooth mobility and failure of the bridge. Even the tooth with a long root and good bone support will fail if subjected to excessive occlusal forces, that is, a patient who exhibits severe bruxism. The forces and effects of occlusion will vary from patient to patient, depending on musculature and occlusal characteristics such as direction of force in relation to the long axis of the tooth and degree of vertical and horizontal overlap. In some cases the use of several abutments splinted together may help to alleviate this problem by providing a greater distribution of the occlusal forces.

5. Poor positioning or alignment of the abutment teeth. Unsatisfactory positioning or alignment of the supporting teeth in relation to the occluding teeth in the opposite arch may force the clinician to compromise in the design of contour and occlusal contact of the bridge. As a result the occlusal direction of forces may be so unfavorable as to produce an early failure of the bridge.

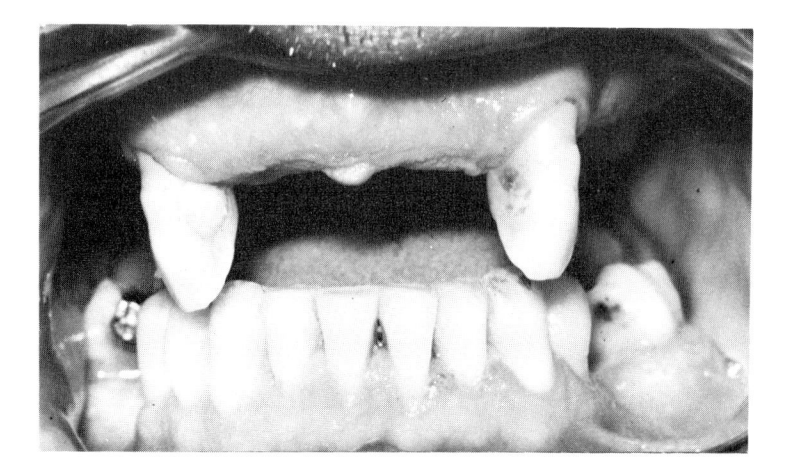

Fig. 4-6. Clinical photograph showing elongated clinical crowns of maxillary canines. Reducing length of such crowns and placing shorter cast crowns provides a more satisfactory crown-to-root ratio.

Occasionally the position of abutment teeth will preclude the ability to obtain adequate retention.

Fixed abutment design. Every abutment tooth does not require a full-crown restoration. Consider the patient who has recently lost a mandibular first molar and has experienced little or no mesial inclination of the second molar. If the periodontal health of the abutment teeth is satisfactory and caries does not involve the buccal surfaces, then a three-fourths crown preparation is the treatment of choice for the retainers. Cases where the second molar is inclined mesially or lingually may be best treated with full-crown preparations to increase retention if a bridge can be constructed at all. Porcelain-bonded-to-metal crowns are indicated if the facial surfaces are extensively involved and appearance is a concern. Remember that even if it does become necessary to use a porcelain-bonded-to-metal crown on the premolar, if it not necessary to cover the second molar with porcelain. In another situation the choices of tooth replacement might be different.

Appearance is of paramount importance in the planning of anterior fixed bridge work (Fig. 4-7). Even the best constructed bridge is considered to be a failure if the patient feels the appearance is unsatisfactory. When a single central incisor or one central and one lateral are missing, poor aesthetics can result because the teeth have shifted so that the spaces are too small or too large to permit tooth replacement of the correct size. In other instances abutment teeth may be positioned so far labially or lingually or the original crowns were so small that it is not possible to satisfy this important aesthetic requirement. Occasionally the malposition of the teeth in the opposite arch preclude the use of a bridge at all. When it is anticipated that satisfactory aesthetics cannot be achieved with a bridge, consideration should be given to the possibility of using a partial denture. For example, if diastemas are desired between the teeth, a partial denture may be the only choice.

Following are advantages of a fixed bridge:
1. They are very stable and comfortable.
2. Chewing efficiency is excellent.
3. People become readily accustomed to them.
4. They cannot be misplaced because patients do not remove them from the mouth.
5. Their splinting action makes supporting teeth more stable.

Following are disadvantages of a fixed bridge:
1. Generally much more chair time is required to complete a bridge.
2. Position of abutment teeth often precludes the construction of a bridge.
3. Generally bridge construction requires more skill and precision than does a partial denture.
4. They are more expensive than a partial denture.
5. If additional natural teeth are lost in the future, they cannot be added to an existing bridge.
6. If changes are necessary in a few months or years, usually the complete bridge is condemned and useless.
7. The placement of a fixed bridge makes proper interdental cleaning more difficult to achieve.
8. Satisfactory appearance may be difficult to obtain.

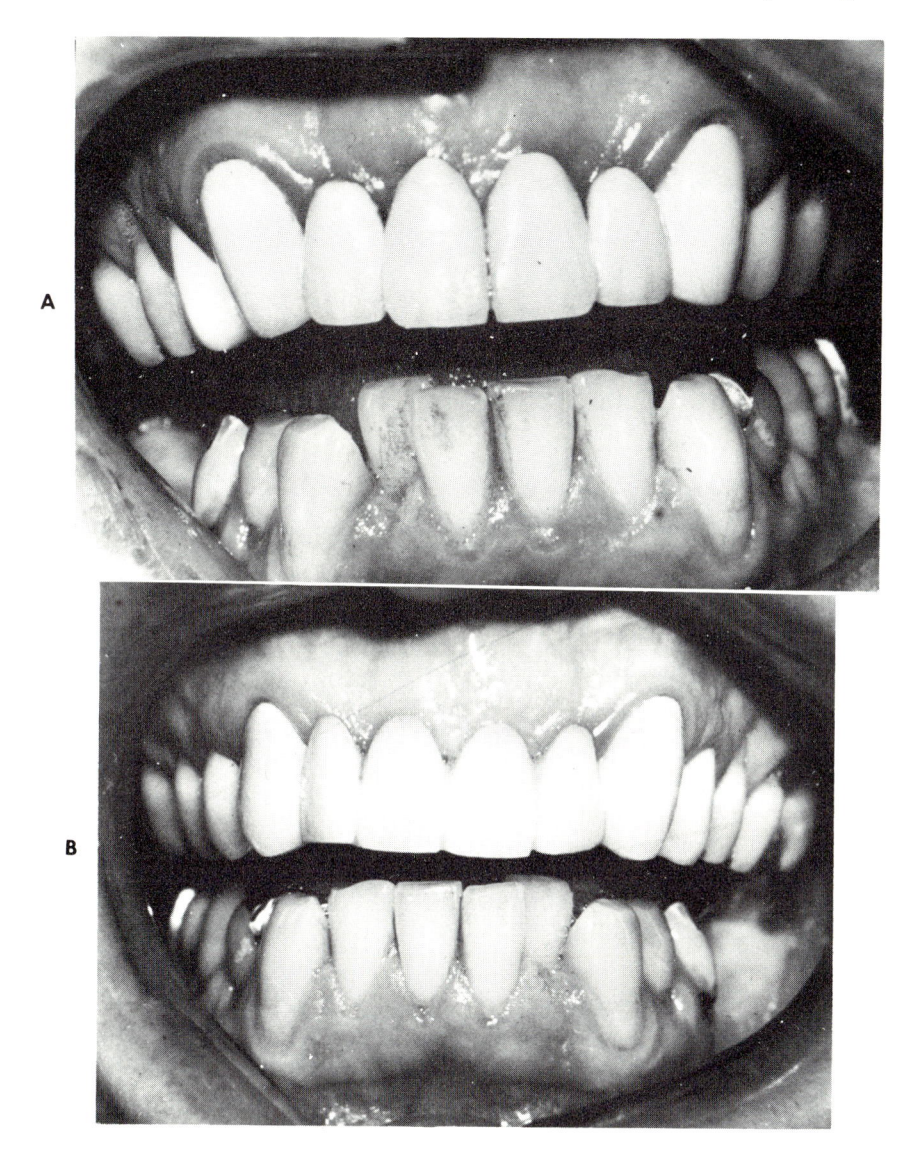

Fig. 4-7. Importance of aesthetics in fixed bridges. **A,** Poor aesthetics produced by artifical-looking teeth in perfect alignment. **B,** Poor aesthetics also. Tooth arrangement is more natural, but contacts are too broad in vertical direction.

Removable partial denture. If circumstances contraindicate the use of a fixed bridge, then it may be necessary to replace missing teeth with a removable partial denture. Fixed bridges are contraindicated when the remaining teeth need cross-arch support, when appearance and tooth alignment considerations dictate, and when there are inadequate posterior teeth to prevent overclosure.

Following are indications for the placement of partial dentures:
1. Obviously, appearance is one of the major reasons for replacing missing anterior teeth.

2. In some cases the patient is unable to masticate his food satisfactorily with his remaining teeth.
3. Some patients are masticating satisfactorily, but the remaining teeth are becoming loose because of excessive occlusal forces. Partial dentures will tend to minimize the occlusal forces on the remaining teeth by distributing some of the load to the artificial teeth, which are partially or completely tissue supported.
4. In other cases the placement of a partial denture will prevent posterior bite collapse by stabilizing the remaining teeth in occlusion, which in turn helps to maintain the proper relationship and prevent temporomandibular joint pathology.
5. In still other cases, partial dentures may prevent excessive bone loss in the opposite arch. For example, patients who wear full maxillary dentures that occlude against only six retained mandibular anterior teeth frequently experience severe loss of their maxillary anterior ridge because all the force of chewing is concentrated in this region. A properly constructed and maintained mandibular partial denture replacing the posterior teeth will help prevent this, providing, of course, that the patient wears the partial denture.

Many dentists feel partial denture construction is the most challenging aspect of dental treatment planning, since tooth loss often results in decreased vertical dimension, inadequate space, overerupted teeth, and poor tooth-to-tooth and tooth-to-ridge alignment. Frequently such cases can only be treated by partial denture construction if they can be treated at all. Sometimes a noncarious periodontally healthy tooth may require a full crown to serve as an anterior rest or to provide the proper retentive contour so that the rest of the treatment plan may be completely successfully. The available options make partial denture treatment planning very complex.

Following are advantages of partial dentures:
1. The fees are less than for fixed bridges.
2. Frequently the abutment teeth do not require preparation for crowns.
3. If additional natural teeth are lost in the future, usually they can be added to the existing partial denture. They cannot be added to a fixed bridge.
4. Repairs to a partial denture are much more readily accomplished and are not as expensive as are fixed bridge repairs.
5. They do not interfere with interdental cleaning or make the practice of home care difficult as fixed bridges might. Ready access is provided to the remaining natural teeth, since partial dentures can be removed before brushing.

Following are disadvantages of partial dentures:
1. Some patients experience a problem getting used to them. Some patients never wear their partial dentures.
2. As a rule, partial dentures do not increase the stability of the supporting teeth. As a matter of fact, in some cases they may make the supporting teeth looser.

It is not possible to discuss all of the individual considerations of fixed and removable partial denture treatment planning. However, it is important to stress that the clinician must not consider teeth as individuals but as integral parts. Frequently this may mean that finalization of the treatment plan is delayed until it is determined if a questionable strategic tooth can be saved.

Full denture. Some practitioners regard full dentures with a great deal of distaste, stressing their inferiority to the natural dentition in comfort and chewing efficiency. Other dentists become quite emotional when a patient requests a full denture: they wring their hands, condemn dentistry for having failed miserably, and sadly inform the patient that he or she will be a dental cripple for life. Generally all this is utter nonsense. Some people actually receive a great deal more satisfaction from full dentures than they received from their natural teeth. A considerable number of patients have suffered for years from the poor aesthetics of their natural dentition and are delighted with the vastly improved aesthetics they receive as a result of a full denture service. The majority of patients wearing full dentures are able to enjoy life and to maintain satisfactory physiology to much the same extent as they did when they had their natural dentition. Of course, there are patients who have a great deal of trouble with their dentures. Some never do master their use. This is particularly true of the full mandibular denture. Agreed, if a dentist condemns readily salvageable teeth in order to provide full dentures without clearly outlining options to the patient, this is malpractice and represents a grievous failure on the part of the *individual* dentist.

In summary, the full denture is the correct treatment in certain situations:
1. A patient with severe generalized periodontal bone loss is a candidate for full dentures, although this service may be delayed in some cases, providing the patient clearly understands the options and their prognosis.

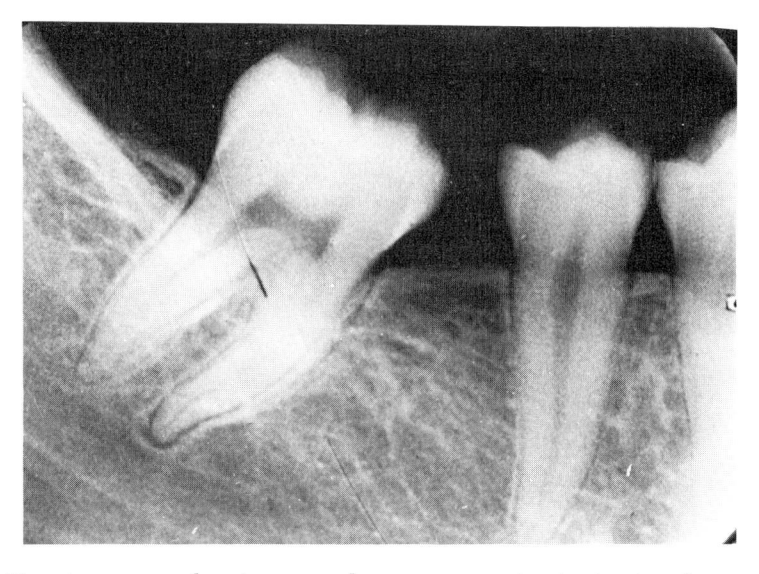

Fig. 4-8. Roentgenogram showing second permanent molar tipping into first permanent molar space 18 months after extraction of first molar. Orthodontic uprighting of second molar would permit construction of more satisfactory bridge.

2. Full dentures will generally be indicated if a patient has lost all or most of the crowns through severe decay activity. Even in these cases, several other options might be possible, depending on the individual situation. The use of overdentures and subperiosteal implants has increased in popularity over the past few years, and these treatments may also be considered in treatment planning.

Orthodontics. Occasionally in the correct situation teeth can be moved orthodontically to take the place of teeth that have been lost or to improve their position prior to restorative treatment. In patients who have lost the 6-year molars, the second or third molars may be moved forward to eliminate the edentulous space between the second premolar and the second molar. Uprighting of a mesially tipped second molar is a relatively simple mechanical procedure that the general dentist should be familiar with and use if necessary to broaden his treatment alternatives (Fig. 4-8).

THE DIFFICULT CASE

It is essential that all practitioners recognize at the outset that a particular case is difficult. Once recognizing this, the clinician can either immediately refer the case to someone who has more expertise or, if he is competent to do the work himself, can carefully devise a plan considering all the ramifications. All too frequently, practitioners realize the difficulty of a case only after rendered treatment has failed.

As a general rule the more complicated the treatment plan the more difficult the case. Habits such as severe gagging or a severely restricted oral opening may render the case almost unmanageable (Fig. 4-9). Gross maloc-

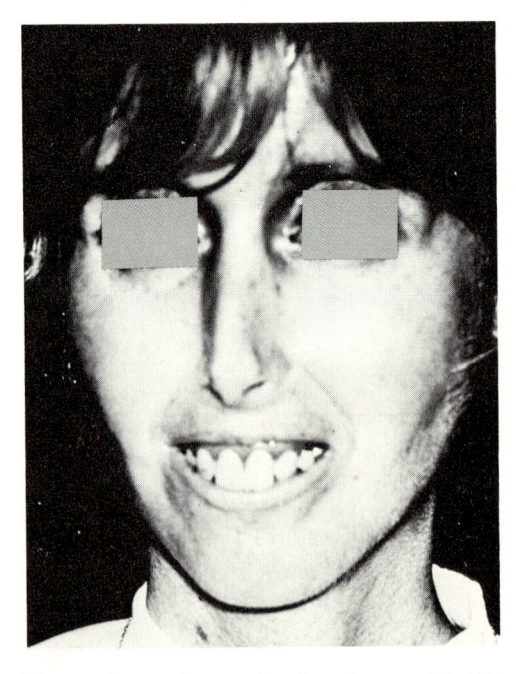

Fig. 4-9. Woman suffering from advanced scleroderma. Rigidity of lips greatly decreases access and makes dental care and home care much more difficult to render.

clusions as well as malalignment of teeth can be very problematic to solve. Closed bites and open bites will require either surgical orthodontic procedures or perhaps a complete change in the occlusal scheme using full mouth reconstruction procedures. A bruxism case requiring tooth replacement or multiple crowns automatically is categorized as difficult as are all temporomandibular joint and myofascial pain syndrome patients. Satisfactory appearance may be extremely difficult to achieve in patients with high smile lines, where there is insufficient space for proper-sized tooth replacement, or where gingival recession is marked. The key to successful treatment of a difficult case is to evaluate the attitudes and desires of the patient. Poorly understood or unreasonable expectations on the part of the patient will render a normal situation very difficult and may lead to needless legal complications.

THE TRANSITIONAL CASE

Some patients represent a gray area; that is, conditions are not so bad that all the teeth should be extracted immediately and full dentures placed. On the other hand, conditions are so bad that extensive work is not warranted in order to save all or most of the teeth. Such patients may have advanced generalized periodontal disease or gross rampant caries. At any rate the in-between status needs to be recognized. Treatment measures include the completion of acrylic partial dentures with wrought gold wire clasps to which teeth can be readily added as they are lost. Overdentures also may be used in this way. The transitional case is discussed in detail in Chapter 14.

TREATMENT PLANNING FOR INDIVIDUAL TEETH

This section purposely follows the case treatment planning because treatment of individual teeth very much depends on the treatment approach to the overall oral problem. The subject of treatment of individual teeth in interdisciplinary cases prompts the restressing of the fact that the general practitioner should serve as overall coordinator of the team. In this way he is able to ensure that the treatment of individual teeth is apropos to the general plan. Without this coordination, treatment will be haphazard and poorly designed; for instance, unrestorable teeth have been subjected to root canal therapy and crowns have been constructed for teeth that are hopelessly involved with periodontal disease.

How can the student practitioner consistently avoid these pitfalls? The answer is *by using an orderly sequential approach*. First, a decision must be made for each tooth regarding *extraction* or *retention*. When the decision is borderline or unclear, the tooth should be indicated for further evaluation. Thus the three possibilities for each tooth are extraction, questionable or borderline cases, or retention.

Which teeth should be extracted?

Although the primary goal of the dental profession is to preserve the natural dentition, there are specific indications for tooth extraction. Nor is the practitioner doing either himself or the patient a favor by hesitating to condemn teeth that really should be extracted. Of course, competence in prognosis, that is, knowing which teeth will likely respond successfully to treatment, comes only after several years of *alert* clinical practice.

Following are indications for extraction:
1. The pulp of the tooth is inflamed or nonvital, and successful endodontic treatment is not possible.
2. So little of the tooth tissue remains that restoration is not possible.
3. Root pathology is present: fracture, perforation, or external resorption.
4. The tooth is hopelessly periodontally involved.
5. The tooth is impacted and chances for successful eruption are small.
6. Third molars that require treatment in a patient who has a full complement of healthy teeth. Frequently it is not possible for the patient to clean these teeth adequately. In addition, distal pockets are very frequently found on such teeth, particularly in the mandible, and elimination of these particular pockets is very difficult to achieve.
7. The tooth is so malposed that it hinders the implementation of a satisfactory treatment plan (Fig. 4-10).
8. The prognosis on a nonstrategic tooth is guarded, and its removal will not modify or jeopardize the treatment plan. Nor will the tooth be useful in the future. An example would be a grossly overerupted lower third molar with a short conical root in a patient who is missing the other three third molars but has a full complement of healthy teeth (28).
9. The overall treatment plan may dictate the removal of a specific tooth for reasons other than those mentioned above.

Questionable or borderline teeth

The most critical decisions of treatment planning frequently revolve about the borderline teeth. It is obvious that healthy teeth should be retained and hopelessly involved teeth extracted. However, it is often difficult to be absolutely certain of this, except in extreme situations. Much of the time the criteria of what constitutes a hopeless periodontally involved tooth is relative. A tooth may be questionable as an abutment for a fixed or removable partial denture. On the other hand, it may serve to maintain the height of the periodontal bone in a critical area. This is frequently the case in the upper first- and second-molar region in periodontal cases. The first molar may be stable, but after the mobile second molar is removed, the first molar becomes mobile because the distal bone has undergone further resorption following the extraction of the second molar. Furthermore, in cases where there is a full complement of teeth, it is often desirable to keep a compromised tooth in order to maintain the integrity of the arch rather than face the complex decision of replacement.

Treatment planning for retained teeth

Happily, in patients where stabilization (disease eradication) has been achieved over a period of time, teeth do not require any treatment whatsoever, not even a prophylaxis. As such cases are unfortunately the exception rather than the rule, the student practitioner will need to know a great deal about treatment of teeth that are to be retained.

There are several questions that must be considered regarding each tooth

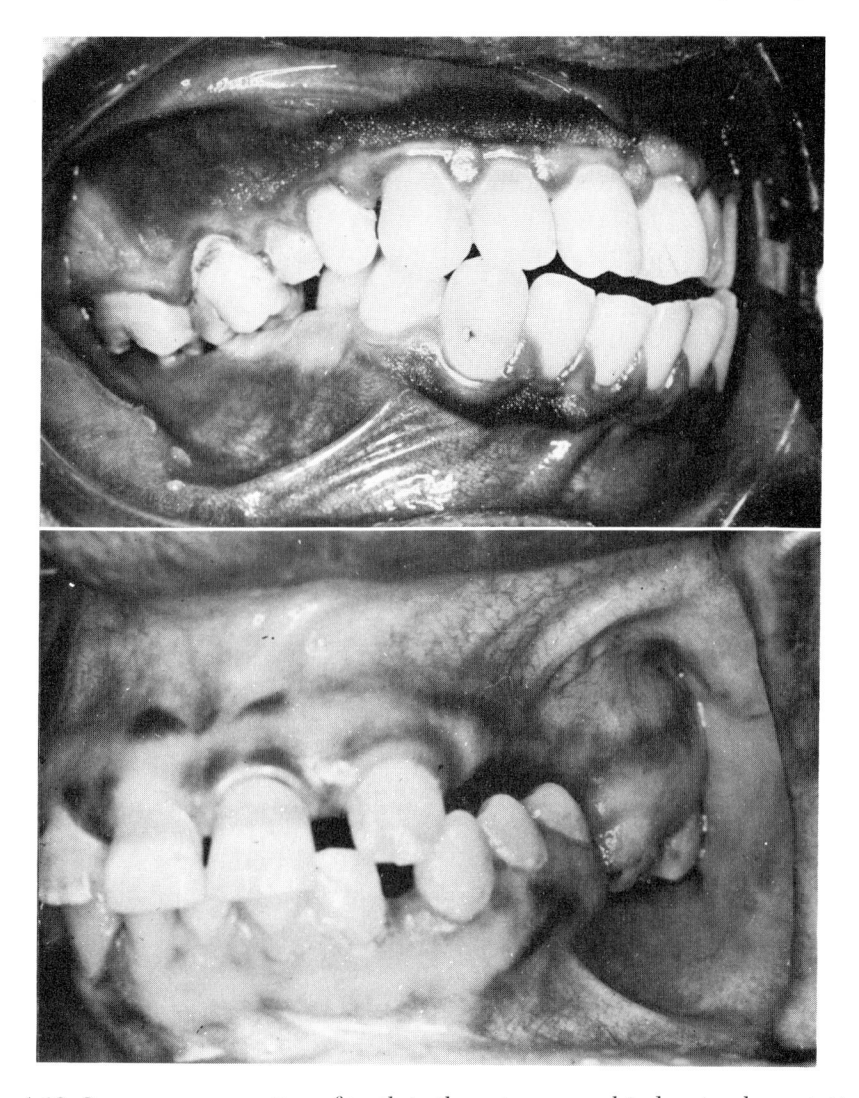

Fig. 4-10. Severe supraeruption of teeth in these two cases hinders implementation of satisfactory treatment plans. Extraction of some of these teeth is indicated unless satisfactory surgical repositioning can be accomplished.

subject to treatment: (1) Is the tooth periodontally healthy? If not, can it or a part of the tooth be returned to health in the future? (2) Can necessary root canal therapy be performed? (3) Can the remainder of the tooth be satisfactorily restored? If the answer to any of these questions is "no," then the tooth should be condemned immediately before any treatment is commenced.

If the answer is "yes" in all instances, then plans can be made to return the tooth to satisfactory health, function, and aesthetics.

Root canal treatment

Assuming that the tooth is not a candidate for extraction and that the periodontal condition, if present, can be treated successfully, the pulpal prob-

38 *Modifying factors in treatment planning*

lem should be considered next. Happily, most teeth can be treated endodontically, and at least 95% of teeth treated by conventional endodontic means respond favorably to treatment. Indications for endodontic therapy include the following: gross pulpal exposures, acute pulpitis, chronic pulpitis, nonvital pulps, and pulpoperiapical lesions (Fig. 4-11). Acute pulpal disease is evident from the history and clinical examination, but chronic pulpal diseases are not

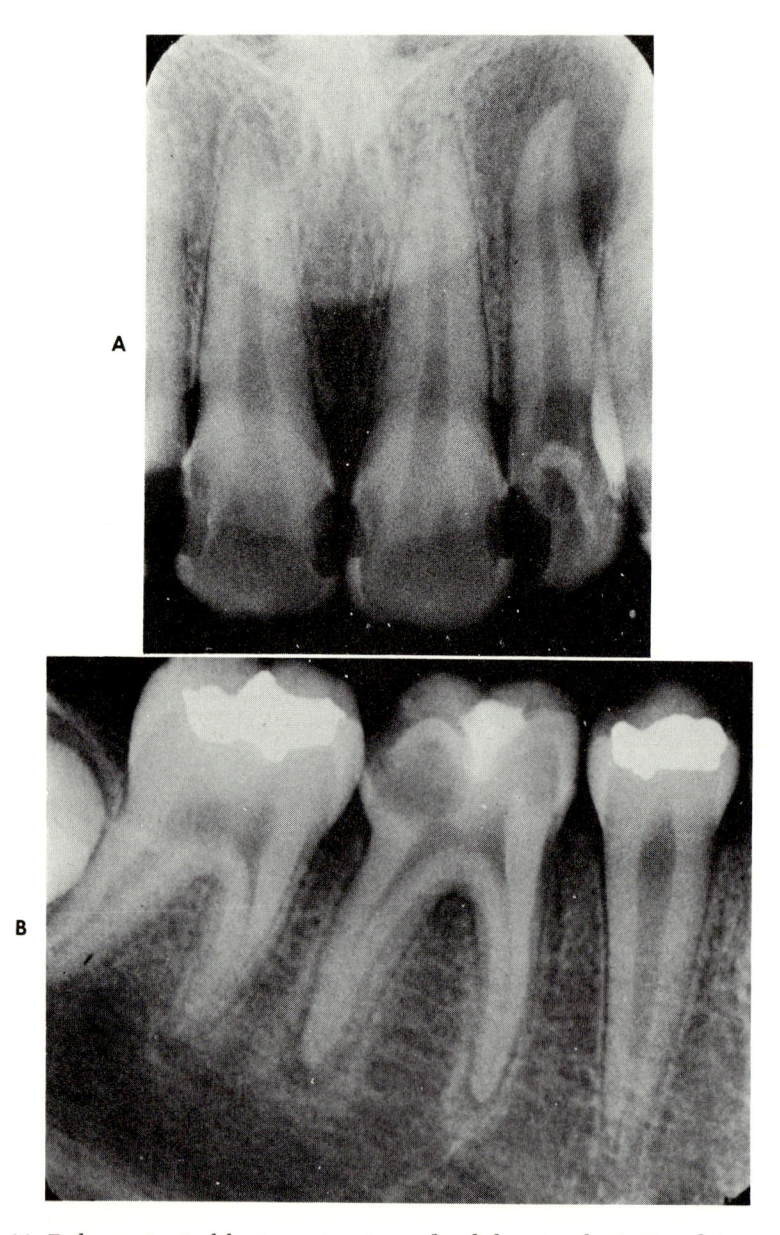

Fig. 4-11. Pulpoperiapical lesions at apices of pulpless teeth. **A,** Rarefying osteitis at apex of upper lateral incisor. **B,** Condensing osteitis in periapex of mesial root and combined rarefying and condensing osteitis in periapex of distal root of carious first molar.

as easily determined. Most often, chronic pulpal disease is associated with a tooth that has had prolonged trauma or contains one or more large restorations.

Roentgenograms, besides revealing possible causes of the pulpal problem such as the presence of deep caries, deep restorations, fractures, and so on, will frequently reveal periradicular changes (Fig. 4-11). The primary acute abscessed tooth will show an increase in width of the periodontal ligament. The secondary abscess, either acute or chronic, as well as the periapical granuloma, cyst, or scar, will show as a radiolucency usually periapical in position. In cases where the irritants are mild, a condensing osteitis may result instead of a rarefying osteitis (Fig. 4-11). A condensing osteitis will show as a radiopacity, or occasionally both processes will be present at once (a rarefying and condensing osteitis) and will show as a radiolucency surrounded by a radiopaque region. (Fig. 4-11).

Unfortunately not all teeth are conducive to endodontic treatment. For instance, so much reparative dentin may have been deposited that the canal may not be negotiable. In other cases the roots may be so twisted or dilacerated that they will not permit the passage of endodontic instruments. If the roentgenogram of a tooth needing endodontics suggests there is not a patent, negotiable root canal, then a final treatment plan based on using this tooth as an abutment is foolhardy. Often the fate of an entire case may depend on the successful endodontic treatment of a single tooth. Hence it is sometimes necessary to determine if the canals of a tooth can be negotiated before planning final treatment.

PERIODONTAL CONSIDERATIONS

Assuming the teeth are not candidates for extraction and that pulpally involved teeth can be treated, periodontal treatment should be considered next. Rules attempting to define what amount of alveolar bone loss constitutes a hopelessly involved tooth are worthless. Any tooth that can function in health should be retained. It is often possible to change the local oral environment so that destructive factors are no longer present. Basically, if the tooth and surrounding tissues can be returned to health and can function, then the tooth should be retained. More important than the millimeters of remaining bone is whether the patient can keep the tooth clean. Periodontal therapy should be looked at from the point of view of modifying the tissues so that the patient can clean the troublesome areas satisfactorily. The patient should be made fully aware of this, since it is foolish to perform periodontal surgery and have a prosthesis placed in a patient with poor oral hygiene. Actually such mistakes can be avoided if proper sequencing is done. As is described in detail in Chapter 10, stabilization (disease elimination) should be achieved first and the patient's performance monitored for a time before the rehabilitative phase is commenced. Unfortunately, prosthetic appliances (bridges or splints) may render proper hygiene more difficult to perform satisfactorily. Then too, partial dentures, though they do not make oral hygiene more difficult to perform, may be injurious to the periodontium if they are not maintained properly in these patients.

Special considerations are required when abnormal anatomic relationships exist. For example, teeth with roots so closely approximated that there is

40 *Modifying factors in treatment planning*

an absence of bone between them may require removal of one or, eventually, loss of both teeth. A similar situation occurs when osseous defects extend into root furcations, which may require root amputation or hemisectioning of the tooth (Figs. 4-12 and 4-13). Most osseous defects can be managed with surgery or root sectioning if there is adequate separation between the roots. However, it must be stressed that heroic procedures performed when the outcome is doubtful should only be used in situations where the retention of a critical tooth is necessary. One must always ask: Is the treatment commensurate with the prognosis? Or will the patient lose the teeth anyway in a short period of time? In other words, has the patient been sufficiently motivated to take care of the mouth?

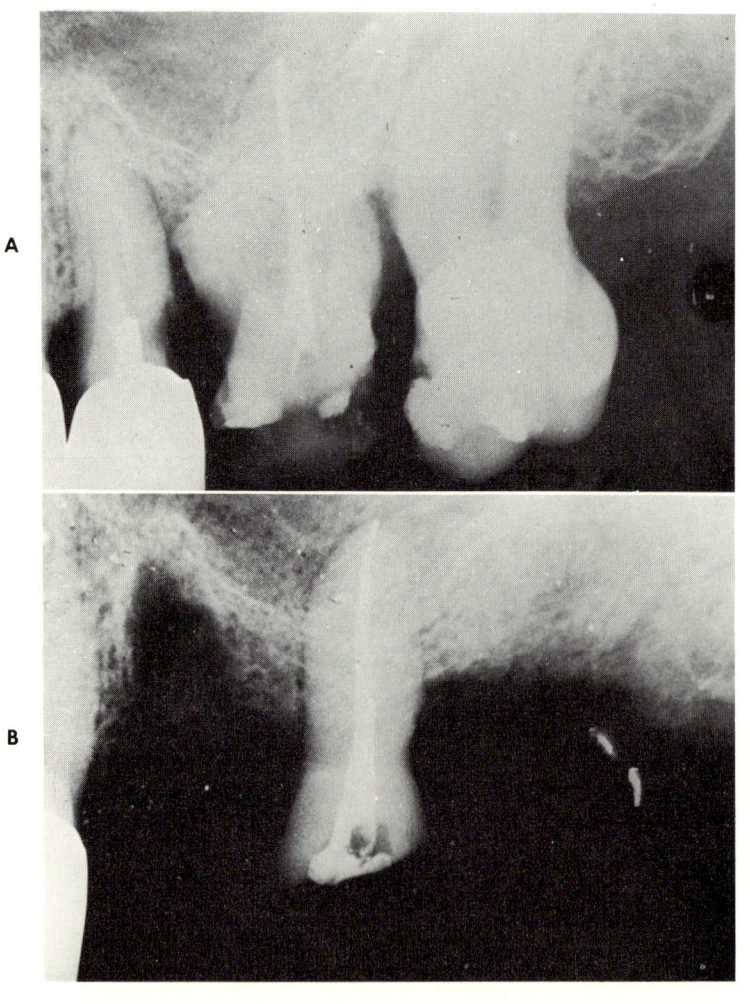

Fig. 4-12. Root amputations. **A,** Periapical roentgenogram showing maxillary first molar that has periodontal involvement of trifurcation area. **B,** Periapical roentgenogram taken after buccal roots have been amputated.

Restoration of teeth

If a tooth is to be restored, it is essential to know the indications and contraindications for each material. Permanent restorative materials currently being used in dentistry include silver amalgams, gold castings, gold foil, composites, silicates, porcelain, and porcelain fused to gold.

Amalgam restorations are the most widely used material. They are easy to manipulate, are relatively inexpensive, and are of adequate strength to resist normal masticatory forces. They have the added advantage of being adaptable for use in relatively inaccessible areas such as root caries. Although amalgam is an excellent material, extremely large restorations usually result in poor contour, lack of proximal contact, and undercondensation, which leads to subsequent failure. In those cases it is highly desirable to use a cast-gold restoration. An amalgam may fracture or need replacement sooner in a bruxism patient than it would in a normal patient. *Gold* is the most commonly accepted material used when sufficient strength is needed to replace lost tooth structure. Cast restorations have the advantage of permitting the establishment of excellent proximal contour and occlusal contact relationships, although the latter advantage is often abused.

It is logical that conservation of tooth structure and maintenance of gingival health is fundamental, especially in situations where extensive tooth structures have been lost. One way of doing this is by the use of pin-retained bases or pin-retained castings. This allows full-crown castings to be used less often and keeps the margins above the soft tissues.

The ideal anterior restorative material has yet to be perfected to the point that it will satisfy the requirements of a permanent restoration. *Composite resin* materials have been shown to be the best materials available, and they are

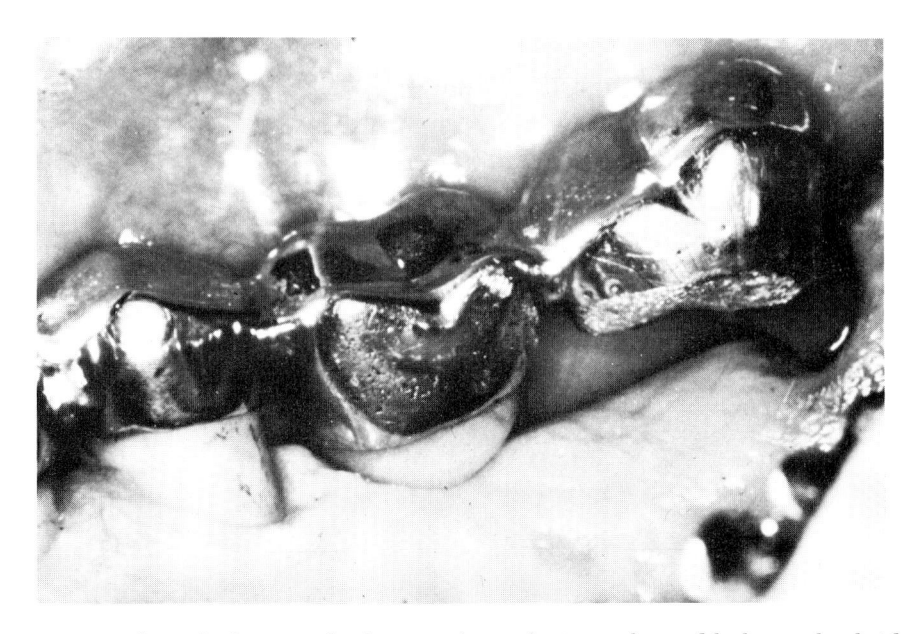

Fig. 4-13. Clinical photograph showing lingual view of mandibular molar bridge abutment with mesial root amputated as treatment for periodontal furcation involvement.

indicated for aesthetic reasons, but only in situations where adequate tooth structure remains. Composite materials are more resistant to wear, less soluble, and more color stable, but are as toxic as the most acidic cement. *Gold foil* has several attractive characteristics. However, it cannot be used for large cavity preparations, and it should not be used where the tooth will be subjected to heavy masticatory forces or where anesthetics are a consideration.

Porcelain-jacket crowns give the best appearance of all the materials. However, their ability to withstand the forces of mastication depends on the bulk of the material, so they may require extreme tooth reduction. *Porcelain-bonded-to-metal* crowns provide excellent aesthetic qualities and the increased strength of a metal casting. Any porcelain-jacket or porcelain-bonded-to-metal crown has several disadvantages. Children and adolescents may require cast-crown restoration because of excessive loss of tooth structure, but because the teeth are not fully erupted or have large pulp chambers it is impossible to achieve an aesthetic and properly contoured result.

Summary

In summary, when treating a single tooth, many considerations are important. A tooth with a small occlusal cavity might be best extracted if the tooth has a hopeless periodontal involvement, while a pulpally involved tooth that is strategic as a terminal abutment might be useless because the canal cannot be negotiated for endodontic therapy.

Flexibility

It is always important to consider alternative treatment plans when attempting definitive treatment planning. Decisions made about which teeth must be extracted, about questionable teeth, and about teeth that are definitely usable may change with treatment. The plan of treatment must retain sufficient flexibility that these possibilities may be taken into account.

5

Medical considerations: renal, endocrine, infectious, bone, joint, and neurologic diseases

Donald A. Falace

    The practicing dentist is confronted daily with patients whose medical problems may complicate his dental treatment. Some of the more common problems encountered are cardiovascular disease, pulmonary disease, allergy, endocrine disorders, hematologic disorders, and psychiatric problems. These problems can generally be placed into one of three categories based on their influence on dental care. The first group comprises those disorders that need only to be identified and do not actually affect dental treatment, for example, a urinary tract infection. A second group of disorders includes those that will allow dental care to continue but with some modification. The classic example is rheumatic heart disease, in which case prophylactic antibiotics must be administered to the patient during dental treatment. In the third category are those problems that may preclude dental care, such as recent myocardial infarction.

    The purpose of this section is to present the dental management and treatment implications of some of the more common medical disorders with which the dental practitioner may be faced in his office. More emphasis is given to chronic disorders that frequently necessitate alteration of the dental treatment plan than to those disorders that are transient and have little effect on dental care. Also, acute exacerbations are not dealt with, as these belong in discussions dealing with emergency care. This material is not intended to be comprehensive, as this would be impractical in a text of this nature. The reader is referred to a standard medical text for additional information.

Material on renal failure, adrenal insufficiency secondary to chronic steroid administration, pregnancy, arthritis, joint prosthesis, and hepatitis adapted from Falace, D. A., and Little, J. W.: Principles of medicine and pathology, rev., Lexington, Ky., 1977, University of Kentucky College of Dentistry.

RENAL FAILURE

Of the 8 million people in the United States with some form of kidney disease, 60,000 die each year as an end result of uremia, the toxic conditions produced by the retention of urinary constituents in the blood. Over half of these individuals are over the age of 55. The onset of chronic renal failure is often undetected and insidious and is not recognized until the later stages. Nocturia and polyuria are frequently the earliest detectable signs. The manifestations of the disease are seen in many organ systems including cardiovascular, gastrointestinal, neuromuscular, hematologic, and dermatologic. As the disease process progresses, conservative medical management becomes inadequate to control the accumulation of toxins. At this point there are two treatment alternatives to prolong life: artificial filtration of the blood via dialysis or transplantation of a kidney. Patients that fall into each category pose specific management problems for the dentist, especially the chronic dialysis patient and the renal transplant patient.

Etiology

Chronic renal failure is a progressive bilateral deterioration of renal function, resulting in uremia (the toxic condition caused by urinary constituents in the blood) and ultimately terminating in death. The rate of progress and severity of the process is dependent upon the underlying primary disease. In many cases the underlying cause is not readily identifiable.

The single most common cause of renal failure is glomerulonephritis (inflammation of glomerular tufts). Glomerulonephritis is a disease process of the kidney manifested by inflammation and variable scarring of the glomerulus. Other causes of renal failure include pyelonephritis (disease resulting from the effects of bacterial infection of the kidney), polycystic kidney disease, renal vascular disease, drug nephropathy, obstructive uropathy, and hypertension.

The most common cause of acute glomerulonephritis is a preceding infection with group A beta hemolytic streptococci. The common pattern is an upper respiratory tract infection with group A beta hemolytic streptococci with subsequent recovery. Then, 1 or 2 weeks later, nephritis becomes evident, manifested by fatigue, anorexia, abdominal pain, edema, and azotemia (accumulation of nitrogenous waste products). The vast majority of patients recover completely from their lesion and have no residual pathology. A small percentage, however, progress to chronic glomerulonephritis and its attendant complications.

Chronic glomerulonephritis is a disease whose pathogenesis is frequently uncertain. It is difficult to say exactly how many cases result from actue poststreptococcal glomerulonephritis, but it is felt that there are relatively few. In fact the majority of patients deny having had an identifiable episode of acute glomerulonephritis.

Pathophysiology

The pathologic lesion that results in the clinical picture of renal failure is manifested in the glomerular tuft, the renal tubules, or the renal vasculature. Any or all of these areas may be affected.

When exposed to chronic inflammatory insult, the glomerular tuft undergoes progressive scarring. This leads to proteinuria or hematuria because of the increased capillary permeability. As the disease progresses, the entire glomerulus may be destroyed.

Occurring independently of or concurrent with glomerular disease, the renal tubules may undergo fibrosis and thickening, resulting in the diminution or loss of ability to concentrate urine.

As with tubular disease, vascular disease may be either primary or secondary. Arteriosclerosis of the renal vessels causes ischemia to the supplied area. This may lead to infarction, glomerular collapse, tubular collapse, and intestinal fibrosis (nephrosclerosis).

Although early renal failure may remain asymptomatic, as it progresses, physiologic changes invariably occur as a direct result of the underlying lesions. Because of the tubular malfunction the sodium pump loses its effectiveness and the excretion of sodium occurs. Along with the sodium, excess amounts of dilute urine are excreted. This accounts for the polyuria and nocturia commonly encountered.

With the loss of the glomerular filtration function, there is a buildup of nonprotein nitrogen compounds in the blood. This is mainly in the form of urea and is called azotemia. In addition to the nitrogenous waste products, other acids accumulate because of tubular impairment, resulting in loss of bicarbonate ions and the inability to synthesize ammonium ions for excretion. The combination of waste products causes acidosis. In the later stages of renal failure this causes nausea, anorexia, and fatigue. Patients may tend to hyperventilate to attempt a respiratory compensation for the metabolic acidosis.

As would be expected, there are several electrolyte disturbances in renal failure. Sodium depletion has already been mentioned. Hyperkalemia may develop in the later stages of progressive azotemia. This becomes particularly evident as the urine output falls significantly.

Renal osteodystrophy develops because of increased phosphate retention, decreased calcium absorption, and increased calcium excretion. In response to the decreased serum calcium level, the parathyroid glands release parathormone, which increases bone resorption and raises the serum calcium level; thus hyperparathyroidism and osteomalacia may develop secondarily to the primary renal disease. Clinically the increased bone resorption may lead to a decrease in the definition of the lamina dura, cystic-appearing bone lesions, bony fractures, and soft tissue calcifications.

Progressive renal failure leads to a decrease in function of bone marrow. This is primarily because of the lack of erythropoietin, which is normally produced by the kidney. The result is a normochromic, normocytic anemia, a qualitative platelet defect, a decrease in the production of white blood cells, and alteration in the normal immune response. All of the pathophysiologic changes that occur are collectively called uremia and are the clinical manifestations of chronic renal failure.

Signs and symptoms

The signs and symptoms of chronic renal failure (uremia) may be manifested in any one of a number of organ systems. Patients with the uremic syn-

46 *Modifying factors in treatment planning*

drome may demonstrate mental slowness or depression. They may become psychotic in the later stages. They also may show muscular hyperactivity. Convulsion is a late finding and is directly correlated with the level of azotemia.

Hyperpigmentation of the skin commonly occurs. It is characterized by a brownish yellow color due to the retention of carotene-like pigments normally excreted by the kidney. These pigments also may produce a profound pruritus. An interesting finding is a whitish coating of the skin of the trunk and arms called the "uremic frost." It is due to residual urea crystals left on the skin when perspiration evaporates.

Renal failure patients demonstrate a variety of gastrointestinal signs. Anorexia and vomiting are common, especially later in the disease. Stomatitis, manifested by oral ulceration, is not unusual. An additional problem is candidiasis, which could lead to a similar clinical presentation. Parotitis may also occur, as well as a "uremic" odor to the breath. These patients frequently suffer from malnutrition and diarrhea.

Bone marrow depression occurs and results in a normochromic, normocytic anemia, decreased white blood cells, and a qualitative platelet defect. In addition, recent studies have indicated a possible functional defect in the factor VIII protein.[10] As a result, hemorrhagic episodes are not uncommon, and purpural or petechial lesions may be noted on the oral mucous membranes.

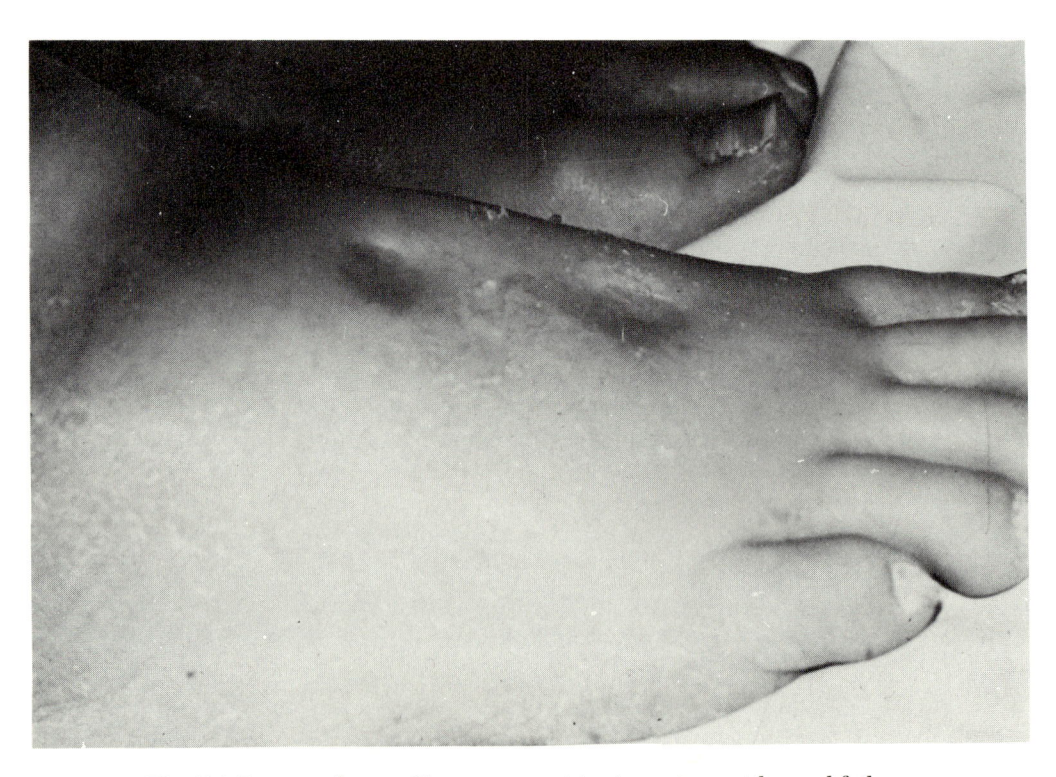

Fig. 5-1. Pitting edema of lower extremities in patient with renal failure.

The cardiovascular problems associated with chronic renal failure include hypertension, which may rapidly progress to encephalopathy. Congestive heart failure with resultant edema is commonly seen (Fig. 5-1). In many cases a nonsymptomatic pericarditis may be found.

Since most of the clinical problems of the uremic syndrome are due to azotemia, the laboratory tests of most interest are those that measure nitrogenous waste products in the blood. The most commonly used test of renal function is that of blood urea nitrogen (BUN). Under normal conditions, the BUN level varies between 10 and 20 mg/100 ml, but may reach levels greater than 60 mg/100 ml in renal disease. The main drawback to the BUN test is its lack of relative sensitivity and the number of factors other than renal function that may affect it. A more sensitive measurement of renal function is the blood creatinine test, which under normal conditions is between 1.0 and 1.5 mg/100 ml. A creatinine level greater than 1.5 mg/100 ml is most often associated with significant renal disease. The creatinine level is not as greatly influenced by extrarenal factors as is the BUN level.

Medical management

Once the diagnosis of chronic renal failure is established, the goal is to prolong life and to improve the quality of life. Conservative medical management is the foundation of treatment and may be all that is necessary for long periods. As the disease progresses, this may become inadequate, and consideration must be given to intermittent peritoneal or hemodialysis or to renal transplantation.

Medical management is directed toward treating specific signs and symptoms. The cornerstone of treatment is to alter the diet to decrease the exogenous protein intake. The level of allowable protein is based on the creatinine clearance, and sufficient quantity must be taken to prevent protein catabolism.[15]

Sodium supplementation is given variably on an individual basis and is constantly monitored. Fluid replacement is a variable requirement, depending on urine output, edema, and weight change. Hyperkalemia is usually seen when urine output falls, and may be treated with a sodium exchange resin. Acidosis is commonly treated with calcium carbonate. An added advantage to this is replacement of calcium. Definitive calcium therapy is accomplished with vitamin D administration. Successful treatment of the calcium deficiency will reverse the osteodystrophic changes. Neuromuscular complications are usually managed by sedatives and hypnotics. In some instances, psychiatric care is necessary.

The cardiovascular problems, congestive heart failure and hypertension, frequently pose treatment difficulties. They are treated with conventional modalities, but usually more aggressively, and the patient must be closely monitored to prevent untoward effects of the medication. The anemia that invariably occurs in chronic renal failure is usually refractive to conservative treatment. No treatment is indicated unless the patient becomes severely symptomatic, develops an infection, or requires surgery. In that event a hematocrit between 25 and 30 mg/100 ml is usually sufficient. Infusion of packed red blood cells is the treatment of choice.

48 *Modifying factors in treatment planning*

Dialysis

As the failing kidneys gradually worsen, the attempt at medical management alone becomes inadequate to prevent azotemia. At this point artificial filtration of the blood may be required in the form of peritoneal dialysis or hemodialysis.

Peritoneal dialysis is accomplished by injecting hypertonic solution into the peritoneal cavity. A period of time is allowed to elapse and then the solution is drawn out. Dissolved solutes, such as urea, are drawn out with the solution. The advantages of peritoneal dialysis are the relative low cost and the ease of performance. Disadvantages include the need for frequent sessions and the significant lack of effectiveness as compared to hemodialysis. Its principal use is in acute renal failure or in patients who require only occasional dialysis.

In chronic renal failure, hemodialysis is more commonly utilized. The technique requires creation of a permanent arteriovenous shunt, usually from the artery to the dialysis machine, where it is filtered and then returned to the vein (Fig. 5-2). During this period, heparin is administered to prevent blood coagulation. The procedure takes several hours, depending on the instrument utilized, and the filtration is much more complete than with peritoneal dialysis.

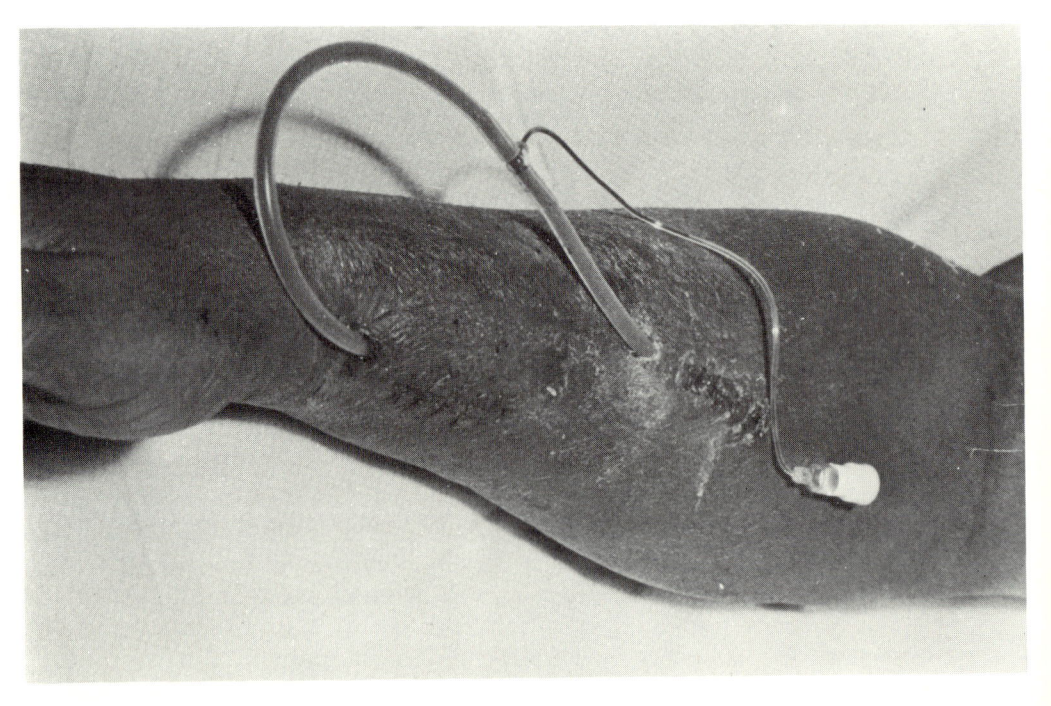

Fig. 5-2. Surgical A-V shunt has been prepared in this renal patient to facilitate hemodialysis. (This particular apparatus is now seldom used.)

Transplantation

An alternative to chronic dialysis therapy is kidney transplantation, although not every patient is a candidate for a transplant (Fig. 5-3). The patient who does undergo a successful kidney transplant has a life that is much improved in quality over the dialysis patient. According to the "Twelfth Report of the Human Renal Transplant Registry," there have been a total of 16,444 kidney transplants reported. Of these, 14,479 have follow-up data available, and 46.8% of the 6781 recipients are alive and well with their functioning allograft.[3] As with any organ transplant, the major problem is graft rejection. Numerous methods have been attempted to suppress rejection, including chemotherapy with cytotoxins and steroids, local radiation therapy, and antilymphocyte globulin. Chemotherapy seems to be the most widely accepted mode of therapy and usually includes prednisone and azathioprine in varying dosages. With these medications the patient is extremely susceptible to infection, and in fact, sepsis is one of the major complications in transplant patients. The exogenous steroid also significantly suppresses normal adrenal function in these patients.

Dental treatment planning considerations

CHRONIC RENAL FAILURE

Consultation with the patient's physician is mandatory prior to treating individuals with chronic renal failure. It is advisable not to render outpatient care if the BUN level is greater than 60 mg/100 ml or the creatinine level is

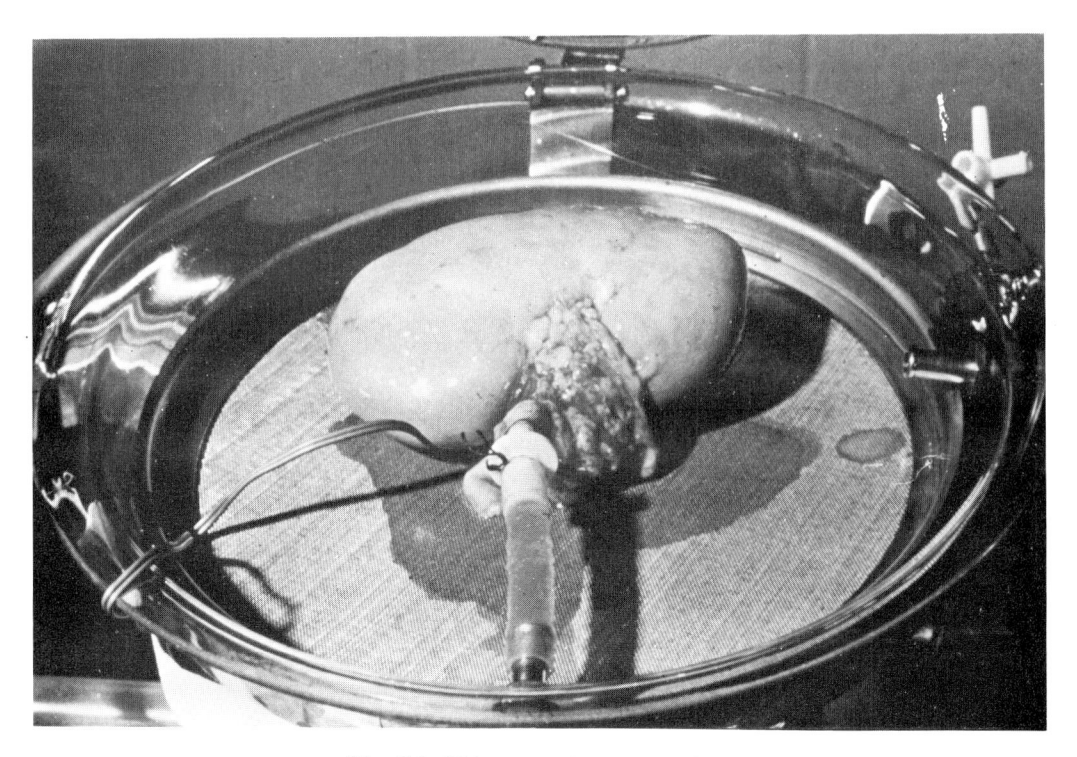

Fig. 5-3. Kidney awaiting transplant.

greater than 1.5 mg/100 ml. Questions concerning this decision must be made in concert with the patient's physician.

If it is decided to treat the patient in the outpatient setting, the blood pressure should be closely monitored before and during treatment. Any excessive readings should be reported to the physician. Because of the potential for bleeding problems, these patients should receive a pretreatment screening for bleeding diatheses. It is advisable to run a bleeding time and a partial thromboplastin time. Abnormalities should be discussed with the physician. In addition to these tests, a hematocrit is advisable, especially if any surgical procedures are contemplated. Few problems will be encountered if the hematocrit is above 25%. Antibiotics are not required prophylactically unless infection is present (e.g., I and D of an abscess).

When surgical procedures are undertaken, meticulous attention to good surgical technique is necessary to decrease chances of excessive bleeding and infection.

The stomatitis that results in oral ulceration can usually be treated symptomatically. A solution of bicarbonate and water rinsed in the mouth, followed by a teaspoon of Syrup of Phenergan, provides topical anesthesia for short periods. It is important to rule out candidiasis as a source of oral infection in these individuals. This may be confirmed clinically using a tongue blade and cytologic tests. The treatment of choice is nystatin.

One of the major problems experienced in treating chronic renal failure patients is drug therapy, specifically those drugs that are excreted by the kidney or those drugs that are nephrotoxic. Table 1 shows some of the more commonly used drugs in dental practice and recommendations for their use.

The goal of dental care for patients with chronic renal failure should be to restore the mouth to the healthiest condition possible and to eliminate all possible sources of infection. Oral physiotherapy training is very important for the maintenance of long-term oral health. It is important to remember that this is a progressive disease that may ultimately necessitate dialysis or transplant, and it is much easier to manage from a dental standpoint the medically treated patient than either the dialysis patient or transplantation patient. Once an acceptable level of oral hygiene has been established, there is no contraindication to routine dental care. However, the practitioner should attempt to enhance the hygiene level through his procedures, and he may include things such as using sanitary pontics when possible.

Dialysis

The same recommendations will apply to managing the dialysis patient, with a few exceptions. Peritoneal dialysis really presents no additional considerations. Such is not the case, however, with hemodialysis. The surgically created arteriovenous fistula or shunt is susceptible to infection (endoarteritis) resulting from a bacteremia. Such an endoarteritis is similar to subacute bacterial endocarditis in the rheumatic heart disease patient in terms of the danger to the patient. Therefore patients with the shunt require the same prophylactic antibiotic coverage for dental procedures as do the rheumatic heart disease patients in order to prevent the infection from occurring. (See discussion on subacute bacterial endocarditis prophylaxis.)

Since hemodialysis aggravates bleeding tendencies by destruction of platelets, it is extremely important to determine the bleeding times before a surgery is performed. If significantly deficient, platelet replacement may be necessary. Heparinization during hemodialysis does not produce residual bleeding tendencies, as its activity only lasts 3 to 4 hours after infusion. Patients just off the machine who present for dental care, however, could be significant bleeders; therefore it is best to avoid dental care on the day of dialysis. If immediate care is necessary, protamine sulfate will block the anticoagulant effect of heparin.

In treatment planning these individuals, it seems prudent to discourage extensive restorative or reconstructive procedures and emphasize a long-term maintenance program that generally would not include replacement of missing teeth. If, however, the patient is very motivated and is adamant about replacing missing teeth, one should certainly consider this as reasonable treatment for this patient.

RENAL TRANSPLANT

If the renal failure patient becomes a candidate for transplantation, the dentist should critically examine the condition of the dentition for potential

Table 1. Drug therapy in renal disease*

Drug	Normal dosage OK	Decrease frequency	Do not give
Lidocaine (dental)	Yes		
Aspirin	Every 4 hours in mild renal failure	Every 6 to 12 hours in moderate to severe renal failure	
Acetaminophen	Yes		Avoid in severe renal failure
Codeine	Yes		
Propoxyphene	Yes		
Meperidine (Demerol)	Yes		
Penicillin	Yes in mild to moderate renal failure	Every 12 to 16 hours in severe renal failure	
Erythromycin	Yes		
Tetracycline			Best to avoid if possible
Diazepam (Valium)	Yes		

*Modified from Bennett, W. M., et al.: A guide to drug therapy in renal failure, J.A.M.A. **230:** 1544-1553, Dec. 16, 1974. Copyright 1974, American Medical Association.

problems to the patient, keeping in mind that any dental care will require extensive treatment modification and drug alteration.

It is advisable to remove any seriously questionable teeth, even though they may be presently functional. These teeth may represent a serious future problem to the patient, and he would be better off without them. Extensive reconstructive work or other time-consuming invasive procedures should definitely be discouraged. The treatment of choice is maintenance of the present dentition in a sound healthy state, although in many cases the patient's future needs may be better served with complete or partial dentures.

Since the transplant patient is usually on high-dose steroid therapy, adrenal suppression will have occurred and will require steroid supplementation above the normal dosage for any dental care. This is to enable the patient to handle the stress created by a dental appointment or procedure. This is usually an individual modification that should be handled by the physician. (See suggested modifications in steroid replacement discussion.)

In addition to steroids, cytotoxic drugs are frequently standard therapy. The combination of these drugs greatly predisposes the patient to infection and sepsis. Therefore antibiotics should be given prophylactically to minimize bacteremia and to avoid postoperative infection at the site of treatment. The subacute bacterial endocarditis prophylaxis schedule may be adequate, but consultation with the physician is advisable.

ENDOCRINE DISEASES
Adrenal insufficiency secondary to chronic steroid administration
ETIOLOGY

Treatment of various diseases with corticosteroids has become commonplace and well accepted. While not curative, the palliative benefits of steroids are extremely useful and serve as powerful adjuncts in the treatment of diseases that are not amenable to other therapy. There are unfortunately numerous serious side effects that accompany chronic steroid therapy. The principal side effect of interest to the dentist is that of secondary adrenal insufficiency.

INCIDENCE AND PREVALENCE

Adrenal insufficiency may be either primary or secondary. Primary disease is due to disorders of either the pituitary gland or the adrenal glands themselves. Primary adrenal insufficiency occurs infrequently, but when it does, the classic presentation is that of Addison's disease. Addison's disease is caused by the progressive atrophy or destruction of the adrenal glands, classically due to tuberculosis. There is also an occasional idiopathic form of destruction that is thought to be on an autoimmune basis.

Secondary adrenal insufficiency is far more common and is due to the chronic administration of exogenous steroids resulting in suppression of endogenously produced steroids. The degree of suppression is related to the dosage and length of time of administration; therefore the lower the dose and the shorter the time of administration, the less suppression would be expected. Steroids are utilized in the treatment of a myriad of diseases such as rheumatoid arthritis, asthma, erythema multiforme, erosive lichen planus, various other dermatoses, systemic lupus erythematosus, "collagen diseases," and autoimmune diseases.

PATHOPHYSIOLOGY

The adrenal glands are located bilaterally at the superior pole of each kidney. They manufacture and secrete at least four hormones, the two principal ones being aldosterone and cortisol. Adrenal function is under the direct control of the pituitary gland, which is regulated by the hypothalamus. When stimulated, the pituitary secretes ACTH, which in turn causes the secretion of cortisol by the adrenal cortex (Fig. 5-4). Aldosterone secretion is mediated by the extracellular fluid volume and sodium.

Aldosterone is a mineralocorticoid whose main function is maintaining normal sodium, potassium, and fluid levels by mediating renal tubular function. Aldosterone is regulated by the renin-angiotensin system of the juxtaglomerular apparatus. The system is stimulated by a fall in renal blood pressure because of decreased blood volume or electrolyte imbalance, specifically a sodium imbalance. The result is a release of renin that activates angiotensin, causing vasoconstriction. Aldosterone also is released and causes sodium retention and potassium excretion. Aldosterone production is inhibited through a feedback mechanism that thus prevents overproduction.

Cortisol is the main glucocorticoid of the body and has a multitude of functions and effects, of which some of the more important are gluconeogenesis, antiinflammatory, and antiallergic. The adrenal glands secrete about 25 to 30 mg of cortisol a day under normal circumstances. The maximum potential output is approximately 250 to 300 mg for a 24-hour period. Of interest is empirical evidence that indicates that the output during medical stress (e.g., pneumonia, surgery) only approaches 60 mg.[5] The normal pattern of secretion is intimately connected with a person's normal sleep-awake sequence. In the average person who works during daylight hours, the level of serum cortisol is highest upon arising in the morning and lowest as the person is going to bed at

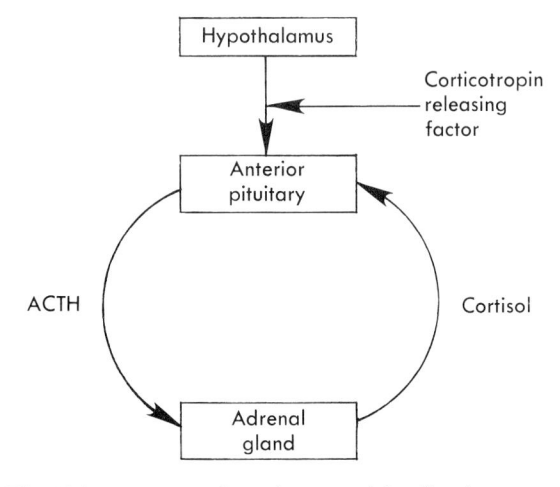

Fig. 5-4. Pituitary-adrenal axis and feedback system.

night. This is reversed in a person who works nights. This normal variation of serum cortisol levels is called diurnal variation.

As mentioned above, the secretion of cortisol is directly dependent upon the level of circulating ACTH. That is, as the steroid level increases, demand is met, and the level of steroid causes the ACTH level to drop. This drop in ACTH then inhibits the production of cortisol and the cortisol level begins to drop. In cases of chronic steroid therapy, the feedback system senses the exogenous steroid and inhibits ACTH production, which in turn suppresses the adrenal glands from producing any endogenous cortisol. The result is adrenal insufficiency secondary to the exogenous steroid administration. Although it is difficult to find uniform agreement concerning when adrenal suppression has occurred, it is generally accepted that significant adrenal suppression will have occurred after 1 month of daily administration of corticosteroid equivalent to 30 mg daily of hydrocortisone. Topically applied steroids may also induce adrenal suppression, although this is variable.[3,12] It appears that treatment of small, noninflamed areas usually will not be a cause for concern. On the other hand, large, inflamed areas requiring similar treatment for a month or longer should be cause for concern, especially if occlusive dressings are used. In this event, one must assume adrenal suppression has occurred.

Almost all cases of adrenal insufficiency secondary to exogenous steroid therapy are reversible, although the longer a person has been on steroids, the longer it takes to regain normal adrenal function once steroids are stopped. Agreement on the exact point of time this occurs is difficult, but generally most people will regain normal function within 9 months, although some severe cases may take up to a year.

Primary adrenal insufficiency is occasionally seen and is represented as the classic presentation of Addison's disease. As would be expected, all adrenal cortical hormones are produced in deficient quantities, and since the main adrenal cortical hormones are aldosterone and cortisol, the disease picture is essentially due to insufficient quantities of these hormones. Lack of aldosterone renders the patient unable to conserve sodium or eliminate potassium and hydrogen ions. The result is a hypovolemic, hyperkalemic, and acidotic indvidual. Cortisol deficiency results in a variety of problems including impaired glucose metabolism, hypotension, impaired fluid excretion, increased ACTH excretion, excessive pigmentation, and inability to tolerate stress. It is evident that this disease can be rapidly devastating if left untreated.

Secondary adrenal insufficiency is due entirely to a deficiency of endogenous corticosteroid induced by the decreased ACTH secretion. It is important to remember that this condition is reversible after the exogenous steroids are discontinued. The rate of return is dependent upon length of time the patient was on therapy and the dosage he received. As with patients with Addison's disease, these patients do not tolerate stress well, which is the main concern during dental treatment.

A frequent treatment modification is that of alternate day therapy; that is, steroids are given only every other day instead of daily. The dose is given to coincide with the patient's normal high serum level, and a 2-day dose is given all at once, the rationale being that since the dose given coincides with the normal high level of concentration, it will not tend to suppress ACTH as much. In addition, on the off day, the adrenal-pituitary axis is allowed to function normally and produce endogenous steroids. The result is less adrenal suppression than is seen with daily therapy. Unfortunately this technique is not uniformly successful, and many patients must return to daily therapy.

SIGNS AND SYMPTOMS

The signs and symptoms of primary adrenal insufficiency all relate to the deficiency of aldosterone and cortisol. Probably the most common complaints are weakness and fatigue and an abnormal pigmentation of skin and mucous membranes (Fig. 5-5). In addition, hypotension, anorexia, and weight loss are frequent findings. If the patient with Addison's disease is challenged by stress, such as infection or surgery, crisis may be precipitated, which is a medical emergency. It is manifested by a severe exacerbation of symptoms, which

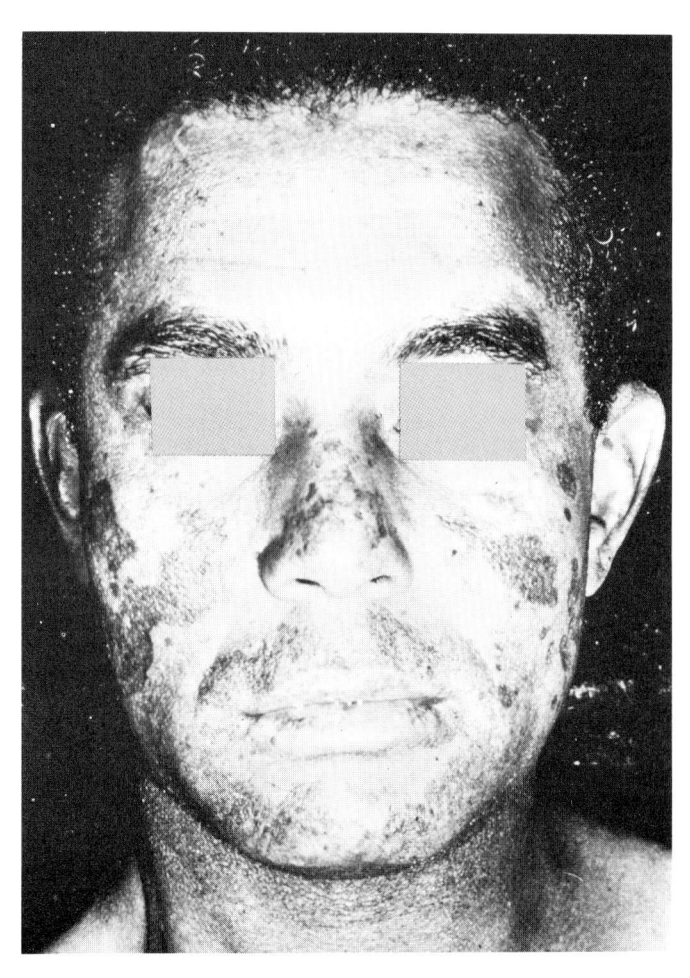

Fig. 5-5. Patient with Addison's disease showing brownish macules on face and deep diffuse tanning of neck region. (From Wood, N. K., and Goaz, P. W.: Differential diagnosis of oral lesions, St. Louis, 1975, The C. V. Mosby Co.)

includes severe hypotension, nausea, vomiting, weakness, headache, dehydration, and hyperpyrexia. If not treated rapidly, the patient will die.

Adrenal insufficiency resulting from chronic steroid administration usually does not in and of itself present any symptoms unless the patient is stressed and does not have adequate circulating cortisol to cope with the stress. In that event, an adrenal crisis may be precipitated. This can usually be prevented by increasing the amount of steroid received to cover the period of stress. It is important to recognize symptoms of diseases usually treated with steroids to prevent untoward reactions.

More commonly, the patient who has been on long-term, high-dose steroid therapy may begin to demonstrate signs and symptoms of hyperadrenalism or Cushing's disease. The person with Cushing's disease may complain of weight gain, round or moonlike facies (Fig. 5-6), a "buffalo hump" on his back, abdominal striae (Fig. 5-7), and acne. In addition, he may be hypertensive and may demonstrate heart failure. Healing may be impaired, and he may also be depressed or psychotic.

MEDICAL MANAGEMENT

The person with Addison's disease is usually treated with glucocorticoids, mineralocorticoid, and occasionally androgens. These are given in maintenance doses and will vary from patient to patient. Successfully treated pa-

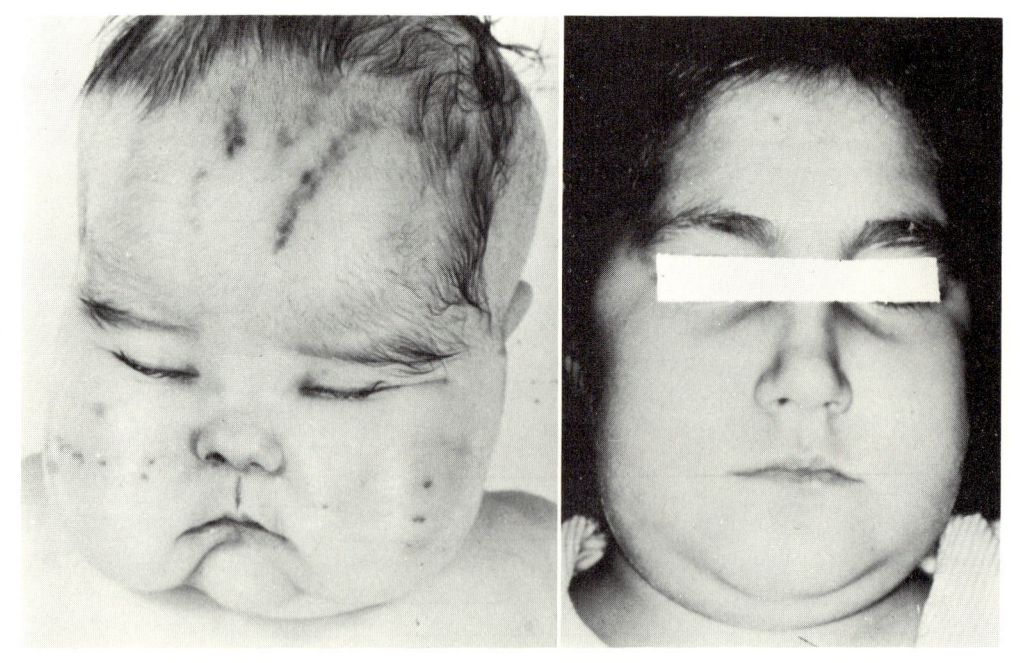

Fig. 5-6. Two patients with Cushing's disease demonstrating rounded face and obesity. A, Congenital Cushing's disease. B, Acquired Cushing's disease. (A courtesy Dr. Stephen Raibley, Maywood, Ill.; B courtesy Dr. James Little, Lexington, Ky.)

Renal, endocrine, infectious, bone, joint, and neurologic diseases 57

tients usually live normal lives, and the principal problem involves increasing steroids to cope with stress.

Acute adrenal crisis requires immediate treatment. Therapy is based on fluid and electrolyte replacement, administration of glucocorticoids, and resolving the underlying stress that precipitated the event.

Patients who acquire Cushing's disease require alteration of the steroid dosages to minimize the signs and symptoms of the disorder.

A variety of glucocorticoids are available for use, and the practitioner may encounter a number of these in his patients. Table 2 is a comparison of the strengths of the various glucocorticoids in common use.

DENTAL TREATMENT PLANNING CONSIDERATIONS

The planning of the technical phase of dental treatment need be no different for individuals with adrenal insufficiency than for the normal healthy patient. However, the medical management during dental treatment is extremely important inasmuch as an error in judgment or an omission of needed therapy could prove to be fatal.

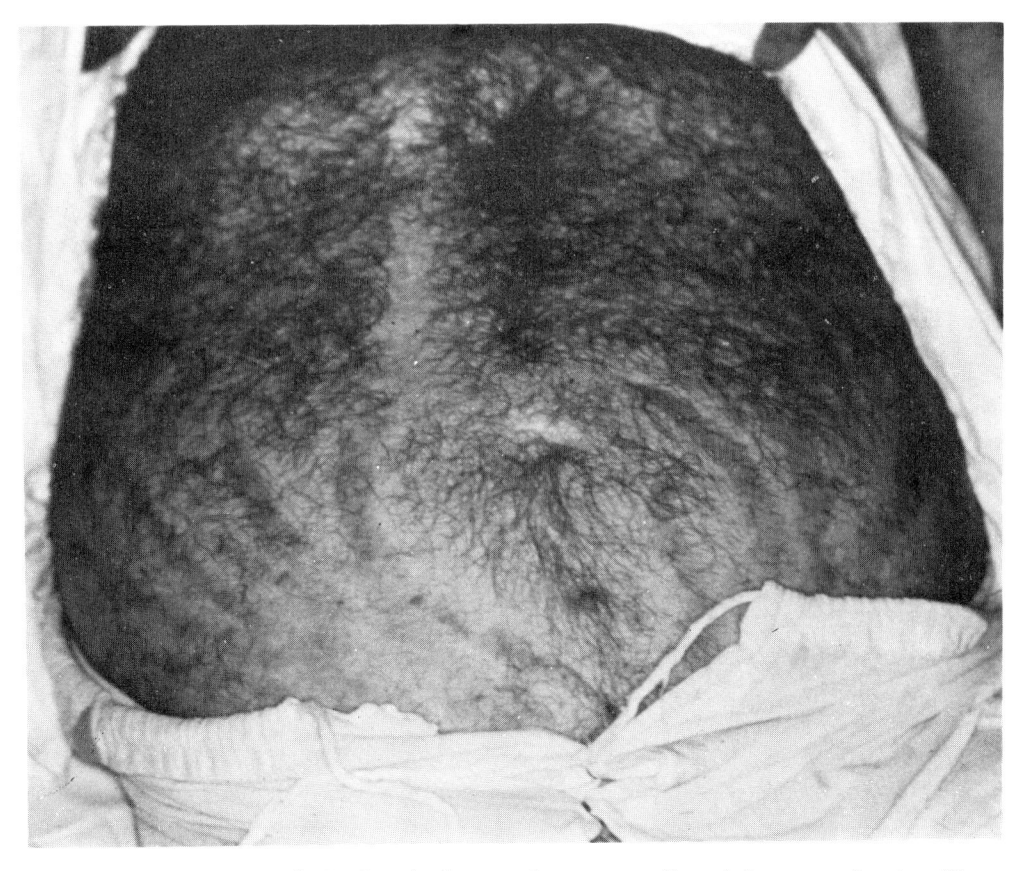

Fig. 5-7. Patient with Cushing's disease showing swollen abdomen and striae. (Courtesy Dr. James Little, Lexington, Ky.)

Table 2. Potency/dosage comparison of various steroid preparations*

Compound	Antiinflammatory potency relative to cortisol	Equivalent dosage to hydrocortisone
Hydrocortisone (cortisol)	1	30 mg
Cortisone	0.8	36 mg
Prednisolone	4	7.5 mg
Prednisone	4	7.5 mg
Methylprednisolone	5	6 mg
Dexamethasone	25	1.2 mg

*Adapted from Goodman, L. S., and Gilman, A., editors: The pharmacological basis of therapeutics, ed. 4, London, 1970, The Macmillan Co., p. 1627.

The following suggestions are to be viewed as general guidelines for managing dental treatment for individuals who are currently taking steroids or have taken steroids in the past year. They are the result of a distillation of many medical opinions. *They are not intended to be definitive,* and may well need to be modified by the patient's own physician. Consultation and close cooperation with the patient's physician are absolutely essential prior to initiating treatment for these individuals.

Significant adrenal suppression is assumed to have occurred in any patient having taken the equivalent of 7.5 mg or greater of prednisone daily, or its equivalent, for at least 1 month. Patients on alternate day therapy should also be considered suppressed, although less so than with daily dosage.

Other than patients with Addison's disease or patients who have had bilateral adrenalectomy, people generally retain the potential to regain adrenal function after cessation of steroid therapy, each patient requiring variable lengths of time proportional to dose and duration of therapy. Following is a summary of treatment for renal function after cessation of steroid therapy.

1. Patients currently taking steroids (longer than 1 month)
   a. Taking *less* than 7.5 mg prednisone daily or its equivalent (includes alternate day dosages): this is a gray area, and one is never sure whether suppression has occurred unless laboratory stress tests are performed; therefore to be safe, assume that the adrenals are suppressed and treat as in *b*.
   b. Taking *greater* than 7.5 mg prednisone daily or its equivalent:
      (1) For routine dental care (prophylaxis, restorations, simple elective extraction), double the normal dosage the day of the procedure.
      (2) For major dental procedures (multiple extractions, osseous surgery, fracture reduction), the patient should be hospitalized, with 50 mg cortisone acetate administered intramuscularly the night before, 50 mg cortisone acetate intramuscularly the morning of, 200 mg hydrocortisone intravenously during and immediately after surgery, and 50 mg cortisone acetate intramuscularly the evening after surgery. If the patient is able to take medications orally, administer 10 mg prednisone orally every 6

hours on the first postoperative day, 10 mg prednisone twice a day on the second postoperative day, and then taper toward maintenance. If the patient is unable to take medications orally, administer 50 mg cortisone acetate intramuscularly twice a day on the first postoperative day and taper by one-half each successive day.
      (3) For acute dental care (pulpotomy, I and D, extraction), administer 100 to 200 mg hydrocortisone intramuscularly 1 hour before procedure, then double the normal dose the day after.
  2. Patients not taking steroids presently, but with past history of their administration
      a. If no steroids have been administered in past year and patient is doing well, no steroids are required.
      b. If steroids have been administered within the past year, treat as though adrenal function is suppressed and administer therapy according to appropriate category under *1*.
  3. Topical steroids
      a. Small areas with no inflammation and no occlusive therapy require no steroid supplementation.
      b. With large areas of inflammation and occlusive dressings, it is probable that topically applied steroid preparations have resulted in adrenal suppression, especially if one has been treated longer than 1 month. Treat according to appropriate category under *1* or *2*.

Inadequate steroid coverage during a dental procedure should always be considered a possibility, and the dentist should be alert for the signs and symptoms. The clinical manifestations of acute adrenal insufficiency are hypotension, weakness, nausea, vomiting, headache, and frequently fever. Appropriate treatment should include establishment of an intravenous line with normal saline, then 100 mg hydrocortisone (Solucortef) intravenously immediately. The patient should be placed under the care of a physician as soon as possible.

As a general rule, it is better to be safe than sorry with these patients. For short treatment periods, increases in steroids will not hurt them; therefore it is better to "overtreat" than to get into problems.

Remember: communicate with the patient's physician.

PREGNANCY

The pregnant dental patient poses a unique and difficult set of management problems that involve rendering therapeutic dental care to the pregnant woman without causing harm to the fetus. Fetal injury can theoretically result from dentally related sources including radiation, drugs, and stress. Management goals then should be to minimize or eliminate all potential sources of fetal injury during dental treatment.

Pregnancy also carries risks independent of external occurrences, specifically spontaneous abortion. During the first trimester, spontaneous abortion occurs in about 15% to 20% of all pregnancies. This falls to only 2% during the second trimester, and then again may rise to as high as 10% during the third trimester. Although it is highly unlikely that any dental care would contribute to this untoward event, it would seem wise to avoid the periods of greatest incidence.

Gestation is classically divided into three equal trimesters, each of roughly 3 months' duration, measured from the time of conception. The particular importance of this is to realize that it is during the first trimester that all major organ systems are forming and developing, and thus the fetus is particularly vulnerable to developmental defects. For the most part, the second and third trimesters are concerned with maturation and growth of existing structures.

Dental treatment planning considerations

TREATMENT TIMING

The basic underlying goal of treatment during pregnancy should be to instill good oral hygiene practices to minimize the exaggerated physiologic response to dental disease. This may be done throughout all three trimesters and includes dental prophylaxis (Fig. 5-8).

The first trimester should generally be limited to acute care such as pain relief and infection control. The reasons for limiting treatment during this period are the high incidence of spontaneous abortion and the vulnerability of the fetus during organ and systems formation.

The second trimester is the safest period during which dental care may be rendered. Most of the organ systems have been formed and are now beginning maturation, and the incidence of spontaneous abortion is very low. Even though this is a relatively safe period, we recommend only minimal routine care such as simple restorations (Fig. 5-8). Emphasis should be placed on eliminating potential problems that could occur during the perinatal and postpartum periods, since care during this period is difficult. Extensive, complicated treatment should not be undertaken, but postponed until after delivery.

During the third trimester, acute care only is again recommended (Fig. 5-8). The rate of spontaneous abortion increases somewhat during this time, and in addition, the patient is usually quite uncomfortable; therefore prolonged periods of chair time should be avoided.

An additional complication that may be encountered during this period is supine syncope. Very simply, this is a syncopal episode that occurs when the pregnant patient has been supine for a prolonged period (Fig. 5-9). Physiolog-

FIRST TRIMESTER	SECOND TRIMESTER	THIRD TRIMESTER
Oral hygiene	Oral hygiene	Oral hygiene
Emergency treatment only	Minor elective treatment	Emergency treatment only

Fig. 5-8. Summary of treatment recommendations during pregnancy.

ically, the gravid uterus compresses the inferior vena cava and interferes with blood return to the heart and may result in loss of consciousness. Treatment for this problem is to roll the patient over on her left side, which allows blood flow to resume, and the patient should rapidly regain consciousness. Prevention consists of allowing the patient to assume a semisitting position and to allow frequent position shifts.

DENTAL ROENTGENOGRAMS

Dental roentgenograms are perhaps the single most confusing problem to deal with in the pregnant patient. It goes without saying that it is most desirable not to have any irradiation during pregnancy, since the developing fetus is particularly susceptible to radiation damage. However, should dental treatment be necessary, roentgenograms may well need to be taken to adequately complete treatment. Therefore one must be aware of how to safely proceed with roentgenograms in this situation.

The safety of dental roentgenography has been well established, provided features such as high-speed film, filtration, collimation, and a lead apron are used. Of all aids, the most important in the pregnant patient is the use of a protective lead apron. Studies have shown that gonadal radiation during dental x-rays has been virtually unmeasurable when a lead apron is used.[2] Therefore when contemporary x-ray technique is utilized, including the lead apron, the dentist can safely take those films considered absolutely *necessary* to render adequate dental care.

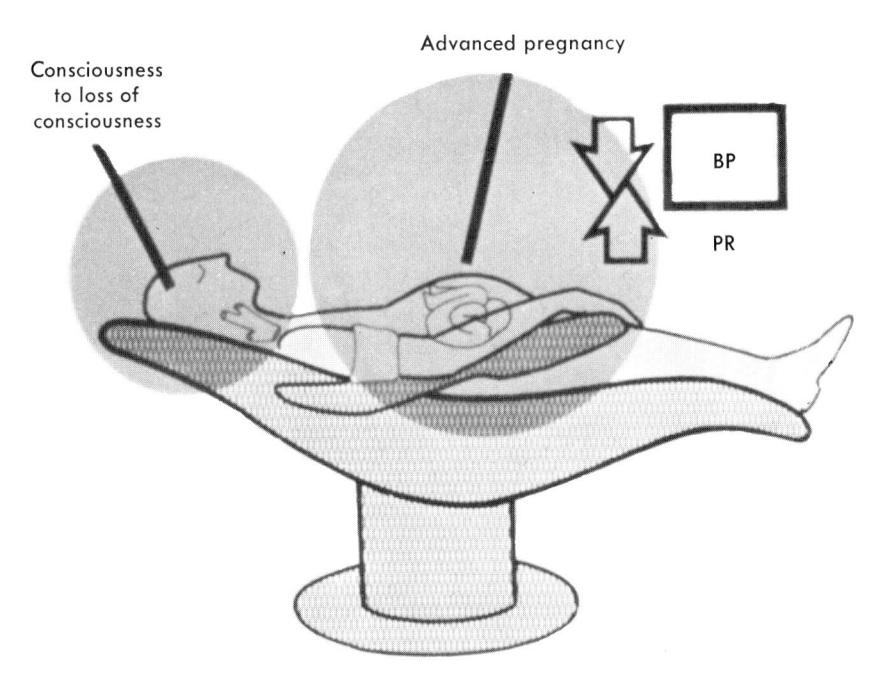

Fig. 5-9. Supine syncope during advanced pregnancy.

Drug administration

The final area of consideration in treating pregnant dental patients is that of drug administration. The principal concern is that the drug may cross the placenta and either be toxic at a given blood level or be teratogenic. In addition, any drug that is a respiratory depressant may cause maternal or fetal hypoxia, which can result in fetal injury or death. It is critical to avoid any period of hypoxia, since the fetus already exists in a low oxygen environment.

Fortunately, with a few exceptions, most drugs in common daily usage in dental practice may be safely used during pregnancy. This is particularly true of the local anesthetics and many common analgesics. Table 3 presents a list of drugs that are commonly used in dentistry and recommendations for their use during pregnancy. It should be emphasized that this is a generalization and that certain physicians may not desire to have their patients exposed to some of these preparations. Conversely, although it is better not to use the drugs designated "no," there may be instances in which their use becomes necessary to complete treatment. An example would be an intravenous sedative for a frightened patient or a patient in severe pain. Also, on occasion a general anesthetic may be necessary to complete treatment. In summary, it means doing whatever you have to do to get the required treatment accomplished and at the same time protecting the fetus to the extent possible. For this reason it is mandatory to consult with the patient's physician to discuss the planned treatment and ask for suggestions or modifications to the treatment.

Table 3. Drug administration in pregnancy

Drug	First trimester	Second and third trimester
Local anesthetic		
Lidocaine	Yes	Yes
Carbocaine	Yes	Yes
Analgesics		
Aspirin	Yes	Yes
Acetaminophen (Tylenol)	No	No
Codeine	Yes	Yes
Antibiotics		
Penicillin	Yes	Yes
Erythromycin	Yes	Yes
Tetracycline	No	No
Streptomycin	No	No
Sedative/hypnotic		
Nitrous oxide	No	No
Diazepam (Valium)	No	No
Barbiturates	No	No
General anesthetic	No	No

Renal, endocrine, infectious, bone, joint, and neurologic diseases **63**

DIABETES MELLITUS

Diabetes mellitus is a metabolic disease caused by a disorder of the beta cells of the pancreas, resulting in a deficiency of insulin. In addition to insulin deficiency, a number of complications are associated with the progress of diabetes mellitus and include microangiopathy, especially of the eye and kidney, arteriosclerosis, and neuropathies.

Since the discovery of insulin in the early 1920s, the major problem with diabetes mellitus has become the treatment of its complications. It has become the number one cause of blindness in this country. Over half the heart attacks today are related to diabetes as well as three-fourths of all strokes. Five out of six gangrenous amputations are due to diabetes (Figs. 5-10 and 5-11, *A*). Diabetic nephropathy is the primary cause of death among juvenile diabetics.[8]

Juvenile diabetes

Diabetes is usually classified by the age of onset into juvenile onset (before age 15) and maturity onset. Juvenile-onset diabetes is the more severe form of the disease and fortunately the less common, comprising only about 15% of diabetics. The cardinal symptoms of juvenile-onset diabetes are those

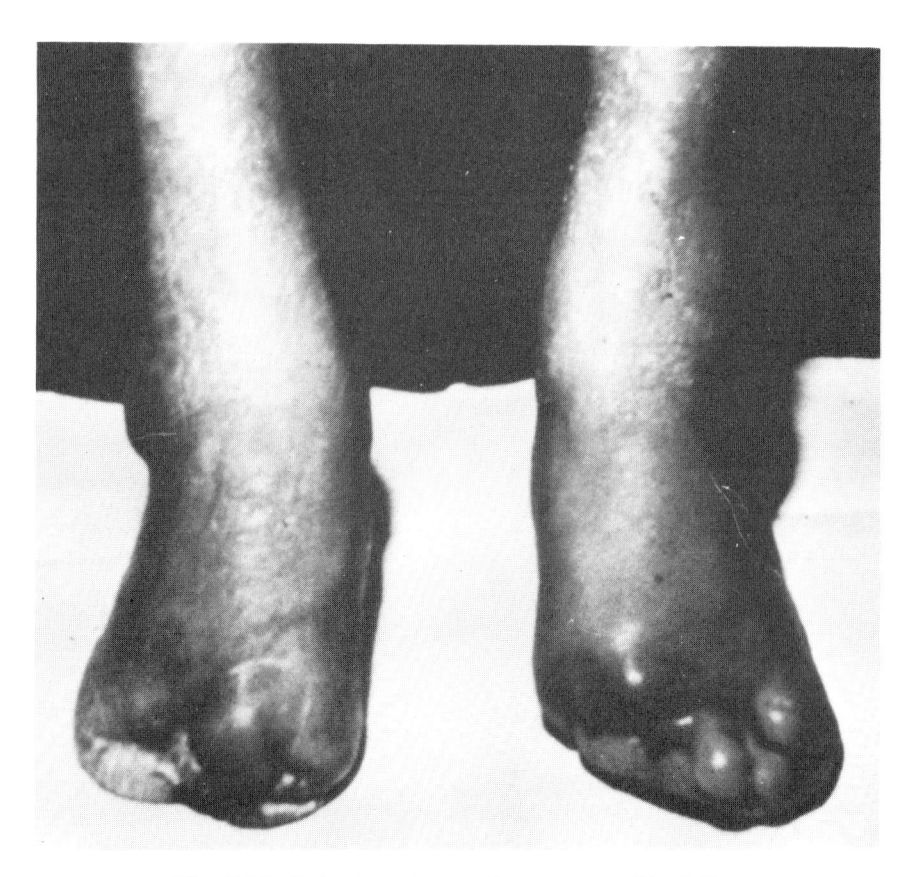

Fig. 5-10. Diabetic patient with gangrene of both feet.

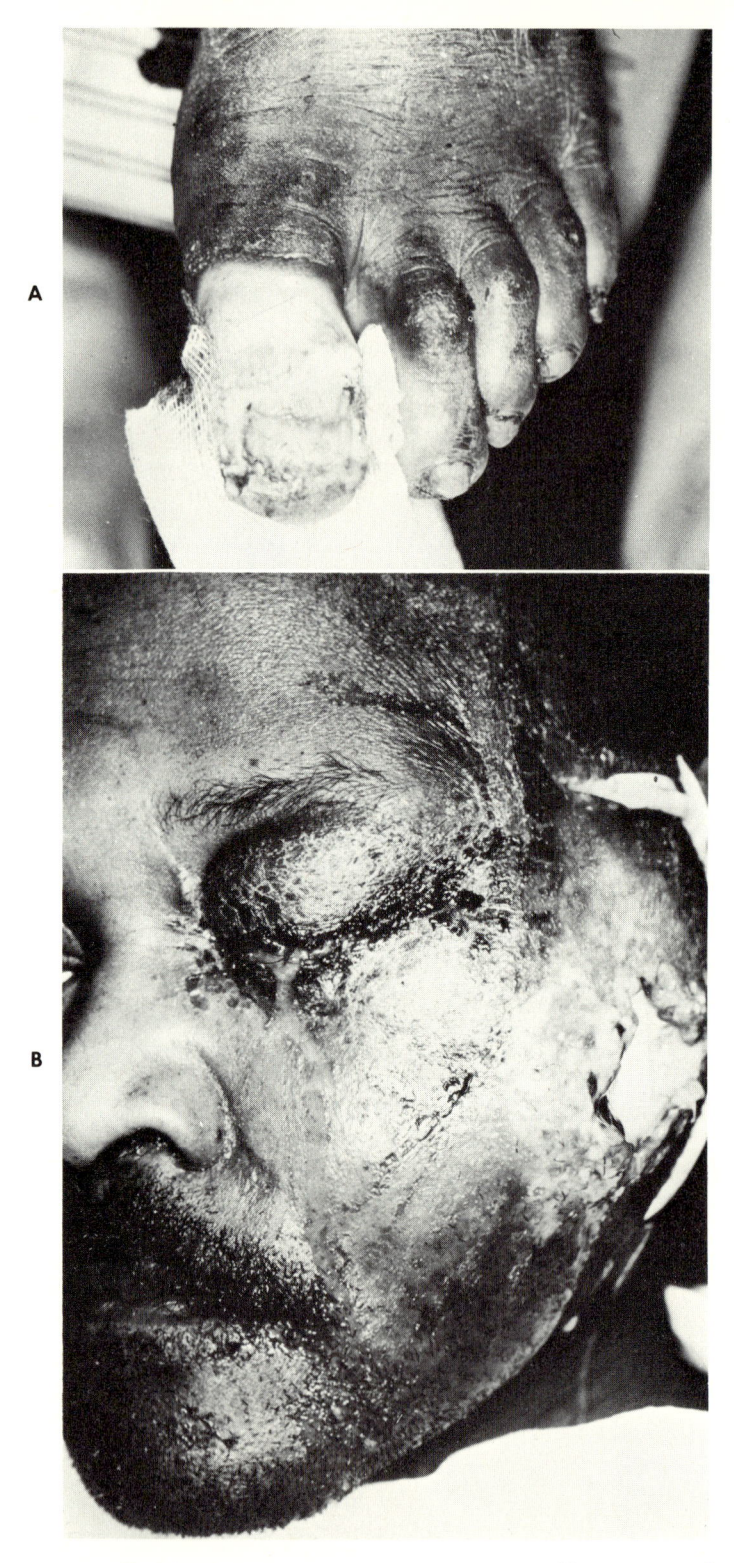

Fig. 5-11. Uncontrolled diabetic patient with **A,** gangrene of large toe, and **B,** massive necrotic and purulent odontogenic infection.

classically associated with the term "diabetes" and include polyphagia, polydipsia, polyuria with nocturia, weight loss, and weakness. This form of diabetes usually has a strong family history for the disease. The onset is frequently abrupt and severe. Ketoacidosis is a frequent occurrence. The juvenile-onset form is usually unstable and almost always requires insulin to control the disease. The complications associated with diabetes are very common in these individuals.

Adult diabetes

The maturity-onset form of the disease generally occurs after the age of 40, but may occur earlier. Some of the cardinal symptoms of the juvenile form may be present but are usually much less severe. In addition, the patient may complain of weight change, visual problems, and paresthesias. These patients are frequently obese. This form is usually less severe and with a slow onset. Ketoacidosis is infrequent. Dietary control alone is usually all that is required to control the disease. Occasionally, oral hypoglycemics or insulin may be required. Complications are much less common in the maturity-onset form.

Laboratory findings

Laboratory diagnosis of diabetes mellitus is varied and depends upon the stage and progress of the disease. The tests most frequently utilized to detect abnormalities in glucose metabolism include urinary glucose and acetone, fasting blood glucose, 1- or 2-hour postprandial blood glucose, 5-hour glucose tolerance test, and cortisone glucose tolerance test. For screening purposes, the postprandial blood glucose determination is of particular significance to the dentist and can be easily accomplished in the dental office using capillary blood via a finger stick and the Dextrostix after ingestion of a standard glucose load. Early or subclinical diabetes may not be detectable except by tests such as the cortisone glucose tolerance test; however, clinical or asymptomatic diabetes is usually detectable using the postprandial blood glucose determination, and detection at this stage may greatly benefit the patient. It should be kept in mind that the early diabetic may demonstrate hypoglycemia instead of hyperglycemia, which is believed to be caused by hyperinsulinism.

Medical management

Medical treatment of the diabetic almost always begins with diet modification. The patient's intake of calories is divided between carbohydrates, proteins, and fats. The diet is tailored to the individual's needs and body weight. In most cases, dietary correction is all that is required in the treatment of maturity-onset diabetes. However, about 35% of individuals with maturity-onset diabetes will require additional treatment, usually insulin, although oral hypoglycemics may be utilized.

Oral hypoglycemics (sulfonylureas) have been utilized frequently in the treatment of maturity-onset diabetes; however, recently they have fallen into disfavor because of the increased incidence of cardiovascular disease associated with their use. The action of these drugs is to stimulate the pancreas to secrete more insulin. (The phenformin group of oral hypoglycemics has recently been removed from the market because of a high incidence of lactic acidosis.)

Insulin is the mainstay of definitive therapy in the juvenile-onset diabetic. There are three basic types of insulin based on duration of action. Regular insulin has its peak action 4 to 6 hours after injection. This type of insulin is used on an acute basis when rapidly changing conditions are present, that is, surgery. Alone it is not useful for maintenance care, although it may occasionally be used with the longer-acting insulins.

The intermediate-length insulins (NPH Iletin, lente) have their peak action 8 to 12 hours after injection. These insulins are characteristically utilized alone or with regular insulin for continued treatment and are the preparations most commonly used for daily maintenance.

Long-acting insulin (ultralente), with peak action 16 to 18 hours *after* injection, is not very useful for daily maintenance care.

Dental treatment planning considerations

The well-controlled diabetic poses very few problems for the dentist. This type of patient should enjoy all the normal technical treatment options and requires no modifications as to type of procedure or technique planned. One additional consideration must be to encourage the optimum in oral hygiene, since evidence seems to suggest that diabetics are more susceptible to periodontal disease than the nondiabetic. Aside from treatment planning considerations, the major problem becomes medical management of the patient while receiving dental care. The major problem is to ensure that the diabetic maintains his normal diet and insulin requirements during treatment. Not uncommonly, the diabetic may take his normal insulin, but because of dental pain or anxiety he may not eat properly. This condition can result in hypoglycemia during dental treatment. Proper management of this problem is the administration of glucose either orally or intravenously. Prevention of the problem is simple but requires awareness on the part of the dentist.

The dentist should ask what type of insulin and the amount of insulin the patient receives. From this information, one can easily determine the time of peak insulin activity and be especially alert for hypoglycemia during the peak action time. It is generally advantageous to schedule morning appointments after breakfast, since the usual insulin peak will fall later in the day.

The uncontrolled diabetic can present serious medical problems and is a contraindication for dental treatment. This patient may have large amounts of circulating glucose and ketone bodies, which after a period of time leads to shock and central nervous system disturbances terminating in coma and death. The patient in pain should be managed with analgesics and antibiotics if necessary and referred immediately for physical evaluation.

The diabetic with an acute orofacial infection is another serious problem. The infection can rapidly become fulminant, and the requirement for insulin and glucose may be severely altered. These patients must be treated aggressively to control the infection. This is usually accomplished medically with high doses of antibiotics and surgically with incision and drainage. During this period the patient may need to be under the case of the physician to regulate his insulin requirements. The more severe cases should be hospitalized (Fig. 5-11, *B*).

INFECTIOUS DISEASE
Hepatitis

The term hepatitis is defined in *Dorland's Illustrated Medical Dictionary* simply as "inflammation of the liver." This may occur as the primary disease process or secondary to another disease. Examples of primary liver disease in which inflammation is the chief finding are viral hepatitis (types A and B), toxic hepatitis, and drug-induced hepatitis. Examples of diseases to which hepatitis is secondary are infectious mononucleosis, secondary syphilis, and tuberculosis. Because of its infectiousness, viral hepatitis is of most concern to dentists, and therefore this discussion will be limited to that particular form of the illness.

Viral hepatitis is caused by at least two distinct viruses and has classically been divided into two types, infectious hepatitis and serum hepatitis. This nomenclature has now been replaced by hepatitis A and hepatitis B, respectively. The older classification was based primarily on the difference in modes of transmission. Hepatitis A was felt to be transmissible only via oral-fecal contamination of food and water supplies or fomites. Many people may contract the disease simultaneously, and this has led to the term epidemic hepatitis. In contrast, hepatitis B was felt to be transmissible only by parenteral contact with infected serum, usually via a contaminated needle. The primary victims were drug addicts and blood recipients. However, it is now generally accepted that there is little difference between the two types in regard to possible routes of transmission. Hepatitis A can be transmitted either by the fecal-oral route or blood, although the fecal-oral route is still the most frequent mode. Conversely, hepatitis B is transmitted not only by blood, but also by saliva, feces, tears, urine, and semen.[11]

The mode of transmission aside, there still remain some significant differences between these two types of viral hepatitis (Table 4). Among these differences, the clinical expression of the disease is important. Hepatitis A has a relatively short incubation period lasting around 2 to 5 weeks. The incubation period for hepatitis B may last from 2 to 6 months. Clinically the signs and symptoms of the two types are frequently indistinguishable; however, type B is associated with greater morbidity and mortality. From the dentist's standpoint, one of the more important aspects of hepatitis B is the occurrence of a nonsymptomatic carrier state that may follow recovery from the disease. During this period the infected person carries the hepatitis B antigen (HBsAg, Australia antigen) in his serum, which is believed to be the infectious agent. This period may last several years, and the carrier must be considered infectious during this time. Approximately 5% to 10% of persons infected with the disease will circulate the HBsAg for up to 25 years.[6]

The chronic carrier state holds some serious implications for dentistry from the standpoint of the patient's and dentist's protection. It should be obvious that it is the practitioner's obligation to protect his patients from infections from other patients or from himself. The other side of the coin, however, is that the dentist must protect himself from infected patients. If a dentist should contract hepatitis B and subsequently become a carrier, it could be a devastating experience both psychologically and economically. There are cases now documented in the literature where dentists have been discovered

Modifying factors in treatment planning

Table 4. Characteristics of hepatitis A and hepatitis B

	Hepatitis A	*Hepatitis B*
Etiologic agent	Type A virus(es)	Type B virus(es)
Route of transmission	Primarily oral-fecal, but possible through blood	Primarily through blood, but possible through saliva, feces, tears, urine, and semen
Incubation period	2 to 5 weeks	2 to 6 months
Age at time of infection	Frequently children or young adults	Infrequent before age 15, but any age possible
Season	Fall and winter	All seasons
Severity	Usually mild	Frequently severe
Effectiveness of gamma globulin	Usually effective	Uncertain
Presence of Australia antigen	No	Yes
Chronic carriers	No	5% to 10% of patients

as being carriers of hepatitis B, have transmitted the disease to their patients, and subsequently have been prevented from practicing dentistry as long as they remained infectious.[13] It should be noted, however, that detection of a carrier has become a very important procedure for health professionals and their patients, particularly in screening potential blood donors. A high index of suspicion must be raised about anyone with a documented past history of hepatitis B. It is fortunate that some relatively sophisticated laboratory screening tests for the antigen are now available at minimal cost. One drawback of the tests at present is the inability to detect very low concentrations of the antigen. This is unfortunate, since it has been shown that extremely small amounts of infected blood, 0.0001 ml, can result in transmission of the disease,[1] and this amount may not be detected by the test.

The signs and symptoms of acute viral hepatitis, both A and B, may include jaundice (icterus), fever, headache, malaise, anorexia, abdominal pain (right upper quadrant), nausea, and vomiting. There may be no jaundice (anicteric hepatitis), as is frequently the case in mild viral hepatitis or during the preicteric phase of hepatitis, which lasts from days to weeks.

Laboratory findings include bilirubin in the urine, elevation of serum bilirubin, elevation of the SGOT (serum glutamic-oxaloacetic transaminase), and positive HBsAg.

MEDICAL MANAGEMENT

Medical management of hepatitis is primarily supportive, as is the case with most viral diseases. It consists of bed rest and encouragement of a nutritious diet. Parenteral fluids are occasionally necessary. In severe cases, corticosteroids are used to control symptoms. Because of the lack of successful methods of treatment, prevention is important.

PREVENTION

Presently there is no absolute method of prevention for either type of viral hepatitis; however, injection of pooled gamma globulin usually contains enough type A antibody to prevent or minimize infections of the type A virus, and it is generally recommended whenever a person is likely to come in contact with infected persons or has already been exposed. In the past, however, there has been no dependable method of minimizing or preventing infection of hepatitis B. However, since the incidence of hepatitis B in the general population is increasing, pooled gamma globulin may contain sufficient quantities of type B antibodies; thus some physicians have begun recommending gamma globulin for prophylaxis against hepatitis B, but the effectiveness of this is still unproven. One promising development is work on a vaccine specific for hepatitis B. It appears to be effective in animal models, and work is now being conducted in humans, so perhaps in the near future total prophylaxis may be a reality.

DENTAL TREATMENT PLANNING CONSIDERATIONS

In planning treatment for a patient with a history of hepatitis, no alterations or limitations are necessary regarding the dental procedures. From the management standpoint, however, it is imperative that certain steps be taken to protect patients, auxiliaries, and the dentist.

1. Differentiation of patients with a history of hepatitis
   a. Attempt to differentiate between type A and type B by history or by contacting the patient's physician.
   b. If type A and if patient is clinically recovered, treat as normal patient.
   c. If type B, attempt to determine if patient is antigen-positive by
      (1) A consultation with patient's physician
      (2) Serum testing for HBsAg (done by commercial lab)*
   d. If patient is antigen-positive or if it cannot be definitely determined (patient refuses test), it should be assumed that the patient *is* positive for type B antigen and treat as outlined in 2.
2. Management of patients with history of hepatitis B and who are or may be antigen-positive
   a. Dentist and assistants should strictly adhere to aseptic technique.
   b. Dentist and assistants should wear masks and gloves.
   c. Handpieces should be either autoclaved or sterilized in a gas sterilizer following use. (Cold-sterilizing solutions are *not* effective.)

---

*At present, this step is not recommended as being necessary for all patients in the high-risk group; however, it would be to the advantage of all concerned if the results of this test were known.

d. Nonautoclavable items (e.g., plastic) should be gas sterilized. (Cold-sterilizing solutions are not effective.)
   e. Chairs should be covered with disposable head covers.
   f. Disposable covers should be placed on top of mobile cabinets before and after use.
   g. All instruments should be cleaned and packaged for sterilization at chairside.
   h. All waste material should be disposed of carefully in a disposable plastic bag and sealed.
   i. Tray set-ups are advisable. Once patient treatment is begun, there should be no reentry into drawers or cabinets. If additional instruments are needed, a circulating assistant should obtain them.
3. Dentist or auxiliary with a history of hepatitis B and antigen-positive (carrier)
   a. At present there is insufficient evidence to prevent a health professional from practicing because of a positive antigen-screening test; however, he or she has a moral, ethical, and legal obligation to protect his or her patients as well as other personnel.
   b. Gloves and masks should be worn at all times during patient contact.
   c. Dentist and assistants should strictly adhere to aseptic technique to prevent transmission from the operator to the patient or other personnel.
   d. There should be periodic retesting for HBsAg.

BONE AND JOINT DISEASES
Arthritis

Arthritis is one of the rheumatic diseases and is characterized by joint pain and stiffness. Rheumatic diseases in general all possess the symptoms of pain and stiffness in some part of the musculoskeletal system. There are a number of other rheumatic diseases including rheumatic fever, bursitis, myositis, and gout (Fig. 5-12); however, this section will be limited to a discussion of arthritis.

Classification of arthritis is difficult, since it is not only a primary disease but may also be a symptom of other diseases. When it occurs primarily, the cause may be obscure or unknown and may follow varying clinical patterns. It is often difficult to differentiate chronic arthritis from acute arthritis. Of the various types of arthritis, only rheumatoid arthritis and degenerative joint disease (osteoarthritis) will be considered here.

RHEUMATOID ARTHRITIS

Rheumatoid arthritis is one of the major crippling diseases. It is a progressively painful and disabling disease that affects 0.1% to 0.2% of the population over age 15. The cause is unknown. The pathologic change is basically chronic inflammation of the synovial membrane of a joint, leading to fibrous adhesions and, ultimately, bony adhesions between the joint surfaces. Enlargement and deformation of the joint also occur.

The typical clinical picture is one of progressively painful, swollen joints, especially of the hands, feet, and knees. Large joints also may be included as the disease progresses. The temporomandibular joint may also be affected. Progressive deformity and limitation of joint motion is the rule, with ulnar deviation of the fingers being pathognomonic. Subcutaneous nodules near joints or pressure areas are relatively common.

Medical management. Since there is no known cure for rheumatoid arthritis, treatment is directed toward symptomatic relief of pain and prevention of deformity and disability. These goals are generally achieved with bed rest, physical therapy, and salicylates. It is not unusual for patients to take 15 to 20 aspirin tablets daily on a regular basis. The dosage is based upon the amount that brings relief of pain without side effects. Because of the chronic salicylate ingestion, qualitative platelet defects may occur in addition to coagulation defects. Therefore the status of platelet function and coagulation function should be determined prior to any surgical intervention. In addition to salicylate therapy, additional drugs may be administered. These include nonsteroid antiinflammatory drugs such as phenylbutazone and indomethacin, gold salts, and corticosteroids.

Some distinct treatment problems may arise in patients taking these drugs, the most serious of which is adrenal suppression secondary to chronic corticosteroid administration. This is a potentially life-threatening problem that must be managed aggressively. Other problems include central nervous system disturbances and headaches with indomethacin and dermatologic disor-

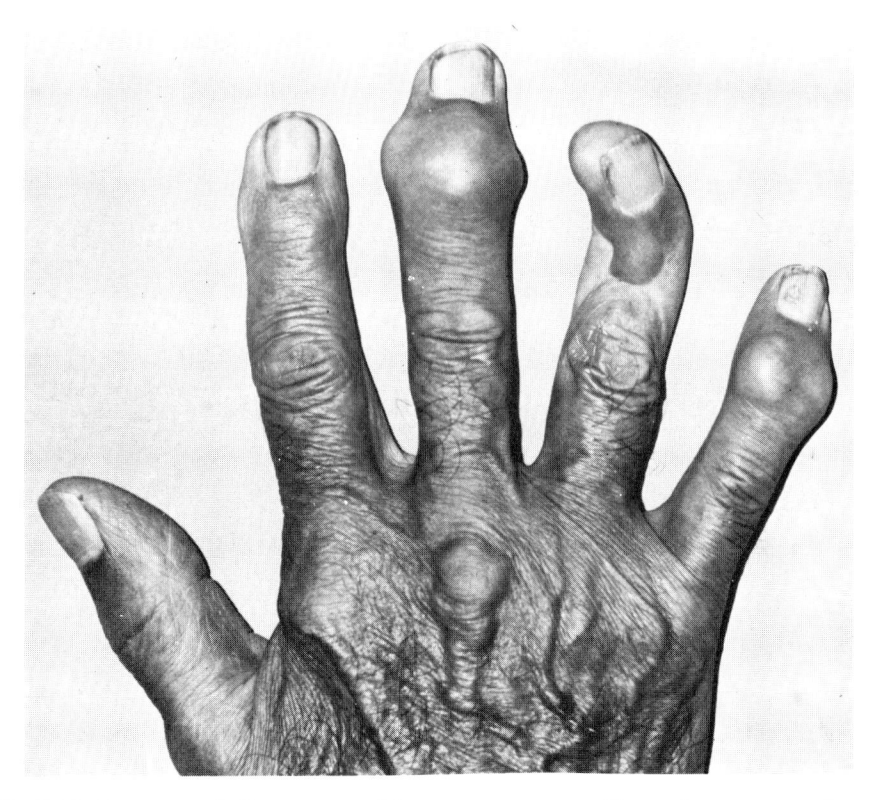

Fig. 5-12. Extensive disfigurement of fingers in patient suffering from gouty arthritis.

ders with phenylbutazone. Gold salts may cause an ulcerative stomatitis and a pruritic dermatitis. In addition to drugs, it may occasionally be necessary to resort to corrective surgical procedures to improve function or deformity; such procedures would include the insertion of a joint prosthesis.

Degenerative joint disease (osteoarthritis)

Degenerative joint disease is differentiated from rheumatoid arthritis in that it is not generally a crippling disease, and the pain and disability associated with it are generally minimal (Table 5). There is no systemic involvement. Osteoarthritis is characteristically a disease of later life and is very common in the elderly, although younger people may also demonstrate the disease. Trauma frequently predisposes to osteoarthritic changes.

The pathologic basis of the disease is a noninflammatory change in the joint characterized by degeneration of the articular cartilage and bone deposition. Over a long period of time a decrease in mobility may occur.

Pain may not be a prominent feature, although when it occurs, it occurs during use of the joint and ceases with rest. Stiffness is common after long immobility of the joint and is often experienced following a night's sleep. However, this quickly disappears with mobilization.

Osteoarthritis does not have the serious prognosis as does rheumatoid arthritis. In contrast, a patient with osteoarthritis may expect some inconvenience and discomfort from the disease, but he does not have the degree of crippling and disability (Fig. 5-13). Some alteration in lifestyle may be necessary, but the degree of change is usually much less than with rheumatoid arthritis.

Medical management. Treatment of this disease is usually limited to rest, physical therapy, and salicylates. Rarely is more aggressive drug therapy warranted. On occasion, when severe deformity has occurred, surgical correction may be necessary.

Dental treatment planning considerations. Most of the dental management modifications are directed toward rheumatoid arthritis, since it is the most severe form with the most complications. Clinical symptoms of other forms of arthritis may be similar, and the recommendations can be adapted to each patient as needed.

Table 5. Characteristics of rheumatoid arthritis and osteoarthritis

Rheumatoid arthritis	*Osteoarthritis*
Joint and systemic involvement	Joint involvement only
Hot, red, swollen, painful joints	Joint pain without inflammation
Subcutaneous nodules	No subcutaneous nodules
Involvement of any diarthrodial joint (including temporomandibular joint)	Involvement of knees, hips, spine, and fingers most commonly (rarely temporomandibular joint)
Rapid onset	Slow, insidious onset

Since pain with multiple joint involvement is the rule, these patients should have short appointments of less than 1 hour, as prolonged immobilization in a dental chair will result in stiffness and discomfort. In addition, physical supports such as pillows or rolls may be needed to support a deformed limb. Frequent change of position may be needed. Patients may be more comfortable in a sitting or semisitting position, as opposed to supine.

Drug therapy may complicate treatment of these patients. Reference has already been made to the potentially fatal adrenal suppression that occurs during prolonged steroid administration. (See discussion on the management of adrenal insufficiency.) Since high dosages of aspirin over a prolonged period may cause platelet and coagulation dysfunction, it is necessary to determine the bleeding time, prothrombin time, and partial thromboplastin time on these individuals prior to surgery. Correction of this problem should be managed in collaboration with the patient's physician.

The dentist should be aware that the patient on indomethacin may demonstrate headache, dizziness, seizures, syncope, or other central nervous system manifestations as a result of its toxic effects.

The use of gold salts may result in a troublesome stomatitis, which is evidence of toxicity of the preparation. This should be reported to the physician. The lesions should be treated symptomatically with agents such as saline or sodium bicarbonate mouthwash, or topical anesthetics, including viscous

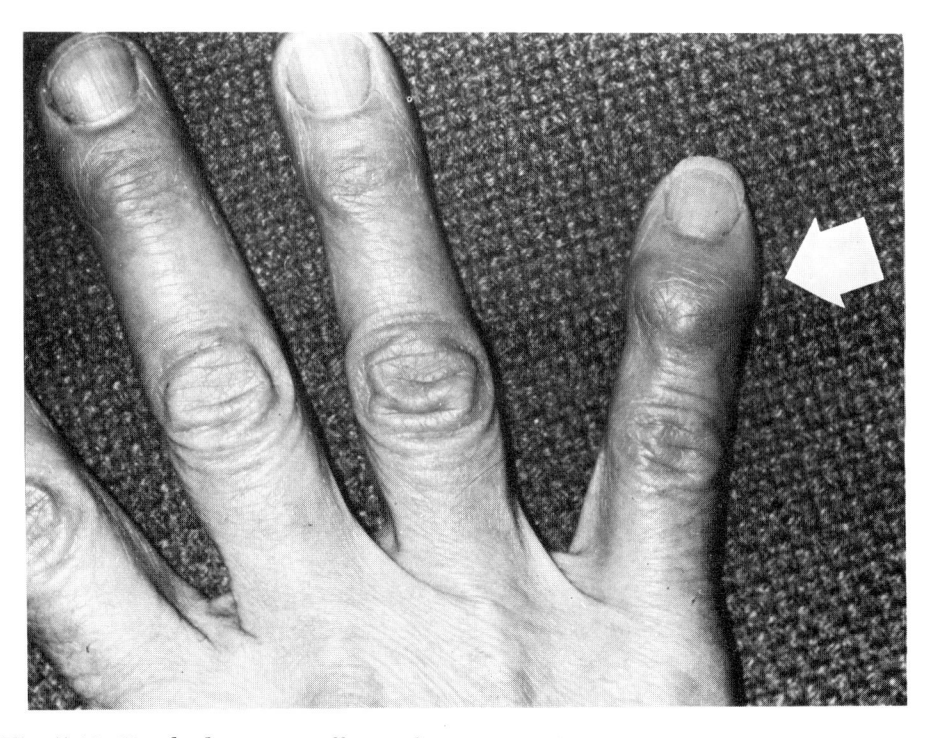

Fig. 5-13. Hand of patient suffering from osteoarthritis. Notice Heberden's node at distal interphalangeal joint (*arrow*) of little finger.

lidocaine (Xylocaine) or promethazine hydrochloride (Syrup of Phenergan).

Actual treatment planning modifications are dictated primarily by the patient's physical limitations. A patient who can tolerate only short appointments or who has limited jaw opening due to involvement of the temporomandibular joint should not be subjected to prolonged, extensive restorative treatment such as crown and bridge. If replacement of missing teeth is considered essential to continued health, it would be better to construct a removable partial denture because the chair time would be less. An additional advantage of a removable appliance is the ease of cleaning, which is an important consideration. If, however, a bridge is constructed, it is advisable to use a sanitary pontic to facilitate cleaning.

The patient who has a hand deformity may have considerable difficulty cleaning his teeth. For this patient one may resort to additional cleaning aids such as floss holders, toothpicks, mechanical toothbrushes, or modified manual brushes. One suggestion for modifying a toothbrush is to place a solid rubber ball on the handle to enable the deformed hand to grasp and manage the brush.

It should be kept in mind that this is a progressive disease that ultimately may lead to marked crippling and disability. Therefore the dentist must be aggressive in eliminating present dental disease as well as potential sources of dental disease. In addition, he must construct restorations or appliances that are easy to clean and comfortable for the patient.

Joint prostheses

In the arthritic patient the goal of treatment is to prevent deformity and loss of function. Unfortunately this is not always possible and function is lost. At this point, surgical correction may become necessary for a small percentage of patients. Of the various surgical procedures, the one that poses potential problems for the dentist is the replacement of a diseased joint with a prosthesis.

There are other indications for a joint prosthesis besides an arthritic joint, including nonunion of a fracture, avascular necrosis of bone of the femoral head, and, occasionally, acute trauma. Most experience to date has been with total hip replacement and knee replacement, although other joints have been replaced, including shoulders, elbows, wrists, and metacarpophalangeal joints. It is estimated that more than 49,000 total hip prostheses are placed annually.[16] From this figure, it is not unlikely that one of these patients may be among the dental practitioner's patients.

One of the biggest problems that faces the prosthetic recipient is that of deep infection around the prosthesis. If unchecked, the infection could result in need for replacement of the unit or total loss of the joint. It is evident that this complication could have catastrophic effects physically, emotionally, and economically. Current estimates of the rate of deep infection around the prosthesis are around 1%.

The infection around the unit may occur either early or late, the early infection invariably being related to the surgery itself. The source of late infection, however, is not as clear. Some authorities feel it is a latent infection resulting from the original surgery. Recently, however, a number of cases have been reported which seem to indicate that late infection may well be due to a hematogenous spread of an infection unrelated to the prosthesis. Some specific cases implicate bacteremia from dental infections and extractions.[4,7]

Dental treatment planning considerations

Although it would be difficult, if not impossible, to differentiate latent infection from metastatic infection, enough evidence exists to reasonably accept the theory of hematogenous spread of infection to a prosthesis. Therefore it is imperative that the dental practitioner take steps to minimize the effects of bacteremia secondary to dental procedures.

Since the principle of hematogenous spread to a prosthesis is the same as that of hematogenous spread to diseased cardiac valves or valve prosthesis in the rheumatic heart disease patient, the same basic antibiotic prophylaxis recommendations should be followed for both. (See discussion on rheumatic heart disease.)

The overall goal of dental treatment of these patients should be the maintenance of a disease-free oral cavity. Preventive measures should be aggressive and may require frequent recall appointments to reinforce home-care procedures. Any acute infections that may arise should be managed immediately and aggressively with antibiotics and medical consultation.

NEUROLOGIC DISEASES
Seizure disorders

A seizure disorder can be a difficult problem to manage medically as well as dentally. The clinical expression of a seizure varies, and may range from a frank convulsion to an imperceptible momentary lapse of consciousness. The cause of a seizure, regardless of the expression, is a paroxysmal discharge of electrical activity in some part of the brain. This discharge may be localized or generalized. When generalized, a convulsion is the result. Epilepsy is a term most frequently associated with recurrent seizures; however, it may also refer to other types of seizures. Since the clinical manifestations of this condition are so variable, there is confusion as to proper terminology. In addition, there are unfavorable historical connotations associated with the word epilepsy; therefore it is preferred to use the term seizure disorder when discussing these conditions.

Etiology

The etiology of seizure disorders is frequently described as either idiopathic or symptomatic. In a large majority of cases the seizures are idiopathic; that is, there is no demonstrable lesion or disorder attributed to their cause. Their onset is most frequent in childhood or adolescence.

In contrast to the idiopathic form of the disorder are the seizures that do have a demonstrable cause and are frequently seen in later life. Examples of conditions that may cause seizures are intracranial tumors, head trauma, cerebrovascular disorders, metabolic disorders, high fevers, and toxic disorders. In some cases, even though the apparent cause of the seizures is removed, the seizures may continue.

TYPES

Grand mal seizure. As previously mentioned, seizure disorders may be clinically manifested in a variety of forms or types of expressions. Probably the most familiar type is the grand mal seizure or convulsion. Frequently this seizure is preceded by a prodromal period or mood change varying from minutes to hours, during which time the patient may sense the approaching seizure. Immediately preceding the seizure the patient may experience a brief period of strange or unusual feeling or sensation such as a peculiar epigastric sensation or an unpleasant odor. This is termed the "aura" and is actually the first part of the seizure. Following the aura, the convulsion itself occurs with a loss of consciousness, the epileptic "cry" due to tonic (rigid) contraction of the diaphragm and respiratory muscles, and tonic contraction of the trunk and extremities, which results in cessation of respiration and cyanosis. This phase lasts about 30 seconds. This is followed by clonic (repetitive beating) movements. During this period the tongue or cheeks may be bitten and a blood-tinged froth may appear at the lips. The patient may also be incontinent of urine. After about a minute the clonic movement begins to subside and the patient relaxes and begins slow, heavy breathing, but remains unconscious. The patient cannot be aroused during this flaccid coma stage, which may last up to 30 minutes. Consciousness usually is regained, and the patient enters the postictal period (after seizure), which is characterized by confusion, fatigue, and deep natural sleep that may last from minutes to hours. It should be kept in mind that although this is the usual sequence of a grand mal seizure, it may be interrupted at any stage. The frequency of grand mal seizures ranges from once or twice during an entire lifetime to several per day. Several years may lapse between seizures.

Status epilepticus. A severe complication of grand mal seizures is a condition called status epilepticus. This is simply repetitive seizures that occur without the patient regaining consciousness between them. It is a serious complication and can be fatal unless treated rapidly. Treatment consists of maintaining an open airway, ventilating the patient, and administering intravenous diazepam (Valium) until the seizure is controlled. Concurrently a search for the cause of the condition is sought and treated appropriately.

Petit mal seizure. The petit mal seizure can be characterized as a brief cessation of consciousness commonly lasting 5 to 10 seconds. The patient's eyes may flicker and assume a blank stare, and he will suddenly stop whatever he may be doing. The lips and hands may demonstrate minor movements. The termination of the seizure is abrupt, with the patient having no recollection of the seizure or of the lost period of time.

Psychomotor seizure. A third type of seizure is the psychomotor seizure, which is preceded by an aura similar to that of the grand mal seizure. This is then followed by an alteration of consciousness, frequently strange visions or hallucinations, and autonomic motor activity. Attempts to restrain individuals during this period may result in violent aggressive behavior.

Focal seizure. Another frequently seen seizure is that of the focal type. These seizures are the result of an isolated focal discharge in the brain usually causing movement limited to one part of the body. Occasionally the focal seizure can progress to a generalized convulsion, but the true focal seizure is usually limited. An example of a focal seizure is the clonic movement of a single limb. A specific type of focal seizure is the *jacksonian motor seizure*. This focal seizure is peculiar in that it is a progressive seizure that may begin in the fingers and toes, then involves the whole limb, and then "marches" over the remainder of that side of the body. It characteristically occurs unilaterally.

Medical management

Medical treatment of seizures begins by attempting to identify their cause. This is done by physical exam, roentgenograms including angiography and ventriculography, laboratory analysis of blood, urine, and spinal fluid, and electroencephalogram. If a cause is discovered, correction of the disorder is accomplished if possible. Some causes may not be correctable such as an inoperable brain tumor. Even in treatable cases, seizures may continue because of residual brain damage. In cases of untreatable or unknown cause, drug therapy is indicated. It should be noted that not all patients are responsive to drug therapy.

Treatment of grand mal seizures and focal motor seizures is frequently accomplished by phenobarbital and diphenylhydantoin (Dilantin). Primidone (Mysoline) is also frequently used. Drug therapy must be individualized and is titrated gradually and progressively until the level of desired control is achieved. Because of drug tolerance the dosages may need occasional regulation. Psychomotor seizures may also respond to these drugs but are sometimes difficult to treat, and they may require larger dosages for control.

Petit mal seizures do not respond to the drugs used to treat grand mal, psychomotor, or focal seizures. The drugs most frequently used for petit mal control include the oxazolidinediones, trimethadione (Tridione) and paramethadione (Paradione), and phensuximide (Milontin).

Dental treatment planning considerations

In planning dental care for individuals with seizure disorders, two aspects must be considered: the medical management during treatment and actual treatment planning modifications.

Medical management is based primarily upon the past medical history. The pattern, frequency, and type of seizures the patient experiences must be determined. This information will forewarn the dentist as to what he may expect during his treatment. Also, it must be determined if there are any causative factors associated with the seizure such as loud noises or specific smells. If so, these must obviously be avoided. Determination of drug therapy and the degree of control must be ascertained. If the seizures are well controlled by the present drug therapy, the dentist must ensure that the patient continues that schedule throughout treatment. Voluntary discontinuance of anticonvulsive drugs is one of the most common causes of recurrent seizures. If the patient is not well controlled by drugs and continues to have frequent seizures, consultation with the physician is indicated. It may well be that the patient needs to be medically reevaluated and placed on different therapy prior to dental treatment.

After these precautionary steps have been taken, the next consideration is to be aware that the patient may still have a seizure while dental treatment is being rendered. Thus it is mandatory that the dentist be prepared to deal with it. The grand mal seizure is the most dramatic form of seizure activity and has the greatest probability for serious complications; therefore this discussion will be limited to that entity.

If a grand mal seizure does occur during dental treatment, the patient may well inform the dentist that he is about to have a seizure. This is especially true of a person who has frequent attacks. The basic duty of the dentist is to protect the patient during the seizure and to keep him from injuring himself. It is probably advisable to keep the patient in the chair and loosely restrain him. No effort should be made to totally prevent the erratic motor movement but merely to prevent self-injury. Should the patient vomit during the seizure, efforts should be made to turn the patient on his side and to suction the vomitus. A frequently made recommendation is to place a padded tongue blade between the teeth to prevent biting of tongue and cheeks (Fig. 5-14). The recommendation has some merit if it can be accomplished early, prior to the tonic phase; otherwise the patients teeth may be clenched and damage can be done by trying to force a tongue blade between tightly clenched teeth. Also, one must be careful not to force the tongue back into the pharynx with the tongue blade, as this will further compromise respiration. During the flaccid coma period, one should ensure that a clear airway is maintained so that oxygen can then be administered. After the seizure is terminated the patient should be allowed to sleep undisturbed until he voluntarily awakes.

As previously mentioned, status epilepticus is the succession of seizures without the patient regaining consciousness and is considered a medical emergency. Should this occur, treatment is by slow intravenous infusion of diazepam until the seizure is controlled. The patient should be transferred to a hospital or physician as soon as possible, as the condition may recur.

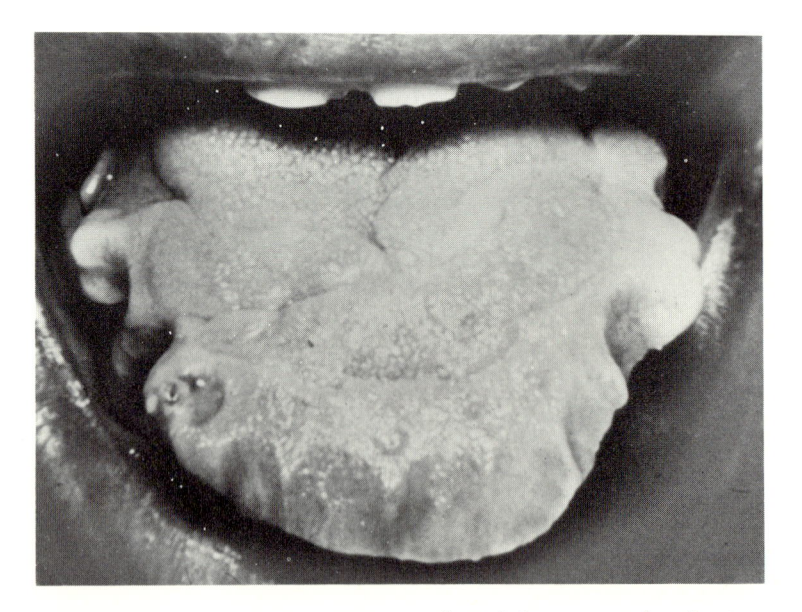

Fig. 5-14. Extensive trauma to tongue inflicted during grand mal seizure.

In planning treatment for these individuals, the most important consideration is the frequency and degree of control of the seizures. Again the grand mal seizure holds the most significance. If a patient is well controlled and has been free of seizures for a period of years, one may feel safe in planning similar procedures as for the patient who does not have a seizure disorder. However, the patient who actively has recurrent seizures presents a different problem. For many of these patients, treatment in a hospital setting could be desirable. The dentist may elect to treat on an outpatient basis if the seizures are not too frequent.

It is advisable to limit care of these individuals to preventive measures and control of active disease through endodontics, plastic restorations (amalgam, composites), and extractions. Treatment such as crown and bridge should be kept to a minimum unless necessary for health or for patient desire. Should crown and bridge treatment be elected, the use of porcelain is questionable because of expense and ease of fracture. A satisfactory substitute would be acrylic, which is cheaper and easier to replace in the event of a fracture. An additional method is to construct copings on abutment teeth and then construct bridges over these. The bridge is then cemented with a temporary type of cement so that removal of the bridge is facilitated in event of the need for replacing facings or new solder joints.

Removable appliances are usually contraindicated in a patient with frequent seizures, since these appliances are easily fractured or dislodged and can cause airway obstruction. In some cases, however, partial dentures can be modified by increasing clasp length and thickness, reinforcing the thickness of acrylic, and relieving areas of occlusal stress. If proper modifications are made, a removable partial denture can be used in selected cases.

Complete dentures again pose a problem, since the same problems exist as with a partial denture. In severe epileptic cases the patient would only be allowed to use the dentures for eating. This is indeed a difficult problem with which to deal, and each case must be evaluated individually.

REFERENCES

1. Barker, L. F., Shulman, N. R., Murray, R., et al.: Transmission of serum hepatitis, J.A.M.A. **211**:1509, 1970.
2. Bean, L. R., Jr., and Devore, W. D.: The effect of protective aprons in dental roentgenography, Oral Surg. **28**:505-508, 1969.
3. Bergan, J. J.: The twelfth report of the human transplant registry, J.A.M.A. **233**:788, 1975.
4. Brand, R. A.: Late hematogenous infection in total joint replacement, J. Iowa Med. Soc. **65**:388-390, 1975.
5. Bybee, D.: Personal communication, 1977.
6. Council on Dental Therapeutics: Type B (serum) hepatitis and dental practice, J.A.D.A. **92**:153-159, 1976.
7. Cruess, R. L., Bickel, W. S., and von Kessler, K. L.: Infections in total hips secondary to a primary source elsewhere, Clin. Orthop. **106**:99-101, 1975.
8. Ellenberg, M.: Diabetes: current status of an evolving disease, N.Y. State J. Med. **77**:62-67, 1977.
9. Gruenberg, J. C., and Mikhail, G. R.: Percutaneous adrenal suppression with topically applied corticosteroids. Arch. Surg. **111**:1165, 1976.
10. Kazatchkine, M., Sultan, Y., Caen, J. P., et al.: Bleeding in renal failure: a possible cause, Br. Med. J. **2**:612-615, 1976.
11. Mackinzie, D. L., et al.: Advances in viral hepatitis, Va. Med. Mon. **102**:125-132, 1975.

12. Maibach, H. I., and Stroughton, R. B.: Topical corticosteroids, Med. Clin. North Am. **57**:1253-1264, 1973.
13. Must hepatitis carriers stop treating patients? Med. World News, **16**:19-21, December 15, 1975.
14. Oles, R. D.: Personal communication, 1977.
15. Wang, F.: Conservative management of chronic renal failure, Med. Clin. North Am. **55**:137-154, 1971.
16. Wilson, P. D., Jr., Salvati, E. A., and Blumenfeld, E. L.: The problem of infection in total prosthetic arthroplasty of the hip, Surg. Clin. North Am. **55**:1431-1437, 1975.

6

Medical considerations: cardiovascular, respiratory, gastrointestinal, and hematologic systems, xerostomia, and irradiation

Ellen Eisenberg

DISEASES OF THE CARDIOVASCULAR SYSTEM
Hypertension

Sustained elevation of the systolic and diastolic pressures, coincident with increased mean arterial pressure, constitutes true systemic hypertension. This is most frequently associated with increased peripheral vascular resistance of smaller arteries and arterioles. A sustained arterial pressure of 160/95 mm Hg or greater in a resting supine adult indicates the presence of hypertension. Hypertension may be classified as *primary* or *secondary*. Primary hypertension accounts for approximately 95% of all cases of hypertension. It is also called *essential hypertension*, and its cause is unknown. On the other hand, secondary hypertension is induced by diseases in other organ systems and is uncommon. *Malignant hypertension* is a phase of the disease that appears suddenly as a sustained high elevation in arterial pressure, which is usually fatal.

Essential hypertension

The vast majority of patients with hypertension suffer from the essential variety. Usually these patients experience a progressive rise in blood pressure with age, thus decreasing life expectancy. Damage classically results to three target organs: the brain, heart, and kidney. The danger of cerebral vascular accident is imminent, as well as coronary ischemic disease and congestive heart failure. Months or years may pass, however, before the patient becomes symptomatic. Clinical symptoms may include dizziness, headaches, general malaise, epistaxis, and dyspnea. Because of the lack of symptoms in the early stages of hypertension, it is essential that dentists record blood pressures routinely for all adult patients. This is doubly necessary because many patients do not receive annual physical examinations.

Medical management. Management of essential hypertension is directed at lowering the blood pressure, alleviating symptoms, and minimizing potential complications such as brain, heart, and kidney damage. Antihypertensive agents act in one way or another to inhibit the quantity or the actions of the catecholamines. Propranolol is a beta adrenergic blocking agent. Methyldopa inhibits norepinephrine synthesis. Rauwolfia alkaloids inhibit norepinephrine storage in the adrenergic nerve ending vesicles. Guanethidine blocks norepinephrine release from sympathetic nerve endings. Monamine-oxidase inhibitors block catecholamine degradation, thus reduced quantities are actually released. Hydralazine is a vascular smooth muscle relaxant that decreases arterial resistance without major adrenergic blockade. Diuretic agents, especially the thiazides, increase sodium excretion by the renal tubules and thus decrease extracellular fluid volume. Antihypertensive agents are utilized either alone or in varying combinations to lower the arterial pressure to more physiologic levels.

Dental treatment planning considerations. Taking the blood pressure for each patient as well as recording it in the dental chart is essential. It is imperative to ensure that persons having previously undiagnosed hypertension receive a complete physical examination by an internist and that appropriate treatment is instituted. For the patient who is known to have hypertension, blood pressure must be recorded at each visit to determine whether the current reading is compatible with the stress of the anticipated dental procedure. During particularly stressful and prolonged procedures such as oral surgery, it may be advisable to take the blood pressure at several different times. The patient's physician should be consulted before dental treatment is undertaken if the current readings are worrisome.

Most of the dentist's efforts should be aimed toward the maintenance of patient tranquility. The patient will do best when he is well rested; therefore morning appointments are preferred. Premedication with sedatives or tranquilizing agents administered intravenously or orally prior to appointments may be beneficial for the nervous hypertensive patient. Prevention of pain is of paramount importance. Local anesthetic injections with vasoconstrictors should be employed to assure profound anesthesia during the complete procedure. Careful aspiration technique and slow administration of the injection must be performed. Nitrous oxide analgesia generally produces concurrent elevation of blood pressure and so is contraindicated. Physician consultations are required when prolonged surgical procedures are anticipated in persons having poorly controlled hypertension. Extensive oral surgical procedures on such patients probably would be best accomplished in the hospital instead of in the private office.

Since sodium retention is a side effect of many of the antihypertensive drugs, diuretics are prescribed concurrently to enhance sodium elimination. Unfortunately this tends to predispose the patient to orthostatic hypotension; that is, patients raised rapidly from a supine to a sitting position will suffer a hypotensive episode that will cause dizziness and even syncope. For this

Cardiovascular, respiratory, gastrointestinal, and hematologic systems

reason, such patients who have been in a supine position in a dental chair should not be brought rapidly to a sitting position. Rather they should be gradually raised to a sitting or standing position in increments.

Persons having poorly controlled hypertension should not be denied dental care, but minimization of pain, stress, and chair time is strongly recommended. Thus an extensive reconstructive treatment plan may need to be altered to one involving less arduous removable partial dentures. Endodontic therapy would usually be recommended instead of extraction because stress and the chance of bleeding are minimized, as well as the future need for crown and bridge. Indeed, the requirement for modified scheduling and stress minimization, especially in the poorly controlled hypertensive dental patient, favors conservative dentistry such as disease control and relatively short, uncomplicated procedures. Thus extensive periodontal and oral surgical procedures should be avoided if possible. When these cannot be avoided, hospitalization and physician cooperation are indicated.

Secondary hypertension

Secondary hypertension accounts for approximately 5% of all cases of hypertension. A detailed discussion of each predisposing disease state is beyond the scope of this book. The major disease states producing secondary hypertension are adrenal gland hyperfunction (hyperplasias and pheochromocytomas), unilateral renal disease, elevated intracranial pressure, pituitary tumors, coarctation of the aorta, eclampsia, polycythemia, periarteritis nodosa, peripheral neuritis and ascending myelitis, diencephalic syndrome, and thyrotoxicosis. It is readily apparent that a consultation with the patient's physician must be obtained prior to the development of a treatment plan or the initiation of any dental work in patients who suffer from any of these diseases.

Ischemic heart disease

Ischemic heart disease is the most prevalent variety of heart disease and is attributed to insufficient coronary circulation secondary to coronary artery atherosclerosis. Angina pectoris and myocardial infarction are the two principal clinical syndromes of ischemic heart disease.

Angina pectoris

Angina pectoris is a symptom of compromised coronary circulation. Characteristically the patient describes it as a substernal tightness or pain that may radiate down the left arm or down both arms. Occasionally the pain may appear to be in the back, the neck, and even the left angle of the mandible. The discomfort or pain is rapidly ameliorated by vasodilators such as nitroglycerin.

Episodes of angina pectoris are precipitated by sudden demands for increased cardiac activity, such as physical exertion, emotional stress, or a heavy meal. Existing atherosclerotic narrowing of the coronary arteries produces a phenomenon of *relative* myocardial ischemia in such situations. Hypertensive patients often experience angina as well, since left ventricular oxygen requirements are raised in working against the increased pressure. Pulmonary hypertension, hyperthyroidism, and cardiovalvular disease may also produce angina. Attacks of angina are significant for two reasons: (1) they signal the presence of a serious disease, and (2) progressive diffuse myocardial fiber necrosis accompanies the severe pain.

Medical management. Adjustment of the patient's lifestyle is one of the most important aspects of management. In addition, the following vasodilatory drugs are useful both to prevent and to alleviate attacks of anginal pain: papaverine, aminophylline, the nitrites, and beta blocking agents such as propranolol. Coronary bypass surgery is performed in selected cases.

Dental treatment planning considerations. Treatment-associated stress should be minimized or eliminated for the angina patient. It is important to determine the frequency, intensity, and duration of attacks, as well as the degree of exertion required to precipitate an attack. It is also necessary to determine the present emotional state of the patient. A history of hypertension or myocardial infarction will require further assessment of the patient. The patient's cardiologist should be consulted even before treatment planning commences.

The basic approach to dental treatment for the angina patient is reassurance and elimination of pain. The patient should bring his medication to each appointment. The appointments should be reasonably short, and procedures should be as atraumatic as possible. If indicated, preoperative sedation, such as a short-acting barbiturate, may be prescribed with the physician's consent. If necessary, a 0.6 mg tablet of nitroglycerin administered sublingually may be used in conjunction with a tranquilizer or barbiturate. Narcotic analgesics raise the pain threshold and so may be useful as well. Parasympathomimetic agents such as atropine are contraindicated, since they tend to increase the heart rate. Local anesthetic injections should be employed for all potentially painful procedures. Ancillary medications should be administered only after clearance is obtained from the patient's physician. Procedures requiring general anesthesia must be performed in the hospital.

Dental emergencies involving pain or bleeding episodes must be treated promptly so as to provide patient comfort and relief. This helps to prevent occurrence of an anginal spasm. Should the patient complain of precordial or thoracic pain during routine dental treatment, immediate discontinuation of the procedure is required. All further dental service at that appointment must be postponed, and a fresh nitroglycerin tablet should be immediately administered sublingually, or nitrite should be given by inhalation. A second dose of nitroglycerin may be given if relief is not experienced after the first tablet. Generally these patients are familiar with the quantity of tablets required to alleviate their distress, and if the usual dose proves unsuccessful, myocardial infarction must be considered.

It is wise to treatment plan for short appointments and simple procedures although tolerance for lengthy procedures will vary from patient to patient. The stress of time-consuming fixed prosthodontics may be eliminated by treatment planning for a removable partial denture instead. Even extraction may be preferable to the repeated stress of endodontic treatment for the very anxious hypertensive patient. Extensive procedures such as multiple extractions and plastic revisions are best spread out over several appointments and done under local rather than general anesthesia. Extensive periodontal surgery should not be considered for the patient with severe angina, and extensive procedures to improve malocclusion should be discouraged. Selective grinding and removable partial dentures are about all that should be attempted in this regard. It follows that the more severe the anginal problem, the more limited dental treatment should be and the closer the collaboration with the physician.

Myocardial infarction

Coronary artery occlusion may occur suddenly and totally in a single branch because of thrombus formation in an atherosclerotic vessel or as a result of sudden hemorrhage into an atherosclerotic plaque. Rarely, embolism may be the cause. At any rate the coronary occlusion leads to acute ischemia and progressive degeneration of the deprived area of the myocardium. Pain and often death ensue. Immediate fatalities may be caused by acute arrhythmias such as ventricular fibrillation. Cardiac tamponade is a threat in the first week or so following the attack. Survival past 10 days is indicative of a fairly favorable prognosis. This is because inflammation of the acute variety is succeeded by macrophage immigration and elimination of necrotic material by the end of the first week and the beginning of the second. The "soft infarction" site becomes fibrotic during the third week, and repair progresses with the maturation of collagen.

Patients susceptible to myocardial infarction are those with a history of hypertension, angina pectoris, atherosclerosis, and increased demand for oxygen, especially smokers, diabetics, and obese individuals. Signs of coronary occlusion are crushing, persistent, precordial pain that may radiate but is not relieved by nitroglycerin. It is not necessarily precipitated by stress, and can occur during rest or sleep. Ashen facies, cyanosis, cold sweat, pallor, nausea, and vomiting are seen. Left-sided heart failure, due to left ventricular or ventricular septal infarction, may result in pulmonary edema. Shock can occur.

Medical management. Medical treatment in the acute phase of the disease basically involves pain relief with morphine or with tranquilizers if pain is less severe. Rest is essential during convalescence when collateral circulation is being established. Adequate oxygenation is essential during this period. Anticoagulants are employed during the 2 weeks following acute myocardial infarction, and in some cases on a permanent basis. Survival of the patient past the initial 3 or 4 weeks is related to the location and extent of myocardial damage and scarring. Prognosis depends on several factors such as the presence of cardiac failure, arrhythmias, emotional profile, age of the patient, presence of other systemic diseases, and prior infarction history. Periodic electrocardiogram studies and careful monitoring by the cardiologist are essential follow-up procedures for these patients.

Dental treatment planning considerations. Infarction patients may be treated with analgesics for relief of dental pain during the acute convalescent period. For a month thereafter, all dental service of an elective nature must be deferred. After the first 3 weeks of convalescence, incision and drainage procedures for abscesses may be performed.

It is important to establish that the patient actually suffered a myocardial infarction. This is frequently necessary because diseases such as acute indigestion may mimic a myocardial infarction. The physician should be consulted if the patient is sketchy or uninformed about his history.

Dental procedures for the patient with a history of myocardial infarction should be as atraumatic as possible. Local anesthesia with epinephrine is indicated for all potentially painful procedures and should be administered in adequate amounts. Sedation can be prescribed (with the consent of the cardiologist) for the apprehensive individual and is especially desirable prior to fairly extensive surgical procedures. Nitrous oxide analgesia is contraindicated, since it is associated with a blood pressure rise, hypoxia, and prolonged excitement. An elective general anesthetic should not be given until at least 6 months have lapsed. Patients taking anticoagulants must be carefully evaluated when procedures that induce bleeding are contemplated. This requires consultation with the patient's physician. A prothrombin time maintained at no more than one and one-half to two times that of the control is desirable for the avoidance of excessive bleeding, and the physician can gradually titrate the anticoagulant dosage down to achieve this, if necessary, in preparation for dental surgery. Surgical procedures should be kept relatively simple, and hemostatic adjuncts such as sutures, pressure dressings, and absorbable gels should be utilized.

Essential dental treatment can be planned for the cardiac patient, especially with judicious management and cooperation on the part of the physician. If the patient has recovered and is not displaying progressive signs of decompensation or angina pectoris, he can receive ideal dentistry, provided that procedures are carried out with minimal stress.

Congestive heart failure

Cardiac decompensation or congestive heart failure is the failure of the heart to supply blood to the tissues according to their metabolic needs. The condition is due to the decreased ability of the diseased myocardium to pump blood. Chronic excessive workload, as seen in severe valvular heart disease or primary cardiomyopathy, eventuating in decreased contractility, is responsible for the hemodynamic manifestations, namely, forward failure (diminished stroke volume) and backward failure (systemic venous congestion). Compensatory mechanisms such as cardiac hypertrophy and dilatation occur early in an effort to achieve greater contractility of the compromised myocardium. Catecholamine secretion may be increased; stroke volume and systemic blood volume are augmented as well. As heart failure progresses, however, compensating mechanisms become depleted and become themselves an additional burden on the heart. Consequently, tolerance for exertion decreases.

Left-sided heart failure may be the result of mitral or aortic valvular pathology, hypertension, or myocardial disease secondary to insufficient coronary arterial blood flow. Pulmonary edema is the most prominent manifestation of this syndrome and is caused by pulmonary vascular congestion and increased circulatory pressure. Right-sided heart performance is relatively normal despite the almost invariable clinical manifestations of right-sided heart failure.

Cardiovascular, respiratory, gastrointestinal, and hematologic systems 87

Right-sided heart failure is seen in *cor pulmonale*. In this condition, as in left-sided heart failure and obstructive lung disease, compromised pulmonary circulation restricts adequate cardiac function. Effects are those that ensue from systemic venous congestion and oxygen deprivation. Chronic passive visceral congestion leads ultimately to hepatic parenchymal necrosis and cardiac cirrhosis, splenic fibrosis, kidney failure, and secondary erythrocytosis.

The clinical signs and symptoms of advanced congestive heart failure include dependent edema, dyspnea and orthopnea, cyanosis, clubbing of the fingers, and lack of exercise tolerance (Figs. 6-1 and 6-2). Irritability due to cerebral hypoxia may also be seen.

MEDICAL MANAGEMENT

A tripartite approach is taken in the medical management of the heart failure patient. Objectives include the reduction of cardiac workload, enhancement of myocardial contractility, and control of fluid retention. These are accomplished through physical and emotional rest, weight reduction, restricted sodium chloride and caloric intake, smaller meals, and curtailment of strenuous activity. Additionally, various therapeutic agents may be prescribed. Sympathomimetic amines such as epinephrine, dopamine, and isoproterenol strengthen myocardial contraction. Diuretic medications, such as the very popular thiazides, mercurials, spironolactones (aldosterone antagonists), and furosemide or ethacrynic acid, mobilize excessive fluid. Digitalis is effective in heart failure caused by hypertension and valvular or ischemic heart disease because of its positive inotropic action. Prognosis is assessed generally by the

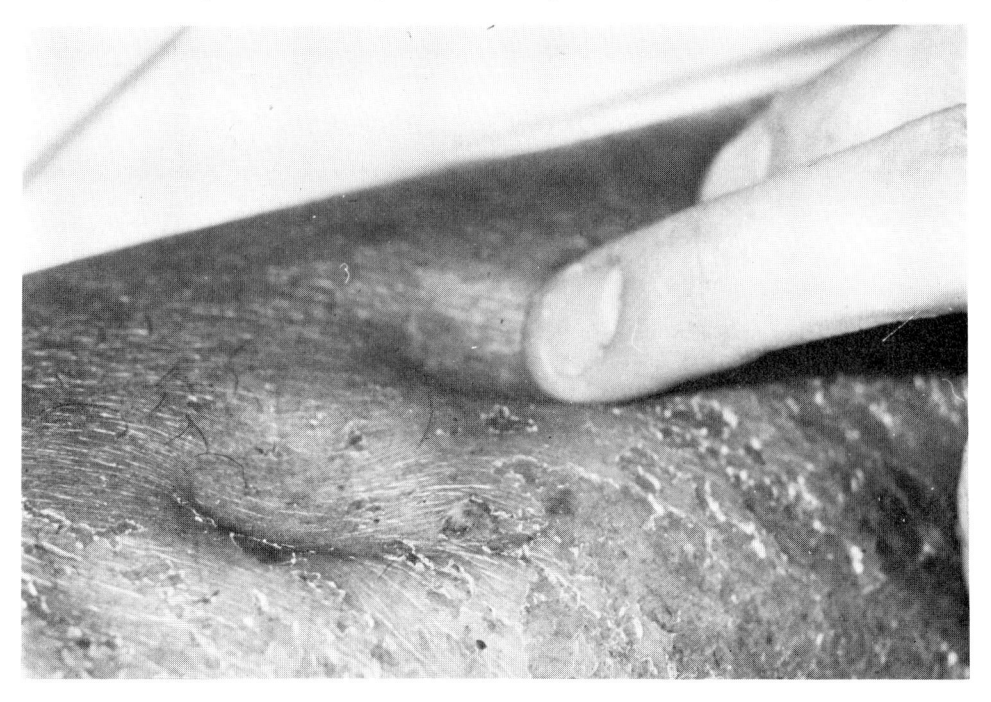

Fig. 6-1. Pitting edema of lower extremities of patient suffering from congestive heart failure.

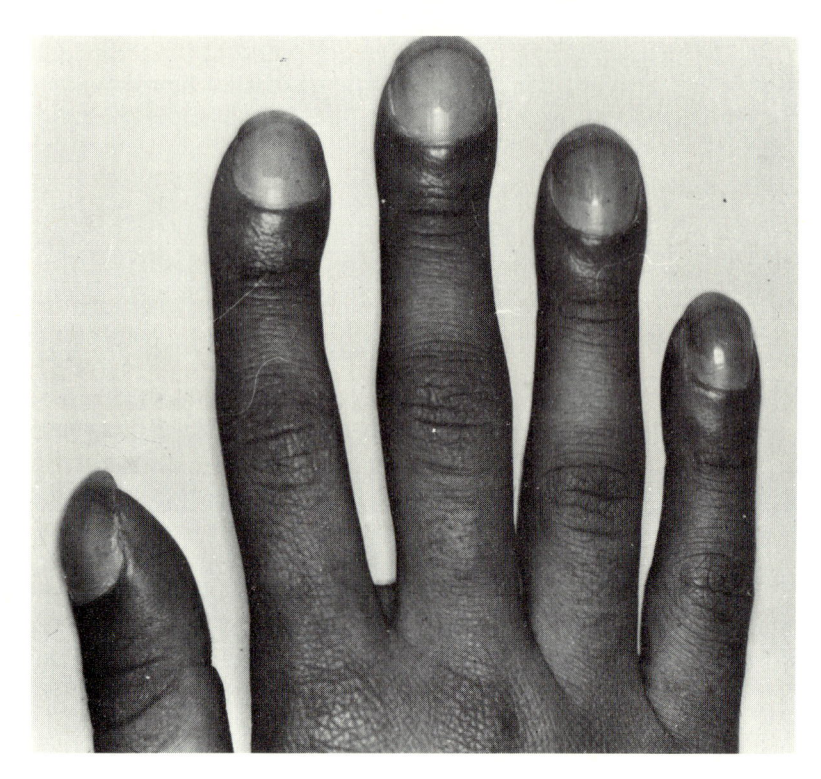

Fig. 6-2. Clubbing of fingers and "watchglass" nails in chronic congestive heart failure patient.

patient's response to treatment. As a rule, patients demonstrating improvement with dietary modification of sodium intake with or without digitalis tend to have a better future than those requiring additional therapy.

Dental treatment planning considerations

Early signs and symptoms of cardiac decompensation can be elicited from the history, follow-up questioning, and observation of the dental patient at the initial visit. These findings in conjunction with the physician's advice permit the division of heart failure patients into three groups as far as restrictions for dental treatment are concerned:

Group 1. If cardiac compensation has been established through medical intervention and dyspnea occurs only with routine exercise but not at rest, dental treatment planning may proceed with no major modifications. However, special attempts should be made to minimize stress during dental treatment.

Group 2. For patients who experience dyspnea with less than routine exercise but not at rest, a physician consultation is required. Frequency of visits will be commensurate with a need for decreased chair time. Accordingly, less extensive procedures to maintain oral health are planned, and where a choice exists, more conservative services are rendered. Appointments scheduled early in the day with the patient well rested and fed a light meal prior to the visit are conducive to comfort. Chair positioning should favor the seated rather than supine approach in order to decrease the possibility of orthopneic discomfort. Local anesthetics are indicated, and vasoconstriction can be used. Depending on the tolerance of the patient for moderately lengthy dental procedures, advantages are weighed for treatment planning of either removable or fixed prosthodontics. Should the patient require a short-span tooth-borne replacement for edentulism, a fixed prosthesis may be the treatment of choice. On the other hand, removable partial dentures are acceptable substitutes for procedures anticipating extensive fixed prosthodontics that would require an inordinate number of lengthy appointments.

In a well-compensated cardiac patient, minor extractions and preprosthetic surgery can be performed in stages when more than one quadrant is involved. Preoperative sedation can be administered with advice and consent of the cardiologist. Periodontal treatment requiring stabilization of teeth should be accomplished using temporary-permanent techniques (i.e., continuous-extracoronal wire and acrylic splints, intracoronal amalgam and wire A splints, conjoined resin acid-etch preparations, and orthodontic appliances) rather than permanent fixed splinting procedures, which are considerably more exacting and time-consuming. Occlusal therapy of a conservative, non-reconstructive nature is permissible. Periodontal surgery can be performed provided the procedure is brief. Oral hygiene instruction, scalings, and prophylaxis are the most desirable modalities of periodontal treatment. Endodontics is, where possible, acceptable; if periodontal surgery and dental heroics are found to be necessary to save a single, questionably restorable tooth, extraction is preferable. Operative dentistry and caries control should be undertaken in order to maintain the existing dentition. Lengthy visits employing quadrant dentistry are discouraged.

Group 3. Congestive heart failure patients who are dyspneic at rest are probably not able to be treated on an outpatient or private basis, and their treatment should be confined to palliation. Extractions can be postponed and substituted for by antibiotic and analgesic medications and pulp extirpation until myocardial compensation is achieved. Sedative dressings can be placed in lieu of definitive restorative dentistry for painful carious teeth, and endodontics can be deferred. Predisposition to nausea and vomiting is experienced by many patients maintained on digitalis and related drugs. It is therefore advisable to exercise treatment precautions similar to those indicated for patients with hiatal hernias and peptic ulcers in order to obviate stimulation of gagging and vomiting reflexes, which could result in aspiration of regurgitated material.

The operator is familiar with his own speed and capabilities. This must be taken into consideration when treatment planning for decompensated or artificially compensated patients according to the mandate for shorter, relatively atraumatic appointments.

Rheumatic heart disease and bacterial endocarditis

As a late inflammatory complication of group A beta hemolytic streptococcal infection, acute rheumatic fever may occur. Rheumatic fever is characterized by a spectrum of lone-standing or multiple combinations of chorea, rash, subcutaneous nodules, polyarthritis, and carditis. The presence of at least two of these together is generally diagnostic of rheumatic fever. Despite the fact that allergic responses to microbial antigens on the part of the host most often enhance immunologic defense against an invading microorganism, in the case of rheumatic carditis it is currently theorized that antibodies (antistreptolysin O) elaborated to the cell-wall antigens of beta hemolytic streptococci are cross-reactive with human myocardium. Thus gross valvular lesions such as fibrous leaflet thickening, stenosis, chordae tendineae contraction, and commissural verrucae are produced by a hypersensitivity "bystander"-type of antibody-antigen reaction. Mitral insufficiency and stenosis are the most classic cardiac manifestations of chronic (subclinical) rheumatic fever (Fig. 6-3). The other valves can also be affected. As the disease progresses and valvular deformities become more exaggerated, clinical manifestations of left and right cardiac decompensation with pulmonary edema and systemic congestion will present.

Acute rheumatic valvulitis has the potential to resolve without scarring and deformation of the valves; in most cases, however, and in recurrent cases, the fibrinoid verrucae *will* produce fibrous bridging across the valve commissures and will shorten, thicken, and fuse the chordae tendineae. Cardiac murmurs, attributed to turbulence of blood flow across the scarred myocardium, are auscultatory signs of valve disease. Patients who have sustained a

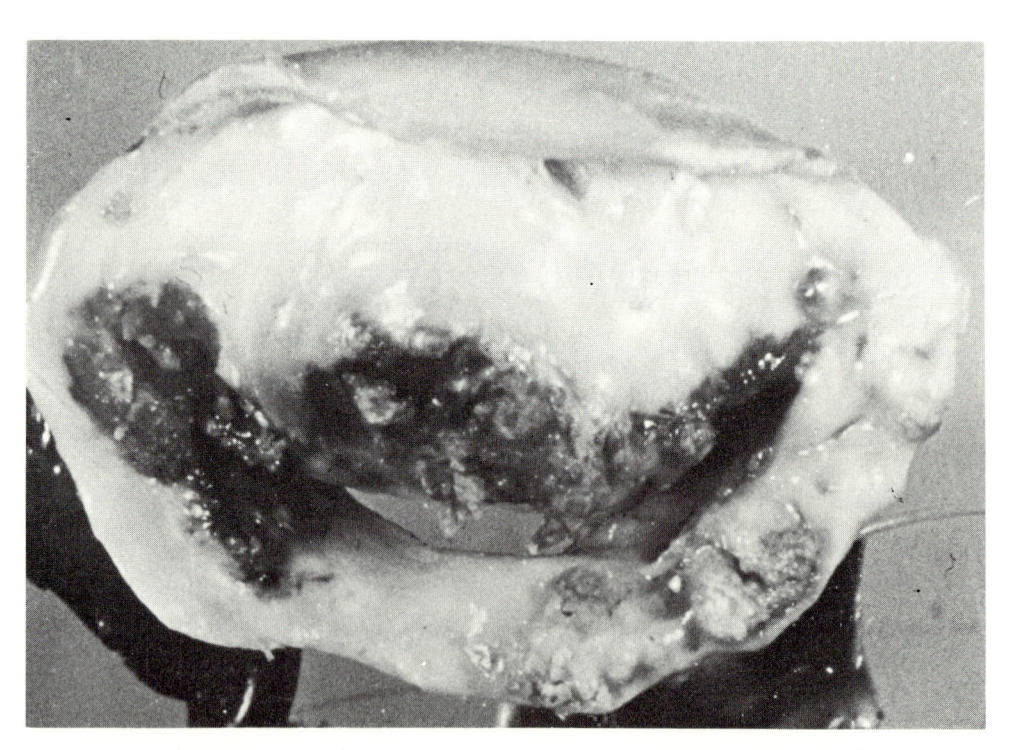

Fig. 6-3. Mitral stenosis secondary to rheumatic heart disease. This patient suffered from episodes of bacterial carditis. Note the many vegetations present on damaged valve. (Courtesy Dr. Stephen Raibley, Maywood, Ill.)

bout of rheumatic fever are particularly prone to recurrences; damaged valves are susceptible to acute and subacute bacterial endocarditis (Fig. 6-3).

MEDICAL MANAGEMENT

Apparently any pathologic bacterium or mycotic organism is capable of producing an endocarditis. Diagnosis is based upon the following signs and symptoms: petechiae of the hands, oral cavity, and feet; chills; sweating; fever; Janeway lesions; cardiac murmurs; arthralgias; splenomegaly; Osler nodes; prior cardiac disease; cardiac decompensation; and positive blood cultures. Indeed this is a very grave disease state that is pathologically attributed to valvular destruction and systemic septic embolization of valvular vegetations (thrombi). Prophylactic therapy with antibiotics is imperative for prevention of recurrent rheumatic fever and bacterial endocarditis. Currently, continuous penicillin or sulfadiazine chemoprophylaxis is instituted to prevent streptococcal infections that have the capacity to produce recurrences of rheumatic fever. Medical opinions vary as to the optimum maintenance schedule of antirheumatic prophylaxis, but it is believed that a reasonable regimen calls for continuance of chemoprophylaxis for at least 5 years after the last acute attack and until 25 years of age. Indefinite maintenance should be applied for those patients who have had carditis. Exposure to bacteremias in susceptible patients mandates additional antibiotic coverage.

DENTAL TREATMENT PLANNING
CONSIDERATIONS

At the history-taking visit it is essential to establish whether the patient has had rheumatic fever, and this can be elicited by using the modified Jones criteria (chorea, carditis, polyarthritis, subcutaneous nodules, erythema marginatum, fever, preceding infection with *Streptococcus* organisms). Simply asking "Have you ever had rheumatic fever?" is insufficient. Patients reporting a heart murmur must be further questioned about a rheumatic fever history, since murmurs may be functional or organic. Suspicion of a positive rheumatic fever history calls for referral of the patient to a physician for confirmation or denial, prior to the undertaking of any dental treatment, in order to determine whether rheumatic heart disease is present. Should the diagnosis prove positive, responsibility lies, then, within the physician's judgment as to whether a long-term prophylaxis is necessary. Supplementary antibiotic coverage to prevent alpha hemolytic streptococcal bacteremia and valvular vegetations consequent to dental manipulations in the rheumatic heart disease patient is prescribed in addition to continuous, low-dose prophylaxis.

Penicillin remains the preferred antibiotic in rheumatic fever, valvular disease, and bacterial endocarditis prophylaxis by virtue of its effectiveness against gram-positive bacteria such as viridans streptococci, which are the primary offenders in infections of dental origin.

Premedication with penicillin or, if that is contraindicated, erythromycin *must* be instituted before surgical procedures are performed such as dental extractions; periodontal scaling; curettage; gingival, mucoperiosteal, or osseous surgery; endodontic therapy; operative or prosthetic dentistry where gingival manipulations or injections are performed; preprosthetic plastic procedures; and incisional or excisional biopsies.

According to the current findings of the Committee on Prevention of Rheumatic Fever and Bacterial Endocarditis of the American Heart Association, the following chemoprophylactic regimens are suggested for dental manipulations likely to cause gingival bleeding and surgical procedures involving the upper respiratory tract.[1,2]

Regimen A is either parenteral-oral or oral and employs penicillin. For adults, intramuscular injection of aqueous crystalline penicillin G (1 million units) combined with procaine penicillin G (600,000 units) is given 30 to 60 minutes prior to the procedure, and penicillin V (500 mg) is administered orally every 6 hours for eight doses following the procedure. This parenteral-oral combined regimen is particularly useful in the case of a dental patient with valvular disease who requires definitive emergency treatment, that is, incision and drainage or extraction.

Regimen A oral administration is used in the following manner: For adults and children over 27 kg, penicillin V (2 g) administered orally 30 to 60 minutes prior to the procedure, and 500 mg administered orally every 6 hours for eight doses following the procedure, is recommended. Children under 27 kg are to be given 1 g penicillin V orally 30 to 60 minutes prior to and 250 mg orally every 6 hours for eight doses following the procedure.

Regimen A for patients allergic to penicillin employs erythromycin. For adults, 1 g erythromycin administered orally 1.5 to 2 hours before the procedure is supplemented by 500 mg administered orally every 6 hours for eight doses following the procedure. Children are given 20 mg/kg erythromycin orally 1.5 to 2 hours prior to the procedure and 10 mg/kg every 6 hours for eight doses following the procedure.

For patients with prosthetic heart valves (or as an alternative regimen for patients with valvular disease of a congenital, rheumatic, or acquired nature), regimen B, employing penicillin plus streptomycin, is preferred. Parenteral-oral sequence for adults is as follows: aqueous crystalline penicillin G (1 million units) mixed with procaine penicillin G (600,000 units) plus streptomycin (1 g) is administered intramuscularly 30 to 60 minutes preceding dental manipulations; penicillin V (500 mg) is administered every 6 hours for eight doses following the procedure. For children, identical time schedules are adhered to, with intramuscular injection of aqueous penicillin G (30,000 units/kg) mixed with procaine penicillin G (600,000 units) plus streptomycin (20 mg/kg). Oral postsurgical doses are the same, except for children under 27 kg, in which case the recommended oral dose of penicillin V is 250 mg every 6 hours for eight doses.

For patients requiring regimen B who are allergic to penicillin (or regimen A patients allergic to penicillin), 1 g vancomycin administered intravenously over 30 to 60 minutes prior to the procedure and erythromycin 500 mg administered orally every 6 hours for eight doses following the procedure are suggested for adults. For children, vancomycin (20 mg/kg infused intravenously over 30 minutes to 1 hour prior to the procedure) with erythromycin (10 mg/kg every 6 hours for eight doses following the procedure) is the regimen of choice.

For regimen A or B, prolonged healing may warrant additional doses of antibiotics. Also, regimen B or oral erythromycin may be substituted for regimen A (at the discretion of the dentist or physician) for patients receiving continuous oral penicillin prophylaxis.

Congenital heart disease

Although many of the structural defects in the heart or great vessels are not acknowledged until low tolerance for exercise, susceptibility to respiratory infections, or heart murmurs are demonstrated, they are present from birth and derived from developmental error.

Idiopathic errors in development occur as well as those errors attributed to teratogenic agents such as rubella and thalidomide; many defects are incompatible with life or will lead to an early demise. The broad categories include cyanotic and acyanotic congenital anomalies. Cardiovascular shunts are right-to-left (venous-to-arterial) in cyanotic anomalies and left-to-right (arterial-to-venous) in acyanotic anomalies.

Tetralogy of Fallot is the most common cyanotic defect in which survival is seen beyond 2 years of age. Surgical correction is advisable for almost all patients. These patients are susceptible to subacute bacterial endocarditis and other complications, including paroxysms of cyanosis. Interventricular septal defects, patent ductus arteriosus, and coarctation of the aorta comprise the most frequently seen acyanotic heart defects and are generally amenable to surgery. Uncorrected defects predispose these patients to endocarditis and other complications.

DENTAL TREATMENT PLANNING CONSIDERATIONS

Patients with congenital heart disease (other than uncomplicated atrial septal defects) must be prophylactically covered with penicillin or erythromycin prior to *any* dental treatment that could produce bleeding. The therapeutic regimen is identical to that of the rheumatic heart disease patient (see recommendations). It is important (according to the symptomatology of patients with cyanotic heart defects) to be prepared to limit treatment planning to disease control and oral hygiene instruction in order to minimize the possibility of stress-induced cyanotic dyspnea due to abrupt reduction in pulmonary blood flow (especially in tetralogy of Fallot). Dental treatment should be reserved in severe, uncorrected cases for the hospital inpatient operating room, should major dental rehabilitation be required, and *only* in close cooperation with the physician.

Intracardiac prosthesis

Patients with successful intracardiac prostheses are unique in that they are surgically compensated for life-threatening or activity-limiting cardiac disease. However, they are tremendously susceptible to endocarditis. The prostheses are held in position by sutures, and should vegetations develop around these sutural-myocardial-valvular complexes, intractable valvular regurgitation may ensue. It is *mandatory* that dental treatment and treatment planning be postponed until a mutually satisfying antibiotic prophylaxis plan is determined by the attending physician, surgeon, and dentist. Hospitalization is preferable. Most acceptable chemoprophylaxis programs for cardiac prosthesis patients consist of combined antibiotic therapy. Massive doses are administered intravenously or intramuscularly (or in combination) over a 3- to 5-day perioperative period.

Definitive dental treatment planning for these patients must be limited to caries and periodontal disease control. Since hospitalization is required for institution of acceptable chemoprophylaxis, the hospital outpatient dental clinic is a reasonable setting for treatment. Extraction of unrestorable teeth should be performed early in the disease control program. Extensive fixed prosthodontics or periodontal procedures are contraindicated. The oral cavity should be maintained with home care methods and conservative scaling and plaque removal. Prolonged endodontic treatment for nonstrategic teeth is not indicated. Since endodontic therapy generally requires multiple-stage procedures, extraction is the treatment of choice.

RESPIRATORY DISEASES

Both the cardiovascular and pulmonary systems are responsible for the physiologic process whereby oxygen is delivered to and carbon dioxide is eliminated from individual cells. This is accomplished through a three-step mechanism involving (1) pulmonary ventilation (atmospheric air is inhaled into the pulmonary alveoli), (2) alveolar gas exchange (the diffusion of oxygen into the blood and diffusion of carbon dioxide out of the blood), and (3) oxygen transport to the tissues by hemoglobin coupled with carbon dioxide return to the lungs. Impairment of any or all of these steps may be the result of cardiac failure or valvular disease, neurologic disturbances affecting the inspiratory-expiratory musculature, physical deformation or injury directly preventing rib-cage expansion and thus lung compliance, or increased airway resistance or obstruction. Dyspnea resulting from airway obstruction may be attributed to emphysema, chronic bronchitis, and asthma. Since maintenance of an adequate airway is imperative, it is essential that the dentist treating the patient with chronic airway obstruction be aware of these conditions and the limitations they impose upon dental management. Acute respiratory diseases will not be discussed here because they do not influence treatment planning per se.

Emphysema

Both emphysema and chronic bronchitis seem to be clearly related to smoking. Air pollution, especially particles of smoke and sulfur dioxide, tends to periodically exacerbate episodes of bronchitis. Viral, bacterial, occupational, and genetic factors have all been implicated, but it is likely that they play a secondary role to smoking in the etiology of these diseases.

Degenerative alterations in the walls of terminal bronchioles, producing a constriction of their lumens, will cause a distention of the associated alveoli and hence emphysema. These changes may occur on a panlobular or centrilobular basis. As a result of these irreversible changes, the total surface available for alveolar gas exchange is decreased. In addition, pulmonary vascular resistance is increased consequent to the destruction of lung capillaries and venules.

Patients with emphysema usually have a history of dyspnea on exertion. Production of sputum is minimal when cough is present. These patients are generally thin and often barrel-chested. Poorly discerned breath sounds and hyperresonance to percussion of the thorax are noted. However, clinical signs of emphysema are not entirely diagnostic. Chest x-ray findings are most helpful in making a diagnosis of emphysema. They show overinflation of the lungs and narrowing of the peripheral vasculature.

Chronic bronchitis

Chronic bronchitis is characterized by mucous gland hypertrophy, increased production of mucus in large bronchi, and a resultant excessive expectoration of sputum. Active infection, inflammation of the bronchial wall, and bronchial muscle hyperplasia all contribute to the decreased lumen of the airway in this disease.

The chronic bronchitis patient typically presents to the physician with a long-standing history of sputum production and a chronic cough as well as years of cigarette smoking. The patient is generally short in stature, obese, and demonstrates wheezing and basal rales, reflected in a decreased ventilatory capacity. These patients experience frequent pulmonary infections that tend to increase the severity of the airway obstruction. Late in the disease, secondary polycythemia and edema may develop into respiratory failure and cor pulmonale. Indeed, radiologic evidence of infective stigmas is seen, as well as cardiomegaly and changes consistent with pulmonary congestion.

MEDICAL MANAGEMENT: EMPHYSEMA AND CHRONIC BRONCHITIS

Once the severity of the disease, functional compromise, and psychological state of the patient have been determined, a program aimed at cessation of smoking and weight reduction is undertaken as early as possible. The patient is closely monitored several times yearly to establish the disposition of the disease state. In the chronic bronchitis patient in particular, antibiotic therapy is instituted during episodes of infection. Portable oxygen is helpful in severely hypoxemic patients. Surgical removal of affected lung areas is sometimes performed in emphysema patients.

Hay fever and asthma

Aberrant, hypersensitive immune responses to otherwise common environmental antigens (allergens), due to overproduction of the antibody IgE, manifest clinically as allergy. Hay fever or allergic rhinitis occurs seasonally and is related to the dispersion of pollen. It consists of the clinical syndrome of ocular pruritus, rhinorrhea, tearing of the eyes, sneezing, and nasal mucosal edema. These patients display dermatologic stigmas of allergy in the form of pruritus and urticaria, and *many will develop asthma eventually.* Since hay fever patients tend to have recurrent episodes of sinusitis, they often develop intranasal polyps secondary to inflammation.

The onset of asthma within the first decade of life is reported in about 50% of cases and is more common in males than females. As the fourth decade approaches, the incidence in males and females is equal. Latent asthma has been reported. There is evidence of a familial tendency in approximately one-third of patients. Emotional stress, infections of the respiratory system, and especially allergic factors tend to interact, giving rise to attacks. Asthmatic patients are predisposed to bronchospasm.

Asthma differs from hay fever in that in asthma the lower respiratory tract is involved, while in hay fever the upper respiratory tract is affected. Asthma is characterized by generalized narrowing of the lumens of the components of the bronchial tree, which varies in degree at different times, either with or without treatment. Hypertrophy of the bronchial musculature is seen.

Panthoracic wheezing and dyspnea on expiration, along with cough, rhonchi, and overinflation of the lungs, varying in duration and occurring in spasmodic patterns, comprise the clinical picture of asthma. Between these "attacks" patients are virtually free of symptoms.

Medical management: hay fever and asthma

Treatment for the hay fever sufferer includes elimination of the incriminating environmental antigen, skin testing, and hyposensitization injections. Antihistamines are generally effective in controlling hay fever, and steroid inhalants may be used supportively in very severe conditions.

Allergic asthma is best prevented by elimination of known antigens. Perennial desensitization injections in allergic patients with asthma are useful. Acute asthma is treated best at onset. Milder attacks are treated with inhalants of isoproterenol mist. More severe, rapidly progressing attacks require subcutaneous injection of epinephrine. Aminophylline, a bronchodilator, may be used with or in lieu of epinephine. Hydration to prevent mucus inspissation is imperative and is accomplished by infusion of intravenous glucose.

Administration of corticosteroids is indicated during episodes when epinephrine or aminophylline is ineffective or recurrence is rapid. Corticosteroids administered on a prophylactic basis have also proven effective for preventing paroxysms of asthma, as well as phenobarbital and ephedrine given orally several times daily during periods of high susceptibility.

Dental treatment planning considerations

Dental treatment planning for patients with chronic obstructive lung disease should include a vigorous program of reinforcement and supportive measures to discourage entrenched smokers. Prohibition of smoking in the dental office and waiting room emphasizes the health concern of the dentist for his patients, supporting staff, and himself, and sets the proper example.

A well-ventilated air-conditioned treatment room will minimize airborne allergens and dust particles in the environment and will benefit these patients. Stressful procedures such as multiple tooth extractions, extensive periodontal surgery, and restorative dentistry are best tolerated by these patients in multiple short visits. Patient chair position should be as upright as is practical for the dentist in order to assure maintenance of the airway. This will also decrease the possibility of aspiration of foreign material, saliva, water, or blood, which would precipitate paroxysms of coughing and mucus secretion, eventuating in acute airway obstruction or lung abscess. All minor surgical procedures should be undertaken with the utilization of high-speed suction and adequate anesthesia. If there are no contraindications medically and if the patient is an excessive salivator, premedication with an antisialagogue may be indicated. Atropine sulfate in 1 mg tablets administered 1 or 2 hours prior to the appointment or 50 mg of methaneline (Banthine) administered 30 minutes prior to the appointment may be suitable drugs.

Patients with chronic bronchitis, emphysema, or asthma are highly susceptible to upper respiratory infections. Thus it seems prudent to promptly eliminate acute periodontal inflammatory conditions, periodontal abscesses, periapical infections, and large, open carious lesions. Antibiotic coverage is recommended when purulent pulp canals are left open for drainage, since aspiration of the exudative material could initiate an acute attack of bronchitis.

Chronic lung disease patients characteristically experience difficulty with expiration. Thus it is best to defer dental treatment procedures demanding the use of the rubber dam, such as endodontics or gold-foil restorations, during episodes of nasal and sinus congestion in these patients. Indeed, each patient with emphysema, chronic bronchitis, or asthma should be empirically assessed for rubber dam tolerance with regard to the airway as early in treatment as possible. Certainly the rubber dam is an invaluable means of protecting the airway from particulate foreign objects such as files, broaches, cotton pledgets, restorative materials, and liquid aspirates, and its use (if possible) in the course of treatment is desirable for these patients in particular.

Nitrous oxide analgesia is contraindicated in the patient with emphysema and chronic bronchitis. However, it is imperative that the dental operatory be equipped with satisfactory oxygen-administering equipment, since the patient with chronic destructive lung disease has a tendency to become hypoxemic.

Since high concentrations of oxygen tend to depress the respiratory center, it is advisable to be prodigious regarding the use of supplementary oxygen in the obstructive lung disease patient. Following this rationale, narcotics and barbiturates are contraindicated.

Respiratory acidosis in obstructive lung disease patients is not uncommon, and syncope, tachycardia, and palpitations may be the reflection of unusually high endogenous epinephrine titers. Epinephrine in local anesthetics is permissible in concentrations no greater than 1:100,000. Intravenous sodium bicarbonate may be indicated if the patient is in respiratory failure.

Since dental procedures can be stressful, asthmatic patients may be susceptible to stress-precipitated asthmatic attacks during the course of a dental appointment. Asthmatic patients should be reminded to bring their isoproterenol inhalants to dental appointments, since mild attacks can generally be controlled easiest at the outset with inhalation of 50 to 150 mg of isoproterenol. Rapidly developing attacks should be treated with subcutaneous injections of 0.3 to 1 ml of 1:1000 epinephrine, which can be repeated, as needed, once every 30 minutes; 50 to 100 mg of sedative may be administered early in the paroxysm to relieve agitation, but this is contraindicated in prolonged, severe episodes. Slow intravenous aminophylline injections (0.5 g) may be given in conjunction with or in lieu of epinephrine, as this is a most effective bronchodilator. This is best administered in an intravenous glucose drip and optimally handled in the hospital emergency room, should the dental office lack the required setup. Steroids are given and are effective in several hours in situations of rapidly recurring attacks; 15 to 80 mg of prednisone will generally produce the desired effect, but this is best undertaken in the hospital.

GASTROINTESTINAL DISEASES

A wide variety of symptoms are reported by patients suffering from digestive disorders. Also, the incidence of *acute* gastrointestinal distress is highest of all organ systems for both sexes at all ages. Symptoms range widely in severity and type and include dysphagia, anorexia, nausea, vomiting, abdominal cramping, diarrhea, constipation, and frequent expulsion of gas. The liver performs many key functions with relation to carbohydrate, protein, and fat metabolism, synthesis of proteins, and most of the blood coagulation factors. In addition, it is responsible for the detoxification of many drugs and endogenous and exogenous hormones. Hepatocellular diseases, both acute and chronic in nature, can lead to compromised liver function on a transient or progressive to permanent basis, respectively. Hepatocellular failure will manifest as ascites and dependent edema (due to hypoalbuminemia), bleeding tendency, ammonia intoxication leading to hepatic coma, failure to remove bilirubin from the blood, jaundice, stigmas of endogenous hormone intoxication (gynecomastia, generalized alopecia, and atrophic testes due to inadequate estrogen inactivation in the male), and drug-induced coma in patients receiving depressant drug therapy. Nevertheless, despite the wide variety of acute and chronic gastrointestinal conditions that may be reported by patients, only a very small number of these will affect the treatment planning and management of the dental patient.

Hiatal hernia (diaphragmatic hernia)

Hiatal hernia is the protrusion of a small segment of the cardiac portion of the stomach through the esophageal hiatus of the diaphragm. Pyrosis (heartburn) is a frequent symptom of hiatal hernia and is caused by reflux of gastric juice into the esophagus; in turn, bleeding may be a consequence of the esophagitis resulting from this phenomenon. Severe pain and prostration may occur secondary to strangulation of the hernia.

MEDICAL MANAGEMENT

Medical management is directed at controlling or decreasing gastroesophageal reflux. This is accomplished by counseling the patient concerning posture and how he may utilize gravity as a preventative measure. Avoiding ingestion before retiring, large meals, and offending foods is also beneficial. Antacids are prescribed when necessary, and weight loss is encouraged. Surgery is indicated in cases of obstruction.

DENTAL TREATMENT PLANNING CONSIDERATIONS

Dental management of the patient should be planned according to symptomatology. It is advisable to schedule appointments 2 or 3 hours after a meal and to position the patient in the dental chair in as upright a position as possible. Since gastric regurgitation has the potential to increase the acidity of saliva, it might be helpful to prescribe frequent noncaustic expectorant mouthrinses; 3% hydrogen peroxide (1 part) in warm water (2 parts) is a suitable rinse. It will effectively minimize decalcification of the dentition and alleviate sour taste or mouth odor resulting from reflux of gastric contents. Oral fluoride supplements may also prove helpful in severe cases.

Peptic ulcer

Peptic ulcers may occur (1) in the lower third of the esophagus (infrequently), (2) in the stomach, and (3) in the duodenum. Duodenal ulcers represent about 80% of all peptic ulcers. While duodenal ulcers are rarely malignant, gastric ulcers have a higher percentage of malignancy. Still, the majority of gastric ulcers are benign (peptic).

DUODENAL ULCERS

The etiology of duodenal ulcers is multifactorial; however, the most constant factor is parietal cell hypersecretion of acid. Drugs such as corticosteroids, caffeine, and alcohol tend to increase acid secretion and have all been implicated to varying degrees. Familial tendency, blood group O, and nonsecretion of erythrocytic mucopolysaccharide into the gastrointestinal tract apparently predispose patients to development of ulceration. Psychogenic factors and diseases such as cirrhosis and pancreatitis are also contributory.

Midepigastric burning and aching relieved by ingestion of food or alkali is the primary symptom pattern of duodenal ulcers. Diffuse abdominal pain, belching, and food intolerance may accompany this.

Medical management. Antacid therapy designed to raise the pH of gastric contents is accomplished through a variety of liquid and tablet preparations, either employed singly or in battery. These consist of nonabsorbable agents such as aluminum hydroxide, magnesium oxide, and calcium carbonate. Anticholinergic drugs reduce gastric acid secretion by parietal cells and also decrease gastric motility by direct action on the vagus nerve. Dietary control through bland foods taken frequently in small amounts and avoidance of alcohol and caffeine is essential. Cigarette smoking is prohibited as well. Adequate rest and sleep are encouraged. Less often, surgery in the form of distal gastric resection or vagotomy is indicated in severe, intractable cases. Irradiation or freezing of the stomach is rarely employed.

Dental treatment planning considerations. Dental treatment planning for the duodenal ulcer patient must include monitoring of hematocrit or hemoglobin levels prior to surgical procedures. This is necessary because unsuspected chronic anemia due to occult bleeding from the ulcer is a potential problem. Tetracycline drugs prescribed for oral infections must be taken more than 1 hour prior to the taking of antacid preparations, since aluminum salts tend to bind most oral tetracyclines in the gut and prevent their absorption. Oral penicillin V is preferable to oral penicillin G when this antibiotic is called for, since gastric hyperacidity partly destroys the action of penicillin G, while penicillin V is acid resistant. Aspirin and aspirin-containing analgesic compounds are to be avoided because of their acidity and their tendency to promote bleeding. Corticosteroid therapy for oral manifestations of serious dermatoses must be substituted for by other antiinflammatory or cytotoxic agents. Preferably, these decisions are made through consultation with the physician.

Dryness of the oral mucosa secondary to anticholinergic therapy warrants the institution of a vigorous program in oral hygiene, since both caries and periodontal disease are fostered by a xerostomic environment. Where the patient has a high caries experience, mild and frequent mouthrinses, oral fluoride supplements in gel form, and full-coverage restorations in preference to large, multisurfaced restorations should be utilized as preventive measures. More frequent recalls for scaling and prophylaxis are necessary. For those duodenal ulcer patients requiring removable prostheses, it is imperative that these be constructed as early as possible in the course of treatment to ensure that the patient is able to masticate properly and thus facilitate the digestive process. The prostheses should be as "bulkless" as possible in order to eliminate gagging.

Gastric ulcers

Gastric ulcers are less common than duodenal ulcers, but generally resemble them pathologically. Unlike duodenal ulcers, they are characterized by decreased or normal gastric secretion by decreased or normal numbers of parietal cells. Thus some believe that gastric ulcers are caused by decreased quantities of mucus. Others believe that the gastric mucosa in these patients is less resistant to ulceration following minor injury.

Symptomatology is diverse and includes nausea, weight loss, decreased appetite, vomiting, food intolerance, and in severe cases, bleeding. Some ulcers are discovered by chance and confirmed roentgenographically. Gastric ulcers (peptic) are not precancerous lesions.

Medical management. Medical management differs from that of duodenal ulcers only in that anticholinergic drugs are *contraindicated.* (Gastric secretion is stimulated by the prolonged gastric emptying induced by anticholinergics.) Surgery is indicated in severe cases that demonstrate perforation, obstruction, or bleeding.

Dental treatment planning considerations. Dental treatment precautions for the gastric ulcer patient differ very little from those applied to the duodenal ulcer patient. However, it is imperative that the former group *not* be premedicated with antisialagogues. These drugs specifically instigate *gastric* ulcers. More conservative dental restorations might be considered practical in the gastric ulcer patient, since dryness of the mouth is not a major finding.

Hepatitis

Acute and chronic forms of hepatitis exist. The acute viral hepatitides (types A and B) are discussed in the section on infectious diseases. Recurrent attacks of hepatitis caused either by alcohol abuse, chemical or drug hepatotoxicity, or drug hypersensitivity may lead to chronic hepatitis if the offending agent is not promptly removed. Repeated subjection to these directly hepatotoxic or allergenic substances, resulting in cholestatic, necrotic, and degenerative inflammatory changes, may eventuate in liver cirrhosis and loss of function. The same is true of patients with chronic *active* hepatitis, a progressive degenerative liver disease that is probably of autoimmune derivation.

MEDICAL MANAGEMENT

Medical attention directed at prompt removal of the offending drug (i.e., halothane, oral contraceptives, chlorpromazine), chemical (i.e., carbon tetrachloride), or antigenic stimulus is essential for patient recovery with minimal liver damage. Chronic active hepatitis is managed mainly with steroids and immunosuppressive agents on a long-term basis. These efforts are directed at arresting or containing the cirrhotic process.

Cirrhosis of the liver

Cirrhosis categorically defines a generalized, progressive, inflammatory disease of the liver that demonstrates extensive hepatocellular necrosis, parenchymal proliferation and regeneration, circulatory alterations, and fibrous scarring. The three forms of primary hepatic cirrhosis are Laennec's (portal, alcoholic, or fatty), postnecrotic, and biliary.

LAENNEC'S CIRRHOSIS

Laennec's cirrhosis is attributed to poor nutrition coupled with chronic ingestion of alcohol. Years of steady alcohol abuse lead to the stigmas of liver destruction. These include jaundice, hepatomegaly, ascites, vascular "spiders," hair loss, palmar erythema, gynecomastia, purpura, and digital clubbing (Fig. 6-4).

Medical management. Medical management stresses strict prohibition of alcohol and institution of a carefully monitored high-protein, high-calorie, salt- and water-restrictive diet. Drugs normally detoxified by the liver are avoided. Anemia is evaluated and controlled.

POSTNECROTIC CIRRHOSIS

Postnecrotic cirrhosis is believed to be attributed to viral hepatitis, chemical hepatotoxicity, or infections mediated by autoimmune hepatocellular injury. Signs and symptoms resemble Laennec's signs, but patients are younger and generally nonalcoholic.

Medical management. Medical management is similar to that of Laennec's cirrhosis, emphasizing drug avoidance, limitation of protein intake, and dietary control. Care revolves around the interception of possible hemorrhage resulting from vascular changes secondary to portal hypertension.

BILIARY CIRRHOSIS

Biliary cirrhosis is rare. Most cases are attributed to bile duct obstruction or intrahepatic chronic cholestasis. An immune etiology has been offered. Patients are mostly middle-aged women. Weakness, pruritus, steatorrhea, hepatosplenomegaly, and jaundice are the signs. Because of the absence of bile, intestinal absorption of lipids and fat-soluble vitamins is impaired.

Medical management. Medical management is aimed at controlling itching. A salt- and fat-restricted diet and controlled liquid intake is prescribed for prevention of edema and ascites. Injected supplements of fat-soluble vitamins (A, D, and K) are given regularly to prevent hypoprothrombinemia and osteomalacia.

102 *Modifying factors in treatment planning*

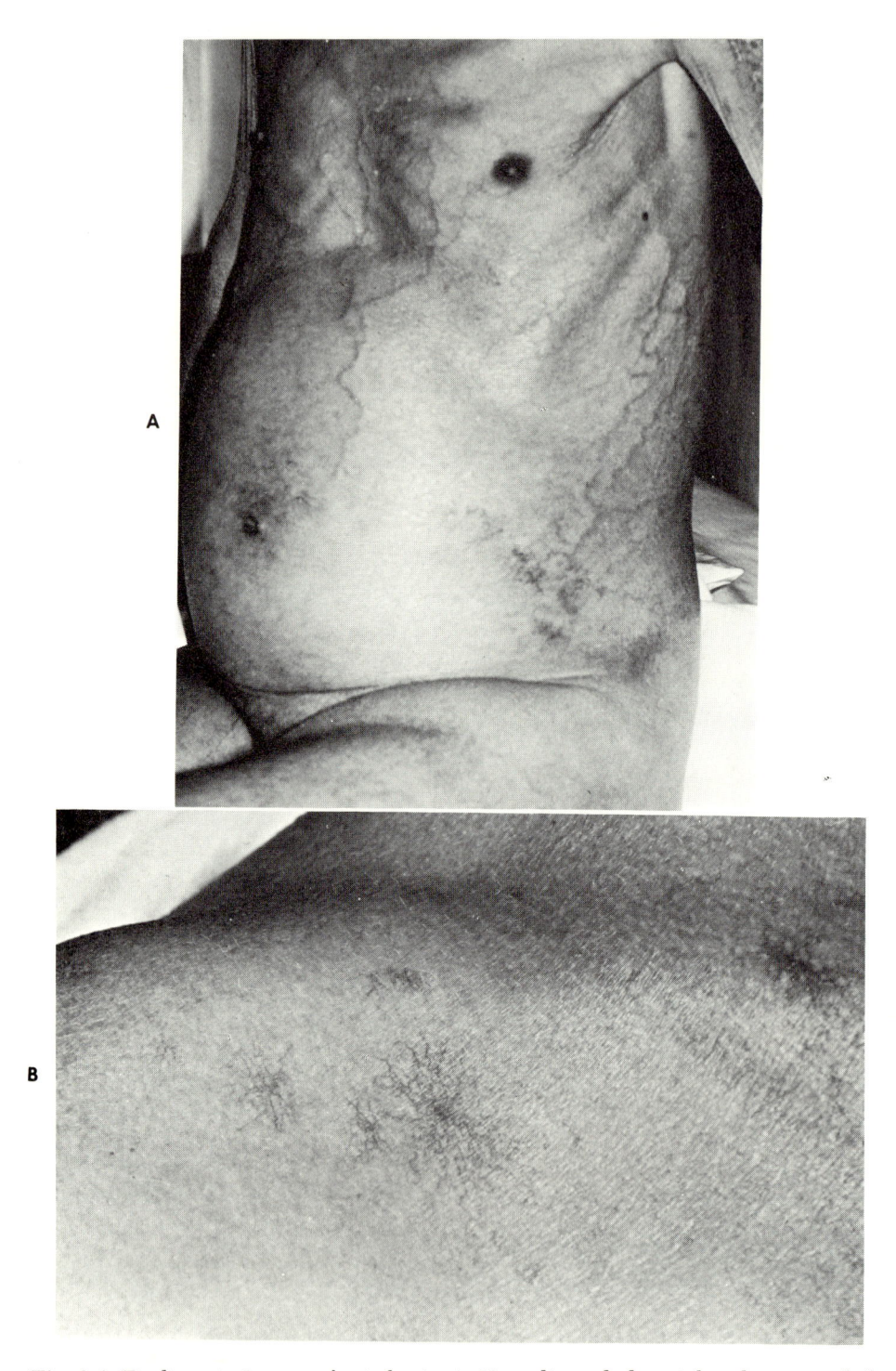

Fig. 6-4. Findings in Laennec's cirrhosis. **A**, Note distended peripheral veins and abdominal swelling caused by ascites. **B**, Note several spider nevi on skin surface. (**A** courtesy Dr. Paul Akers, Chicago, Ill.; **B** courtesy Dr. Michael Lehnert, Burnsville, Minn.)

Dental treatment planning considerations

Dental management of the patient with chronic liver disease is aimed at precautionary measures against drug toxicity and bleeding. Since these patients may possess minimal hepatic capacity to metabolize and detoxify anesthetic and sedative agents, it is advisable to consult the physician regarding the individual risk involved should the patient require surgical procedures or sedative premedications.

As a general guideline, chronic liver disease patients requiring extensive dental treatment or emergency intervention must be worked up hematologically to determine the extent of liver function compromise. Enzymes such as serum glutamic-oxaloacetic transaminase (SGOT) and alkaline phosphatase are elevated in liver damage. The serum levels of these enzymes provide the dentist and physician with a profile of liver function for the patient. Total protein values and the albumin to globulin ratio are upset in states of liver disease. Serum determination of these will add information.

Any bleeding tendency must be assessed and controlled prior to definitive dental treatment planning. Prothrombin time is employed as a means of evaluating the degree of abnormality in clotting.

Prothrombin deficiency (prothrombin time prolonged two to three times the normal 12 to 15 seconds), as well as deficiency of fibrinogen and factors VIII and X, may exist in these patients. Hematocrit should be determined also, since many liver disease patients are anemic. Hypoprothrombinemia must be corrected by vitamin K administration prior to extensive oral surgery. This should be carried out under the auspices of a physician.

Cirrhotics may develop hepatic coma (ammonia intoxication) as the result of excessive ingestion of blood. This is caused by an inability to metabolize large quantities of protein in light of the high protein content of blood. Therefore unavoidable procedures of an oral surgical nature demand meticulous hemostatic measures, oropharyngeal packing, and careful suctioning during and after surgery in the mouth to obviate swallowing of blood. Periodontal surgery, extractions, and unavoidable preprosthetic surgery might best be performed in the controlled environment of the hospital operating room, but only after the patient is serologically and medically cleared for surgery. Where there is a treatment planning alternative of either tooth extraction or endodontic therapy, it is preferable to institute endodontics so as to avoid the risk of hemorrhage. Prior to instrumentation of root canals, it is imperative that antibiotic therapy be instituted to avoid intractable or unmanageable infection.

Periodontal inflammatory disease and active dental caries must be treated as quickly and conservatively as possible for the same rationale. Local anesthesia without general anesthesia or depressant medication is the method of choice for the chronic liver disease patient. General anesthesia should be avoided for routine dental procedures.

Medical advice and conjunctive management are imperative for patients on corticosteroid therapy for chronic active hepatitis. The problems encountered with long-term corticosteroid therapy are discussed in Chapter 5.

HEMATOLOGIC DISEASES

The dental patient with a disorder of hematopoiesis, hemostasis, or the lymphoreticular system requires scrupulously thorough treatment planning designed to intercept and alleviate potential complications. Such complications may be caused by either the disease itself or its medical management. Indeed, initial signs and symptoms of hematopathology may first present in the oral cavity and may be the primary reason why an unsuspecting patient seeks dental care. Deficiency or proliferation of any or all of the cellular or platelet components of the peripheral blood may be reflected in an array of signs and symptoms. It is not within the scope of this discussion to cover in detail all the diseases of the hematologic and lymphoreticular systems, but rather, to discuss the more common pathologic states that warrant consideration in dental treatment planning.

Anemia

Anemia, a decrease in circulating erythrocytes or hemoglobin, is a sign rather than a diagnosis. The underlying cause of this recognized entity must be established in order to determine the degree of concern necessary in treatment planning. Since loss of blood, increased hemolysis, or diminished production of erythrocytes are the etiologic mechanisms of anemia, they provide the system of classification that consequently outlines the rationale of medical management. Laboratory studies are the only means of definitively detecting the presence of anemia, but a carefully taken history and physical evaluation of the patient may strongly suggest its presence in moderate to severe cases and will aid in the interpretation of laboratory results. Hematocrit and hemoglobin determinations are the most practical screening procedures. Should the hematocrit be lower than normal, red cell counts and indices, leukocyte counts, and stained blood smears should be performed. Prior to institution of therapy for anemia, it is crucial to seek out the reason for its presence.

Anemias related to loss of blood

The most common cause of anemia is represented by acute and chronic loss of blood. Gastrointestinal ulcerations, benign or malignant neoplasms, or repeated episodes of menorrhagia may be contributory to chronic iron-deficiency anemia.

Hemolytic anemias

In hemolytic anemias the destruction of erythrocytes exceeds the capacity of the marrow to replace them. There are two etiologic bases of hemolytic anemias that produce fragile erythrocytes: (1) those with extracorpuscular defects (mostly acquired) and (2) those that have intracorpuscular defects (inherited).

Extracorpuscular defects may be acute in onset, such as those derived from infection with malaria, from toxins, venoms, chemicals, or cardiac prostheses. Chronic types are usually immunologically based, such as Rh incompatibility or acquired hemolytic or Coombs positive anemia from repeated transfusions in which "cold" and "warm" antibodies are found. *Intracorpuscular* defects may involve either the membrane, as in hereditary spherocytosis, or the hemoglobin, as in thalassemia and sickle cell disease. Regardless of the etiology, hemolytic anemia of a chronic and severe nature will result in a clinical syndrome of hepatosplenomegaly, jaundice, pallor and atrophy of the skin and mucous membranes, bilirubin cholelithiasis, and malaise. In attacks of acute hemolytic anemia, chills, fever, cardiopulmonary dysfunction, and abdominal symptomatology are characteristic manifestations. Hemolytic anemias do not respond to iron-supplementation therapy and are often asymptomatic except when superimposed infection is present.

Major oral findings in Cooley's anemia (beta-thalassemia) are mainly skeletal, although gingival pallor and icterus are often noted. The marrow hyperplasia frequently will produce an expansion of the jaw bones, which will result in diastemas and open bites (Fig. 6-5, A). Roentgenographic changes include generalized rarefaction with a honeycombed trabecular appearance (Fig. 6-5, B). Large trabecular spaces may be seen in patients with sickle cell disease but are not diagnostic.

Hemolytic anemia of the newborn (erythroblastosis fetalis, Rh incompatibility) is an immune problem that today is detectable and alleviated prior to birth.

Primary teeth developing during times of increased hemolysis showed permanent discoloration because of the incorporation of hemoglobin-breakdown pigments into developing dentinal structures. This is seldom seen today.

ANEMIAS OF DECREASED ERYTHROCYTE PRODUCTION

Decreased erythropoiesis may be caused by iron-deficient states as found in pregnancy, poor dietary intake, and inflammatory diseases. A dietary deficiency of folic acid hampers maturation of erythrocytes, as does deficient cyanocobalamin (vitamin B_{12}) absorption in the gut. The bone marrow may be directly suppressed by cytotoxic chemicals or therapeutic agents, ionizing radiation, disorders of metabolism, and infections.

The hypochromic, microcytic anemia of iron deficiency is the most common variety of anemia associated with a nutritional deficit. Administration of ferrous sulfate will relieve the symptoms and resolve the condition, provided there is no underlying pathologic condition producing chronic loss of blood, such as a gastrointestinal ulceration or neoplasm. Manifestations in the more severe cases of iron-deficiency anemia include loss of appetite and vigor, irritability and neurologic upsets, exhaustion, vertigo and headache, pallor, and generalized oral mucosal atrophy (Fig. 6-6).

Plummer-Vinson syndrome (sideropenic dysphagia) is characterized by hypochromic microcytic anemia of the iron-deficiency type in combination with stomatitis and pharyngoesophageal ulcerations. Patients are usually middle-aged women. Cases of long duration often show changes in the nail beds ranging from concavities to total atrophy. Oral manifestations are xerostomia, lingual erythema and atrophy, erosions, ulcers, and angular cheilitis. Lingual leukoplakia of the dysplastic type is seen, and carcinoma appears with fairly high incidence in the oral and pharyngeal lesions.

Pernicious anemia is caused by nonabsorption of vitamin B_{12}, and the erythrocytes are characteristically of the megaloblastic macrocytic type. Vitamin B_{12} is required by bone marrow to complete erythrocyte maturation. It is derived from the diet, stored in the liver, and is absorbed only in the presence

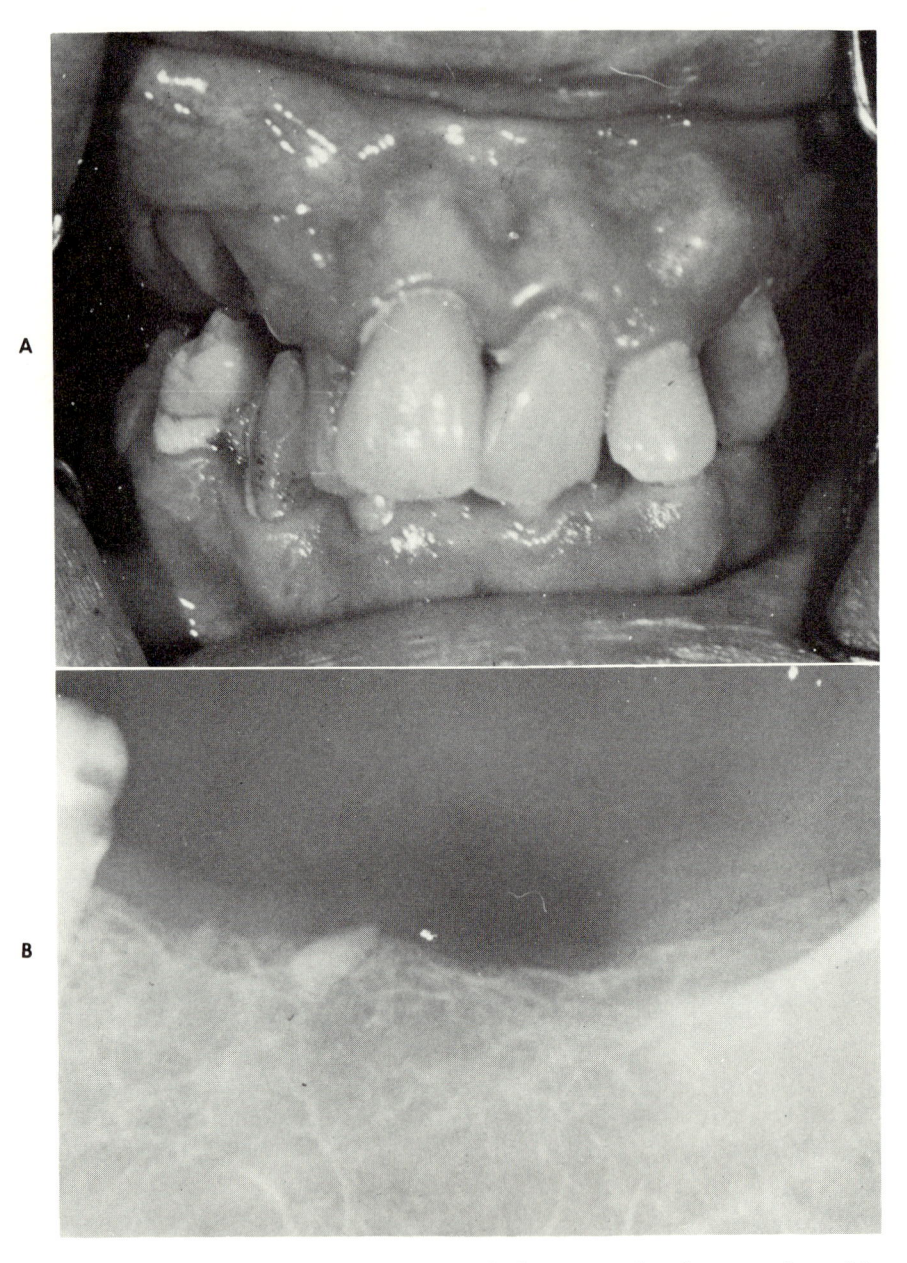

Fig. 6-5. Thalassemia. **A,** Intraoral photograph showing malocclusion and roughly contoured alveolar bone. Malocclusions are common in patients suffering from thalassemia major because of expansion of jawbones secondary to marrow hyperplasia. Gingivae demonstrated pallor in this case. **B,** Periapical roentgenogram of patient in **A** showing "honeycomb" rarefied trabecular pattern of patient with thalassemia. (Courtesy Dr. Gerald Shklar, Boston, Mass.)

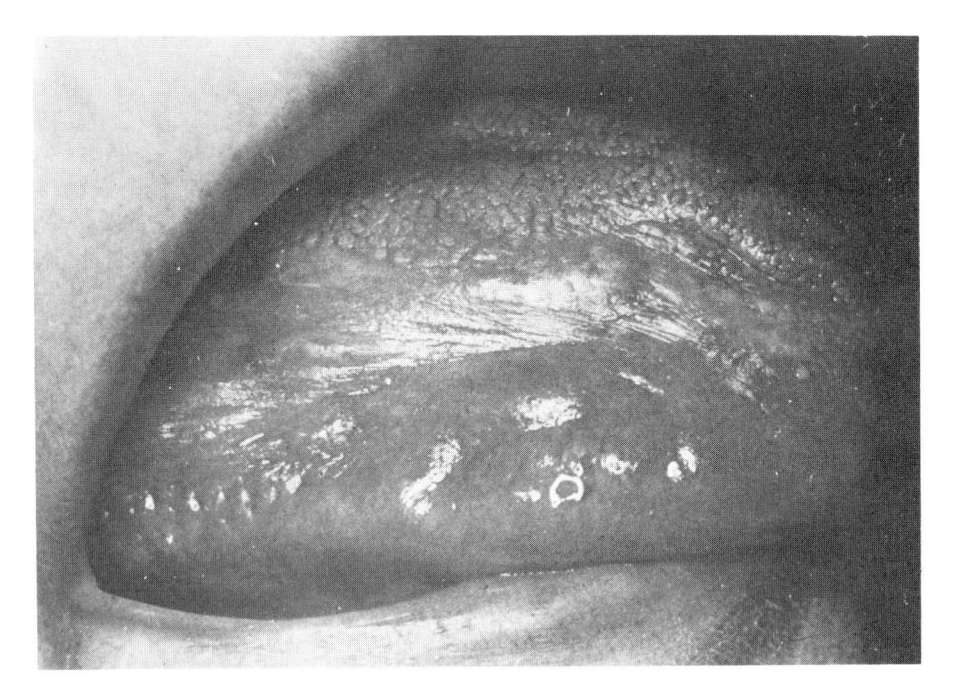

Fig. 6-6. Glossitis in anemia. Note atrophic area on lateral border of tongue devoid of papillae in this patient suffering from iron-deficiency anemia. (Courtesy Dr. Gerald Shklar, Boston, Mass.)

of "intrinsic factor," a glycoprotein secreted by the epithelium of the gastric fundus. Should the secretion of this intrinsic factor be insufficient or discontinued, the absorption of vitamin B_{12} ceases. Once the hepatic stores of the vitamin are depleted, protean manifestations of pernicious anemia become evident because of defective adaptation and rapid destruction of erythrocytes. Achlorhydria secondary to atrophic gastritis, pallor, lassitude, and neuritis are seen. As in iron-deficiency anemia, the majority of patients are middle-aged. Theories concerning an immunologic basis for the disease have been offered, and corticosteroid therapy has produced some beneficial results. Injections of vitamin B_{12} provide the most reliable positive results.

Sprue or folic-acid deficiency is another condition that causes macrocytic anemia. It results from the insufficient absorption of folic acid in the gut or from low dietary intake of the metabolite. The condition is relieved by folic acid supplementation in the diet. Since folic acid (pteroylglutamic acid) is essential for cellular metabolism, cancer chemotherapy with folic-acid antagonists such as methotrexate can precipitate a syndrome that consists of neurologic weakness and disturbances, malaise, hyperpigmentation, anemia, leukopenia, and gastrointestinal upset. Folic-acid deficiency and pernicious anemia have a similar spectrum of oral changes: glossitis, erosions, ulcerations, and gingival inflammation.

Aplastic anemias or hypoplastic anemias result from a primary failure of the bone marrow. The cause may be idiopathic or associated with physical or chemical injury or viral infection. Idiopathic cases comprise about 50% of this type of anemia and appear most often in adolescents. Fanconi's syndrome, a congenital disorder with pigmentation, multiple osteodystrophies, and genitourinary disturbances, also is associated with an aplastic anemia not evident at birth. Pancytopenia is seen often, as well, in aplastic anemias attributed to cytotoxic drugs or chemical agents. Symptoms include weakness, pallor, purpura and frank hemorrhage, oral and mucosal ulcerations, and predisposition to infections. Bronzing of the skin as a result of hemosiderosis develops from multiple transfusions, and hepatosplenomegaly may have a later onset. The diagnosis of aplastic anemia is determined through bone marrow studies, and treatment is essentially supportive. Highly selective use of transfusions and splenectomy in addition to steroid therapy comprise the major treatment modalities. Prognosis is most favorable where a specific toxic agent is implicated and eliminated, allowing for remission of the aplastic process. Most deaths occur within the first 3 years of onset, usually from hemorrhage or infection.

Dental treatment planning considerations for anemic patients

Patients with anemia resulting from *dietary deficiency* or *malabsorption* should be appropriately treated once the diagnosis and cause have been firmly established. Usually, supplementation with the required nutrient will restore the hematocrit to within normal limits and reverse the clinical stigmas of the anemia. Should patients require treatment while in the anemic state, and if the anemia is severe enough to produce mucosal atrophy, erosions, or ulcerations, it is imperative that treatment be limited to atraumatic, noninvasive procedures emphasizing palliation rather than definitive treatment. Bleeding should be avoided so as to prevent shock and dyspnea, and oral surgery and periodontal procedures should be deferred until the anemia is under control. In anemia the periodontal and pulpal tissues as well as the remaining soft tissues of the oral cavity are less resilient to injury; therefore any manipulations in the oral cavity must be undertaken with extreme caution so as to avoid a situation of delayed healing and discomfort for the patient. Local irritants such as sharp cusps, rough restorations, poorly adapted clasps, or broken prostheses must be corrected by polishing and grinding until smoothness is achieved. Conservative periodontal therapy in lieu of more radical surgical treatment is preferred for the anemic patient with moderate periodontitis, the treatment modalities of choice being gentle mouthrinses, nonabrasive dentifrices, and soft toothbrushing as well as limited subgingival closed curettage procedures. Prognosis for endodontic therapy or extractions is unpredictable in the patient with dietary deficiency anemia, since healing and inflammatory responses are either poor or exaggerated. Thus it is recommended that these procedures be delayed until the hematocrit and hemoglobin levels are normalized.

In the patient with *hemolytic anemia*, dental procedures are usually not contraindicated and can be performed with few reservations. Since infection in the patient with sickle cell anemia (who is otherwise living a normal life) can precipitate a life-jeopardizing sickle cell crisis, it is essential to avoid possible infective sequelae by coverage with an antibiotic when endodontically involved teeth are left open for drainage or when acute pulpal or periodontal infections are present. Appointments must be kept short for patients with severe hemolytic anemia, as these patients fatigue easily and become short of breath. This may necessitate a plan for less time-consuming restorative dentistry such as amalgams rather than cast restorations. Removable prostheses or "flipper"-type tooth replacements, which are less demanding of chair time, might be substituted for fixed prostheses. General anesthesia is to be avoided, since hypoxia is a threat. Phenacetin, a hemolysis-inducing oxidant, must not be prescribed as an analgesic for thalassemic patients.

Mucous membrane lesions in patients with Plummer-Vinson syndrome are generally of the ulcerative atrophic and leukoplakic variety. As mentioned previously, in many cases the leukoplakic lesions in this disease tend to demonstrate histologically precancerous epithelial changes. Therefore it is imperative to perform biopsy and tissue examination on these white lesions to determine how they should best be managed. Patients with severe mucosal atrophy and breakdown benefit from gentle mouthrinses with 3% hydrogen peroxide (1 part) diluted in warm water (2 parts), local anesthetic viscous topical preparations, locally applied crushed ice, or a 50-50 mixture of diphenhydramine hydrochloride (Benadryl) in kaopectate rinses. Corticosteroids are to be used only where medical contraindications are not present, and then only in low doses as a last resort for intractable oral lesions. Apparently the oral lesions of pernicious anemia can be alleviated by corticosteroids, since these agents depress the autoimmune reaction to gastric parietal cells.

Dental treatment for the *aplastic anemia* patient (especially where the life expectancy is short and the condition is progressive and severe) must be limited to procedures of palliation and disease control. These should be accomplished using essentially temporary modalities. These patients succumb to infections; therefore infections of dental origin must be prevented or given appropriate attention as soon as they are discovered. Major restorative dentistry, including costly and time-consuming operative procedures, is not indicated for the patient with severe aplastic anemia. Extraction of questionable teeth is preferable to endodontic treatment, and the subsequent ideal of cast-post, core, and full-coverage restorative treatment. If the patient is thrombocytopenic as well as anemic, pulp extirpation under sterile conditions is the treatment of choice over tooth extraction, since bleeding should be avoided. Extractions, where unavoidable, must be performed in a setting where the patient can receive platelets if necessary. Caries excavation and temporary restoration with amalgam or interim restorative materials should be performed where reasonable. Elective procedures have no place in treatment planning for these patients. Physician consultation is required for the patient receiving steroid therapy, as the drug dosage may have to be altered prior to stressful dental emergency manipulation. Mucosal breakdown and susceptibility to infection is the greatest oral problem for the aplastic anemia patient, so the mouth must be kept as clean as is feasible by gentle oral hygiene methods rather than by more long-term, radically oriented procedures. Since neutropenia and thrombocytopenia often accompany aplastic anemia, trauma, irritation, and inflammation caused by local etiologic agents such as plaque and food debris must be eliminated to prevent necrosis at sites of trauma.

Because patients with aplastic anemia are often managed medically with transfusions, making infectious hepatitis a potential hazard, the operator should wear gloves while rendering treatment. Evidently, patients with severe anemia demonstrate poor tissue response and resistance to injury; this must be respected as a treatment-planning guideline.

Polycythemia

Polycythemia is a condition in which an increase in hemoglobin concentration accompanies an increase in erythrocytes. Circumstances capable of depleting body fluid can produce a state of "relative" polycythemia where total hemoglobin is not actually increased. Such circumstances would include diuretic therapy, dehydration, vomiting and diarrhea, and ketoacidosis. True polycythemia may be primary (polycythemia vera, erythremia), stemming from uncontrolled erythropoiesis, or secondary (erythrocytosis), resulting from factors associated with decreased concentration of oxygen in the blood, such as pulmonary obstructive diseases, congestive heart failure, congenital cardiac defects, mitral valve disease, and living at high altitudes. Rarely, erythropoietin-producing tumors are implicated in secondary polycythemia. In secondary polycythemia, successful treatment of the disease of origin reverses the hematologic abnormality.

The erythrocytes of polycythemia vera are most often of normal morphology and function. However, their overproduction augments the concentration of hemoglobin, the viscosity of the circulating blood, and hence the predisposition to hemorrhage and thrombosis that may terminate in death. Leukocyte and platelet counts may be elevated as well, implying possible association with myeloproliferative neoplasia. The cause of polycythemia vera is in question. Onset usually is in the middle or late age range and rarely is seen in children or as a familial disorder. There is a slight male preponderance of polycythemia vera.

Visceral engorgement with blood and marrow hyperplasia comprise the most outstanding pathologic features of the dyscrasia. Extramedullary hematopoiesis may be detected in the liver, and splenic infarcts as well as disseminated thromboses may be seen. Clinical signs and symptoms other than organomegaly include headache, tinnitus, vertigo, malaise, dyspnea, ecchymoses, neurologic disorders, cyanosis of the extremities, dusky complexion, epistaxis, oral petechiae, and gingival bleeding and purple discoloration.

Medical management

Since the major threats are vascular complications, such as hemorrhage and thrombosis, treatment is based on symptomatology and aimed at reduction of blood viscosity. This is accomplished through periodic phlebotomy procedures or induced iron deficiency. Intravenous administration of ^{32}P (to inhibit erythropoiesis) combined with repeated phlebotomies is an alternate modality. Alkylating agents such as chlorambucil have also been employed, but necessitate close hematologic monitoring since they are potentially mutagenic.

DENTAL TREATMENT PLANNING CONSIDERATIONS

Polycythemia vera patients generally show gingival bleeding that is out of proportion to the amount of local etiologic factors of gingival inflammation present in the oral cavity. This is especially true during periods of exacerbation of the polycythemia. With this in mind, dental comprehensive treatment planning should emphasize oral hygiene and nonsurgical periodontal treatment with minimal subgingival manipulation as the mainstay of therapy. Oxidizing mouthrinses are an essential adjunct to oral hygiene practiced at home as well as in the office or clinic, since continuous bleeding adds to the accumulation of oral debris, unpleasant taste, and odor. Dental extractions should be avoided because hemorrhage is an imminent hazard, but where extraction is unavoidable, it is best performed with full knowledge of the patient's platelet count and with appropriate aids for hemostasis at hand. A hospital outpatient or operating room setting is the location of choice for unavoidable oral surgical procedures. Wherever possible, pulp extirpation and endodontic treatment should be chosen over extraction. Operative dentistry should be performed as atraumatically as is feasible, and crown and bridge preparations should maintain the periodontium by keeping the preparations as supragingival as is practicable. Dental or periodontal infections demand immediate treatment with an appropriate antibiotic as well as incision and drainage procedures, since dissemination of infection can trigger a polycythemic crisis and, possibly, death secondary to thrombosis or hemorrhage.

In patients with secondary polycythemia, it is necessary for the dentist to be particularly concerned about the present status of the primary disease state that initially caused the erythrocytosis.

Neutropenia

Depression of the concentration of neutrophilic leukocytes (agranulocytosis, leukopenia) when the total concentration of leukocytes is normal, increased, or decreased constitutes neutropenia. The principal etiologic factors in neutropenia are identical to those responsible for aplastic anemia, and this blood cell dyscrasia may also be found in association with anemia, thrombocytopenia, or both. Drugs, especially antineoplastic therapeutic agents such as antimetabolites and ionizing radiation, as well as aminophenazone and the phenothiazine tranquilizers, are capable of elimination of neutrophils either by arresting stem cell mitosis in the bone marrow or by destruction of mature neutrophils. Hypersensitive immunologic reactions associated with other drugs may accelerate both the destruction and production of neutrophils. Pseudoneutropenia attributed to margination of circulating neutrophils (usually in the lungs) is seen in hemodialysis. Infectious diseases, folic-acid or vitamin-B_{12} deficiency, splenomegalic syndromes, immunoproliferative and hematoproliferative diseases, and hereditary and idiopathic states have been implicated in neutropenia.

Patients with idiopathic syndromes of neutropenia or those receiving drugs capable of inducing neutropenia (patients being immunosuppressed for organ transplantation or with cancer chemotherapy) have markedly decreased resistance to infection. Infection, at first, is caused by organisms comprising the normal flora of body regions. Patients receiving antibiotic therapy repeatedly tend to contract infections with more unusual organisms or antibiotic-resistant organisms.

Cyclic neutropenia, one of the uncommon, idiopathic neutropenic syndromes, occurs in approximately 3-week intervals, persists for many years, and may be related to imbalance in regulation of neutrophil production. Patients with this syndrome rarely suffer potentially fatal infections unless the neutrophil count is lower than 1000 per milliliter. During leukocyte depression periods, a clinical syndrome of fever, malaise, oral lesions, and sore throat is seen.

MEDICAL MANAGEMENT

Medical management of neutropenia related to drugs or physical agents involves discontinuance and further avoidance of the offending preparation. Infection-related neutropenia responds well to treatment of the bacterial, rickettsial, or viral microorganism inducing the disease. In selected cases of neutropenia where congestive splenomegaly is present, favorable response to splenectomy has been reported.

DENTAL TREATMENT PLANNING
CONSIDERATIONS

Patients with neutropenia may develop grave sequelae to major dental manipulations, since their resistance to microorganisms is limited. Patients receiving antimetabolite chemotherapy are most likely to develop oral mucosal breakdown characterized by erosions, ulcerations, and gingivitis. Fusospirochetal necrotizing gingivitis may develop into a gangrenous stomatitis resulting in both oral and facial disfigurement. Therefore while it is mandatory that no oral surgical procedures (including periodontal surgery, tooth extraction, or biopsy) be planned for the patient with severe neutropenia, it is imperative that dental treatment consist of meticulous monitoring and maintenance of the oral cavity so as to circumvent the possibility of fulminating infection by normal oral flora. Immunosuppressed neutropenic patients are not candidates for major restorative denistry, and most of these patients will not be able to wear removable prostheses, since the mucosa is especially sensitive to trauma. Infection with *Candida albicans* is not unusual. Teeth that have been incompletely filled endodontically or those with low-grade pulpal irritation are especially prone to exacerbation. Potential for bacteremia is increased as well. Prior to institution of immunosuppressive chemotherapy, it is advisable for the patient to be seen by a dentist for treatment of potentially problematic teeth or periodontal defects.

In cyclic neutropenia, dental treatment may proceed with few modifications. Treatment should be confined to those periods when the white blood cell count is 1000 per milliliter or greater. Procedures of a surgical nature would be best handled with adjunctive antibiotic prophylaxis to prevent the possibility of disseminated infection.

For patients with mucosal ulcerations, soreness, inflammation, and discomfort, oral hygiene should be limited to gentle rinsing with an oxidizing mouthwash such as 3% hydrogen peroxide diluted in warm water, gauze-sponging of the teeth rather than brushing, and local treatment of superficial candidiasis where applicable. Acute necrotizing ulcerative gingivitis must be treated promptly with oxidizing mouthrinses, gentle superficial scaling, and antibiotic coverage. The patient must be kept well hydrated and nourished on a soft, nonabrasive diet of high protein and high caloric content.

Bleeding disorders

Disorders of bleeding may manifest as petechial or ecchymotic hemorrhages, oozing at sites where minor traumas may have occurred, or as unprovoked hemorrhage. Platelets, the primary physical arm of the hemostatic mechanism, adhere to small blood vessels that have been damaged and create a temporary plug that serves to curtail bleeding. A more stable plug forms with the formation of fibrin as a result of the blood-clotting mechanism. Thus diseases in which excessive bleeding is the major sign may be attributed to (1) platelet deficiency or defects, (2) coagulation system abnormalities, or (3) vascular defects.

PLATELET DEFICITS

Thrombocytopenia, a decrease in the number of circulating platelets, occurs either as a primary idiopathic condition or secondary to a variety of factors. These include myelosuppressive or autoimmunogenic drugs, viral and bacterial infections, replacement or reduction in activity of the bone marrow by inflammatory disease or physical injury, malignancy, and metabolic disturbances.

In young persons, idiopathic thrombocytopenic purpura (ITP) occurs when megakaryocytes are present abundantly in the bone marrow but fail to form platelets. Another ITP mechanism is believed to be antibody related. Antiplatelet IgG has been recovered from the serum of these young patients and is apparently responsible for imparting an abnormal stickiness to the circulating platelets. This predisposes and enhances their entrapment in the spleen. This is the more usual type of ITP and often responds favorably to splenectomy. ITP may develop during the course of or as the initial manifestation of systemic lupus erythematosus and may also be dependent upon heightened capillary fragility.

Spontaneous hemorrhages, gingival bleeding, hematuria, melena, or sudden onset of petechiae may be the first signs and are accompanied by a prolonged bleeding time (Fig. 6-7). Anemia and leukopenia are not present in ITP. Splenectomy and corticosteroid therapy have been the major forms of treatment.

In secondary thrombocytopenia, megakaryocyte production of platelets is impaired. The cause is usually readily identifiable. Conditions that cause "crowding out" of the bone marrow, as well as ionizing radiation, increased destruction of platelets following stasis and sequestration, and platelet lysis (as in bystander hypersensitivity reactions to microorganisms, therapeutic agents, or ingested materials), have been responsible. Secondary thrombocytopenia initially may be treated with transfusion of platelets. Eventually the production of antiplatelet antibodies necessitates discontinuation of that therapy, since the life span of individual platelets is approximately 9 days. Thus repeated transfusions and, consequently, titers of resultant antiplatelet antibody reach prohibitive proportions.

114 *Modifying factors in treatment planning*

THROMBOCYTOSIS AND FUNCTIONAL DISORDERS OF PLATELETS

Thrombocytosis, in which there are excessive quantities of platelets (despite the presence of petechiae, thromboses, and bleeding) and other platelet dysfunctions (characterized by increased bleeding time, dysmorphic platelets, normal platelet counts, and normal mechanisms of coagulation), may predispose to bleeding complications.

Dental treatment planning considerations for patients with platelet disorders. Gingival bleeding of a chronic nature is present in most patients with thrombocytopenic purpura and can best be controlled by oxidizing mouthwashes and atraumatic oral hygiene methods, such as gentle wiping of the teeth, rather than brushing and nonabrasive diets. It is necessary to defer dental procedures when subcutaneous purpura is rampant. Those patients requiring oral surgical procedures in which bleeding will occur must be hospitalized. Physician comanagement is essential, and the platelet count must be elevated to at least 30,000 cu mm in secondary thrombocytopenia. These levels are usually obtained through preoperative platelet transfusion. The patient must be carefully observed for bleeding for at least 2 to 3 days following surgery.

Judicious and conservative periodontal scaling is encouraged for the thrombocytopenic, thrombocytotic, or thrombocytopathic patient, along with oxidizing mouthrinse therapy. Hemostatic agents, including vasoconstrictors

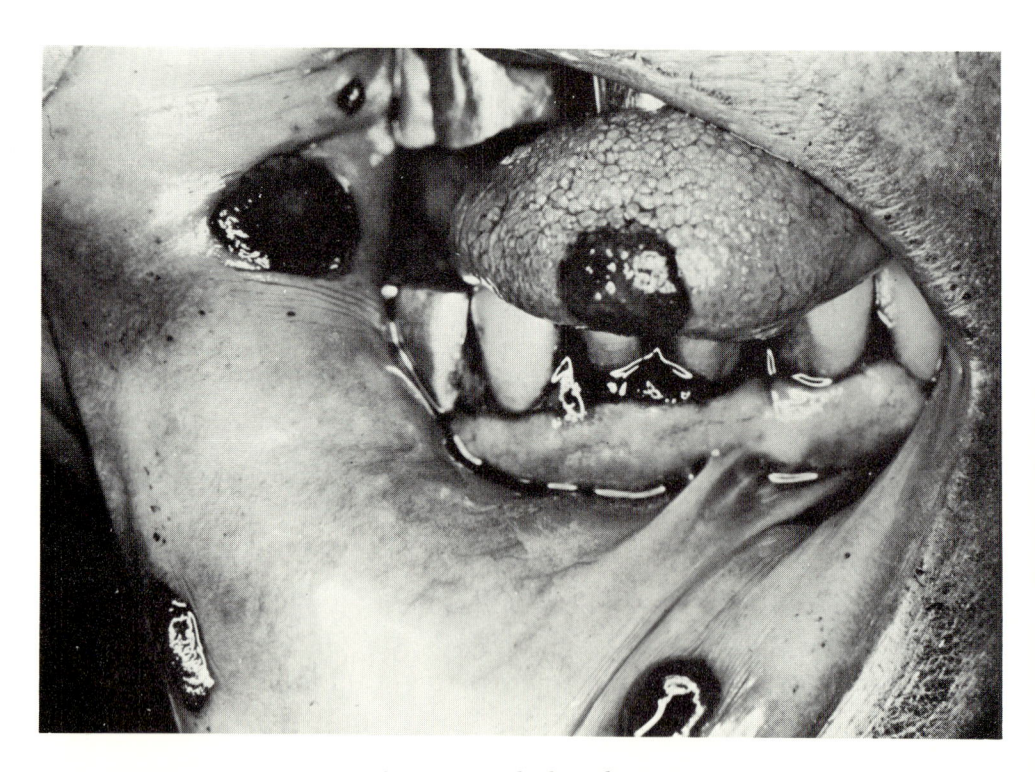

Fig. 6-7. Intraoral picture of patient with thrombocytopenia. Note spontaneous gingival bleeding, four oozing dark clots at other sites of spontaneous bleeding, and area of ecchymosis at right angle of mouth. This patient had petechiae on most skin surfaces.

in local anesthetics, are useful adjuncts for controlling localized bleeding. Extractions are to be avoided whenever possible. When extraction is necessary, Gelfoam, vasoconstrictor, suturing, pressure packing, and postextraction monitoring of the patient will help to minimize the threat of serious hemorrhage. Hospitalization is required in cases in which postoperative hemorrhage is anticipated. Patients receiving steroids for the medical management of ITP present an additional risk for any major dental procedures, and the physician must be consulted prior to institution of any dental therapy. Aspirin-containing analgesics are absolutely contraindicated for patients with platelet abnormalities, since they produce a decrease in circulating prothrombin and thus delay clotting.

Dental treatment should be kept as uncomplicated as possible, with emphasis placed on conservative home-based methods of periodontal disease control and atraumatic, brief restorative procedures. Patients wearing removable prostheses must be advised to leave the prostheses out of the mouth during sleep; ill-fitting prostheses should be replaced. Construction of complete or partial dentures should be reserved for a period of time in which the purpuric manifestations are minimal. Impression-taking and intraoral manipulations must be performed as gently as possible. Endodontics rather than extraction is preferable where a choice exists. Broken or retained roots that are obviously accentuating an inflammatory situation should be removed promptly.

Coagulation disorders

Abnormalities of blood coagulation may be divided into two major groupings: inherited and acquired disorders. In *inherited* disorders, which are less common than the acquired disorders, deficiency of one or more protein factors of the coagulation mechanism appears as the result of sex-linked recessive, autosomal recessive, or autosomal dominant passage. The most commonly encountered hereditary coagulopathies, factor VIII (classic hemophilia) and factor IX (Christmas disease) deficiencies, can be described clinically to illustrate signs and symptoms encountered in the other hereditary coagulation disorders, since deficit of any factor produces a similar picture. The most outstanding sign is massive hemorrhage from trauma, regardless of the degree. Hemarthrosis often occurs without a significant precipitating injury. It is inversely proportional to the level of circulating factor. In classic hemophilia, recurrent and frequent hemarthrosis eventuates in joint destruction. The knee is most often affected, and pain is the initial symptom. Progressively the joint vessels become ischemic, and necrosis or ankylosis may follow. Delayed bleeding from small, "nick"-like cuts is noted and may be attributed to the failure to eventually fibrinize an originally intact platelet plug. Hematomas, petechiae, hematuria, gastrointestinal bleeding, increased menstrual bleeding, and delayed healing of wounds are also seen in the various hereditary coagulopathies.

Hemophilia A (factor VIII deficiency, classic hemophilia)

While this disease is almost always limited to males because it is an X-linked recessive trait, homozygous females may present with it. Survival appears to be related to the severity of the bleeding predisposition and levels of antihemophilia (VIII) factor. Factor VIII transfusions are responsible for the increased life expectancy and more favorable prognosis for these patients who potentially would suffer life-threatening hemorrhage as a result of even minor injury, including dental procedures.

Hemophilia B (factor ix deficiency, Christmas disease)

An X-linked recessive trait, hemophilia B is a much less severe variety than classic hemophilia and is characterized by a deficiency or an abnormality of plasma thromboplastin component. It is distinguished from classic hemophilia only by definitive detection of factor IX deficiency.

Von Willebrand's disease (pseudohemophilia)

Normal platelet counts with diminished platelet adhesion in addition to deficiency of factor VIII (resulting from factor VIII precursor deficit) accounts for the prolonged bleeding and clotting time noted in this disorder. An autosomal dominant trait, Von Willebrand's disease occurs in both males and females, and clinically both sexes show purpura and tendency to hemorrhage. In females, excessive menstrual bleeding is a risk.

Medical management

Laboratory evaluation of the vascular and platelet components of hemostasis is reliably drawn from determination of bleeding time and the platelet count. Extrinsic and common pathways information can be arrived at through determination of plasma thromboplastin time. Intrinsic and common pathways can be assessed for function by partial thromboplastin time determination. These four available tests are a very useful screening battery and should be the preliminary laboratory tests, since with careful history and physical examination they can promulgate a "ballpark" diagnosis. Adjunctive confirmatory studies may follow.

Replacement therapy using intravenous infusion of concentrates of factor VIII (by the glycine or the cryoprecipitate methods), fibrinogen, vitamin K–dependent factors (VIII, IX, X), and prothrombin is the most satisfactory means of treatment. Where factors V, IX, and XI are deficient, plasma is made available. Von Willebrand's disease is usually best managed using cryoprecipitates or fresh plasma.

The regimen of replacement therapy varies with the need for it. Prophylactic maintenance therapy is of restricted use because of high cost and limited availability of the material. Minor bleeding may be managed with several small or one larger daily dose of therapeutic material for a limited period of time. Presurgical preparation or a major bleeding episode requires larger and more frequent doses of replacement therapy for up to approximately 2 weeks or longer. Major bleeding risk procedures such as multiple dental extractions are carried out only in the hospital. Postextraction bleeding is minimized by application of ϵ-aminocaproic acid, an inhibitor of fibrinolysis, in addition to replacement therapy. Supportive therapy, such as arthrocentesis to relieve joint pain, is also employed.

Acquired disorders of coagulation

Deficiencies of vitamin K–dependent coagulation factors may result from hepatic pathology, hemorrhagic disease of the newborn, dietary deficiency or malabsorption, obstruction of the biliary tract, and drugs, notably the coumarin derivatives. These respond to parenteral administration of vitamin K except in cases of liver disease.

Disorders in which destruction of coagulation factors occurs at an abnormally increased rate, such as in disseminated intravascular coagulation (DIC), or disorders in which coagulation-inhibiting factors or malignancy produce coagulopathies (including pathologic proteolysis) are more common than the hereditary disorders and do not respond well to replacement therapy. Rather, treatment of the underlying pathology and supportive measures form the basis of management.

Antibodies to coagulation factors (notably antifactor VIII antibody) may produce hemorrhage. These are demonstrated by specialized tests and are therapeutically handled by steroids, replacement therapy, transfusions, and cytotoxic drugs.

Dental treatment planning considerations

In the patient with hereditary or acquired coagulation disturbances, trauma in the oral cavity caused by toothbrushing, an abrasive diet, or occlusal aberrations may cause some bleeding, ecchymosis, and if extensive enough, frank mucosal breakdown and ulceration. In the hereditary coagulopathies, steady, slow oozing of blood from the gingivae may accompany mild periodontal inflammation. On the other hand, oral surgical procedures may result in a major bleeding diathesis. It is therefore essential to communicate with the patient's physician prior to undertaking any dental treatment (including operative dentistry) in order to determine the need for replacement therapy. Unquestionably, where tooth extraction is planned or other oral surgical procedures are to be undertaken, hospitalization is a requirement. Extensive restorative dental rehabilitation might best be undertaken in the operating room setting with factor replacement administered prior to the procedure. Hemostatic agents such as resorbable gels, local anesthetics with vasoconstrictors, and pressure-dressings will not effectively control hemorrhage without the required coagulation factor.

Purpura, or unprovoked hemorrhage into the tissue, may also be the result of defects of the vasculature (vascular purpura). Causes may be vitamin C deficiency, rickettsial or bacterial diseases, or drug or toxin reactions. Hereditary telangiectatic syndromes are also responsible, as well as conditions where vasculitis is present. The vascular purpura may manifest orally as spontaneous gingival bleeding or as a response to very mild trauma.

The presence of intraoral purpura is of great significance to the dentist, since it may be the first clinical sign of a bleeding disorder. History, including the postoperative course of previous tooth extractions, transfusions, or injuries that have triggered prolonged or abnormal bleeding, familial history, anticoagulant therapy history, as well as tests for capillary fragility, bleeding and clotting time, platelet count, prothrombin time, and partial thromboplastin time, serve as screening parameters for the evaluation of purpura.

Hematologic neoplasms

Acute and chronic leukemias, lymphomas, and myelomas are responsible for approximately half the cancer deaths in young adults and children. Biologic behavior of neoplasms of the hematologic and lymphoid tissues is fairly difficult to predict. However, classification based upon the cell type involved, the peripheral white blood cell count, the clinical progression of the disease, and the tissue of origin attempts to correlate etiology and pathogenesis with clinical course and patient response to available therapy.

LEUKEMIA

Leukemia is produced by either an uncoordinated proliferation of one of the leukocytic stem cell lines or by increased cellular longevity. Theories of pathogenesis include stem cell spontaneous mutation, genetic predisposition, and environmental influences such as chemicals, viruses, and ionizing radiation. Three forms of the myeloproliferative neoplasms exist: myelogenous, lymphatic, and monocytic, and these are categorized as either acute or chronic. Occasionally a rapidly fatal leukemia displaying highly immature, undifferentiated cells may be seen and is classified as a "stem cell leukemia."

Chronic leukemias show more highly elevated white blood cell counts than the acute leukemias; however, the cells in acute leukemias tend to be more primitive ("blast"-like) than the cells in chronic leukemias.

Acute leukemias are abrupt in onset, with fever, malaise, and progressive exhaustion followed soon by a hemorrhagic tendency and susceptibility to bacterial infection. Pain in bones and joints occurs especially in the young patient and is a reflection of neoplastic bone marrow proliferation.

Chronic leukemia is characterized by progressive weakness, loss of weight, or peripheral lymphadenopathy. In addition, splenomegaly, hemorrhagic episodes, and anemia accompanied by exertional dyspnea appear in chronic leukemia, which is appreciably less dramatic than the acute variety. Leukemia patients have an increased susceptibility to bacterial infection.

Diagnosis is confirmed by increased peripheral white blood cell counts, the presence of abnormal blast forms, and differential blood count abnormalities. Anemia and thrombocytopenia are usually seen also. In monocytic leukemia there is a marked predilection for gingival infiltration by leukemic cells (Fig. 6-8). Thus biopsy of enlarged gingival tissues may be of great diagnostic aid.

Medical management. Prognosis, despite therapy and remissions, is generally poor, particularly in the acute leukemias. Radiation and chemotherapy have helped to prolong the life expectancy in the chronic leukemia patient by several years. Most deaths are attributed to hemorrhage or fulminant infection preceded by "blast crisis" where normal leukocytic cells are virtually replaced by immature leukocytic cells and platelet counts, as well as hemoglobin concentration and hematocrit, fall drastically. Cytotoxic agents and antimetabolites and steroids improve the prognosis of the disease by prolonging remission periods. However, these drugs in addition to the leukemic state itself may cause severe hyperplastic gingival inflammation, mucosal ulceration, and widespread necrosis. The patient's immune response, tissue resistance to local irritation, and normal flora are inhibited. As a result, bacterial and mycot-

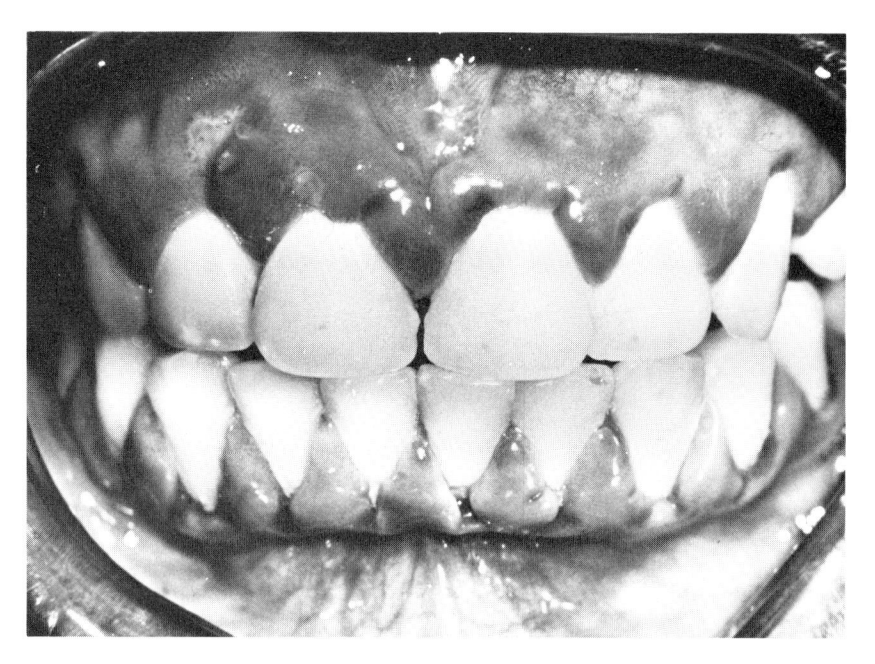

Fig. 6-8. Monocytic leukemia. Note enlarged gingivae with minute areas of spontaneous hemorrhage. Patient's oral home care was moderately good. (Courtesy Dr. Paul Akers, Chicago, Ill.)

ic infections occur especially in the acute leukemias and particularly in those of the stem cell and monocytic forms (Fig. 6-9). Healing is markedly delayed.

Dental treatment planning considerations. The leukemia patient has a reduced life expectancy, a tendency to hemorrhage, a marked susceptibility to infection, and low tissue resistance. These factors mandate a maintenance and palliation-oriented approach to dental treatment. Since the presence of local irritational factors produces exaggerated tissue responses in the face of attenuated immunity, gentle basic oral hygiene must be instituted. Frequent noncaustic mouthrinses with either oxidizing mouthwash (3% hydrogen peroxide in warm water), plain warm water, or warm saline solution (depending on patient tolerance) aid in debridement of loose material, such as food particles, clotted blood, and exudates present on tooth surfaces and interdentally. Wet gauze, rather than a relatively more coarse toothbrush, can be employed to wipe smooth tooth surfaces clean, thus providing less trauma to the adjacent tissues, which might eventuate in hemorrhage, ulceration, or necrosis, and is more comfortable for the patient. Scaling on a supragingival basis is a useful part of the disease control program in that removal of local superficial deposits will reduce the exuberant gingival inflammatory response.

Elective dentistry has no place in treatment planning for acute leukemia patients. Thus if tooth extraction is necessary, the emergency procedure should be carried out in the hospital setting, but replacement of the extracted tooth is not appropriate unless a remission occurs. Since these patients succumb to infections, emergency treatment must include presurgical antibiotic

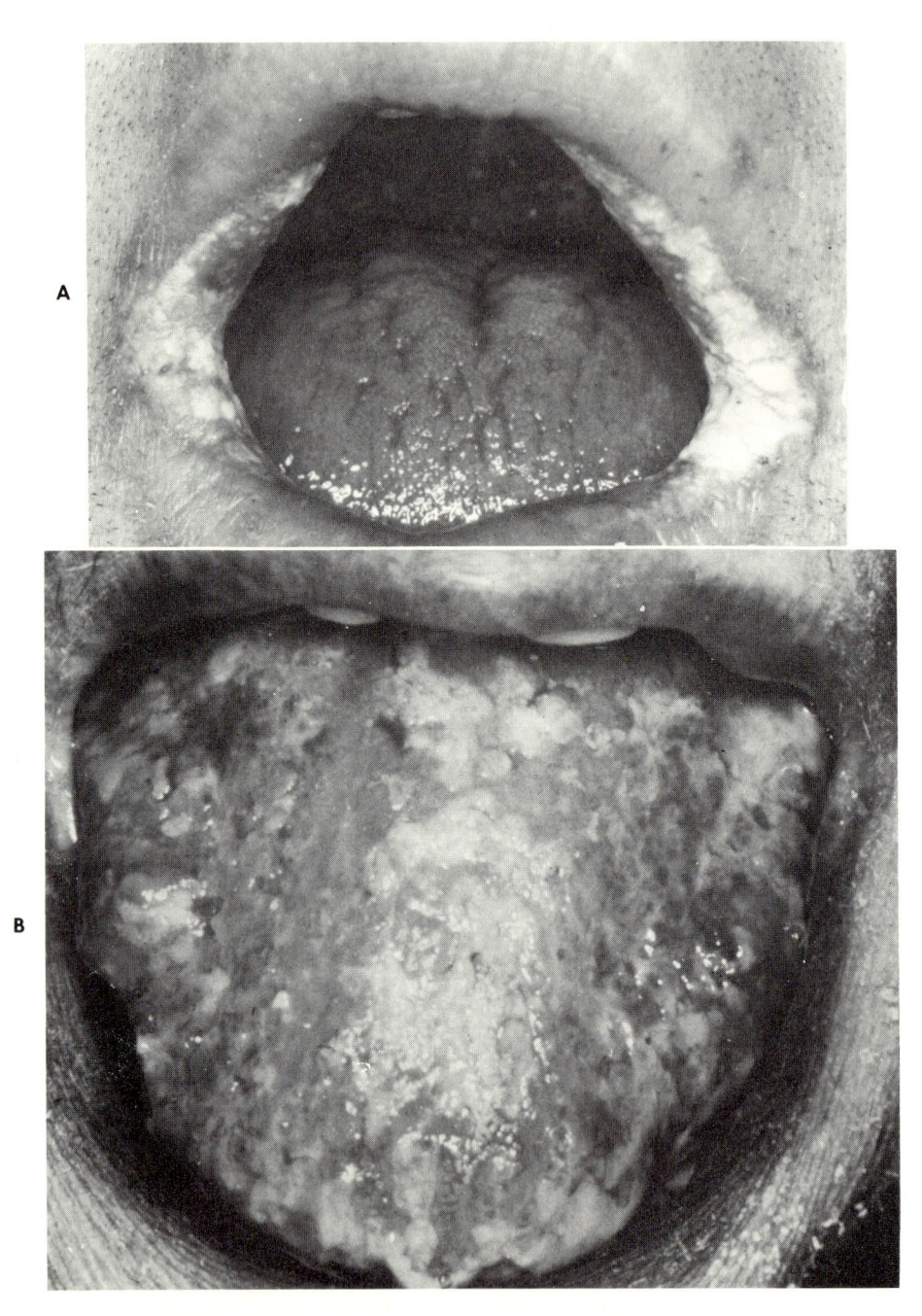

Fig. 6-9. Candidiasis in two patients with leukemia. **A,** Corners of lips. **B,** Dorsal surface of tongue. (Courtesy Dr. Gerald Shklar, Boston, Mass.)

coverage, platelet replacement (should a platelet count reflect the need), and communication with the attending physician. In the immunosuppressed patient, chronic periapical pathology tends to become acute and must be treated aggressively before a fulminating, potentially fatal infection occurs.

During periods of acute, painful oral ulceration and mucositis, candidiasis and acute necrotizing ulcerative gingivitis may also be present. These must be treated locally and the physician contacted immediately so that the need for systemic antimycotic therapy can be assessed. In some circumstances a severe oral response dictates the need for a change in the chemotherapeutic regimen for the systemic disease. Viscous local anesthetic mouthrinses, crushed ice, nystatin (Mycostatin) in oral suspension, or vaginal suppositories for candidiasis dissolved in the mouth in addition to forced hydration and supportive conservative oral hygiene procedures enhance patient comfort. Necrotizing gingivitis requires prompt institution of antibiotic therapy along with oxidizing mouthrinses and gentle debridement of gangrenous tissue and interdental deposits. Of course, follow-up periodontal plastic procedures to improve soft tissue contours deformed as a result of this gingivitis are absolutely contraindicated.

Extractions and incision and drainage procedures must be carried out paying strictest attention to the danger of hemorrhagic diathesis. They should be reserved for the hospital setting after appropriate precautionary measures (platelet count adjustment, antibiotic chemoprophylaxis, and generalized host resistance) are undertaken and assessed. Since many leukemia patients are on steroid chemotherapeutic maintenance, presurgical steroid dose modification may be necessary, and physician cooperation is essential. Chronic patients in remission are candidates for all phases of dentistry. Where the patient will tolerate the procedure and in the chronic leukemia patient in a state of remission, pulp extirpation, endodontic debridement, filling, and antibiotic coverage during the duration of the procedure may be preferable to tooth extraction. Carious teeth may be excavated and restored conservatively with either sedative or amalgam restorations.

Lymphoma

For the sake of thoroughness, a brief mention of lymphoma is included here. Lymphomas are neoplasms of solid lymphoid tissue, in contrast to the leukemias that arise in the bone marrow. Controversy exists as to whether these lymphoid neoplasms are indeed uncontrolled new growths of lymphoid tissue or whether they are initially inflammatory or reactive in nature, presently eventuating in a neoplastic condition. Despite the confusion, if allowed to remain untreated, these lymphoproliferative disorders behave in a malignant fashion, metastasizing widely and resulting in death.

Classification is based upon the cell type involved, that is, lymphocytes, histiocytes, stem cells, plasma cells, or a mixture of cell types. Further categorization is made on the basis of whether the growth pattern is nodular (follicular) or diffuse.

Clinical manifestations of lymphomas in the earliest stages are usually limited to sudden discovery of palpable nodes, often in the cervical region. As the disease progresses, hepatosplenomegaly, malaise, weakness, and anemia may be seen as well as gastrointestinal symptoms, osteolytic lesions, and generalized organomegaly.

Medical management. Prognosis depends on the cell type and tissue patterns seen histologically as well as the progress or degree of generalized involvement at the time of initial evaluation and diagnosis. Chemotherapeutic and radiotherapeutic modalities of treatment can extend remission periods up to 15 years. Thus prognosis is promising. However, patients demonstrating aberrant immunologic responses have a more guarded prognosis.

Dental treatment planning considerations. Lymphoma nodules may present in the oral cavity as either primary lesions arising in lymphoid tissue of Waldeyer's ring or the floor of the mouth or as metastatic lesions. Metastasis to the jawbones will demonstrate a localized radiolucency or a diffuse rarefaction roentgenographically. These or any unexplained soft-tissue tumors in the oral cavity must be investigated and worked up through biopsy study. Dental treatment planning for the lymphoma patient receiving chemotherapy or radiation therapy to the head and neck must be designed to deal with the frequently occurring mucositis. Prior to radiation, preventive measures must be instituted, and these will be discussed in the following section. Mucosal breakdown resulting from chemotherapy is handled in the same manner as was mentioned for the leukemia patient. Certainly those patients under intensive chemotherapeutic control are not candidates for elective dental therapy. Rehabilitative or routine restorative dentistry must be postponed until a time when the oral mucous membranes are no longer iatrogenically friable.

XEROSTOMIA

Xerostomia is defined as dryness of the mouth. It is a relatively common complaint and varies considerably in degree of severity. This sign or symptom may result from primary salivary pathology or may be secondary to systemic conditions. Xerostomia may be classified into four etiologic groups:

1. This group includes diseases either causing ductal obstruction or a reduction in the number of secretory units. Salivary stones and infiltrating tumors are examples of entities that cause ductal obstruction. Examples of conditions that reduce the number of secretory units include aplasia, senile atrophy, infections, immunologic disease (Sjögren's syndrome), and irradiation to the oral cavity, face, or neck (Fig. 6-10).
2. Conditions in this group produce a reduction in salivary production through systemic alterations in electrolyte and fluid balance. Examples are diabetes mellitus and insipidus, dehydration, heart failure, kidney failure, hormonal and vitamin deficiencies, and pernicious and iron-deficiency anemias.
3. Conditions in this group reduce salivary production by influencing the autonomic nervous sytem. The autonomic nervous system is responsible for regulating secretion of both minor and major salivary glands. Flow is increased by parasympathomimetic agents such as pilocarpine and neostigmine. On the other hand, flow is decreased by anticholinergic drugs such as atropine and propantheline bromide (Pro-Banthine). As a rule, stimulation of the sympathetic nervous system inhibits secretions. Hypotensive agents, diuretics, and antihistaminic and decongestant preparations may produce diminished salivary flow. In addition to

pharmacologic agents, the following conditions may also decrease salivation by influencing the autonomic nervous system: brain tumors, neurosurgery, inflammatory neurologic conditions secondary to occupationally encountered dusts and poisons, and physical trauma.
4. This group embraces central nervous system lesions and psychogenic and emotional factors such as fright, agitation, and depression. In addition, pharmacologic agents such as psychotropic drugs, particularly the central nervous system depressants and phenothiazine tranquilizers, are medications that cause xerostomia by direct action on the central nervous system.

Oral findings

Since the minor or accessory salivary glands contribute a significant quantity of saliva, generalized oral mucosal dryness is most likely due to a pansalivary deficiency caused by a systemically influenced condition, rather than a localized salivary gland disease.

In mild, short-term cases the mucosa may appear normal, but patients may complain of itching, burning, or pain of the mucosa as well as dysphagia.

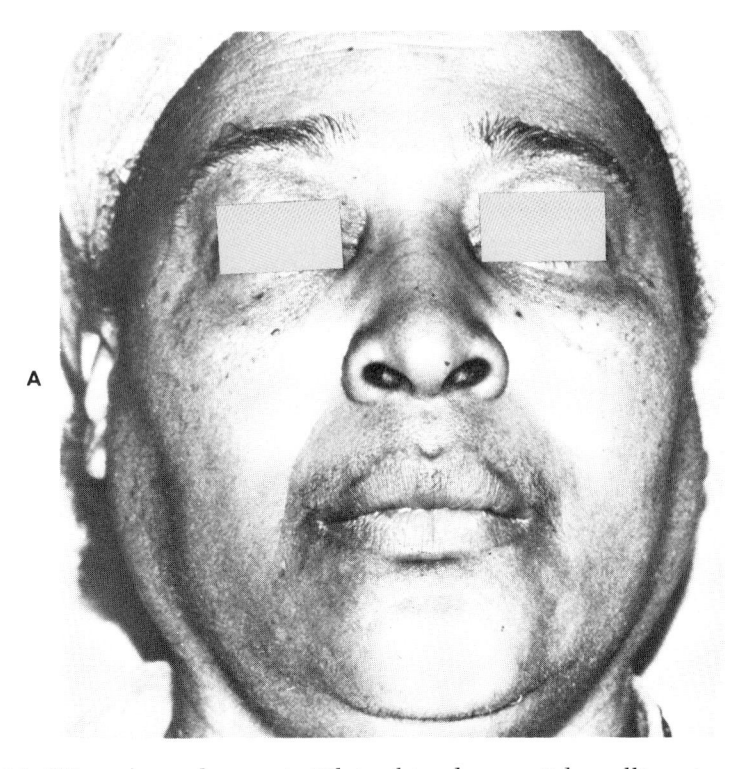

Fig. 6-10. Sjögren's syndrome. **A**, Bilateral tender parotid swellings in woman with Sjögren's syndrome. (**A** courtesy Dr. Paul Akers, Chicago, Ill.; from Wood, N. K., and Goaz, P. W.: Differential diagnosis of oral lesions, St. Louis, 1975, The C. V. Mosby Co.)

Continued

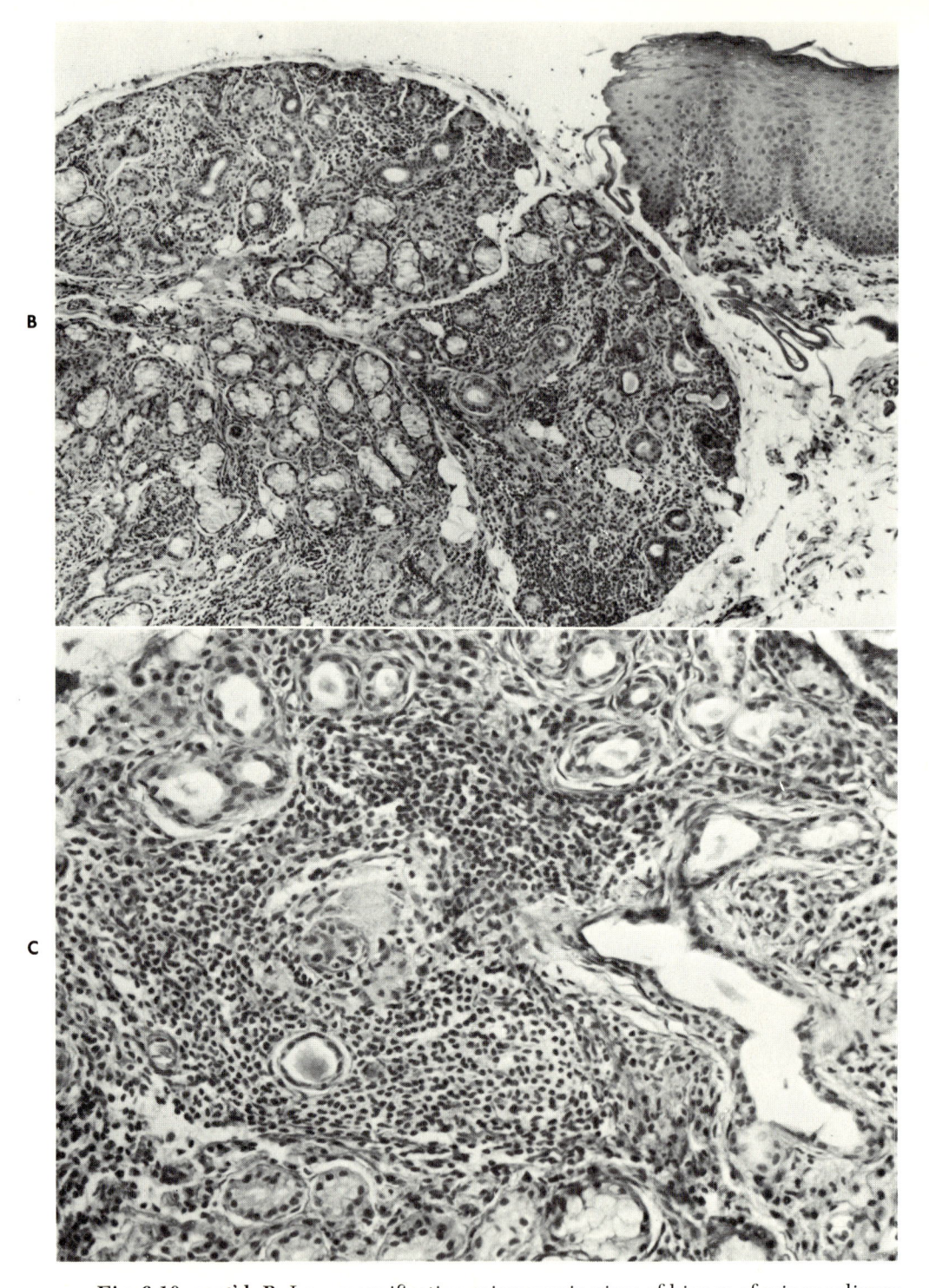

Fig. 6-10, cont'd. **B**, Low-magnification microscopic view of biopsy of minor salivary glands from labial mucosa. Note destruction of many glandular acini and replacement by fibrous and inflammatory tissue. **C**, Higher-magnification microscopic view showing inflammatory stage of destruction.

However, prolonged frank xerostomia will produce marked alteration in the oral mucosa, regardless of etiology. The salivary pool in the floor of the mouth will be missing. The mucosa will have a dull, lusterless appearance. Alternating erythema (smoothness), pallor (roughness), and curdlike debris may be seen on the mucosa. In severe cases the mucosa will show erosions, ulcerations, and fissures. The openings of Wharton's and Stensen's ducts may show redness and possibly purulent discharge, particularly when the glands are "milked." The tongue will frequently be fissured and have painful red areas resulting from the loss of papillae.

Patients with true xerostomia are more susceptible to acute and chronic inflammatory and infectious episodes of the major salivary glands. Bacterial infections are usually retrograde in nature and characteristically produce a purulent exudate from Wharton's or Stensen's ducts. This produces an unpleasant taste and odor and contributes to the overall discomfort. The patient will have a painful, localized swelling over the involved glands and occasionally will have a fever. Speaking may be difficult and may be characterized by a "sticky"-sounding speech.

Marginal gingivitis will be present in both arches and perhaps a severe generalized periodontitis. Rampant caries will usually be apparent, especially at the cervical and incisal regions. These undesirable dental changes occur because of the lack of normal cleansing and antibacterial actions of saliva, resulting in stasis of food debris and increased plaque formation. Patients with full dentures may be unable to tolerate or function with their prostheses. Partial denture wearers may also suffer because of decreased mucosal resiliency.

Dental treatment planning considerations

It is important that the dentist develop a protocol by which the specific cause of the xerostomia may be positively identified in each patient. However, a discussion of the aspects of differential diagnosis are beyond the scope of this chapter.

Once the presence of xerostomia has been established, every effort should be made to prevent and intercept the prospective damage to the patient's oral soft and hard tissues, speech, mastication, deglutition, and psychological outlook. If the cause is known, often it can be removed and the xerostomia will disappear. For instance, other pharmacologic agents may be substituted for offending drugs. Pilocarpine and other parasympathomimetics, as well as corticosteroids, have been somewhat successfully used as short term sialagogues. However, prolonged administration of these agents should be avoided because of their harmful systemic effects.

The patient must be assured that he has the support of the dental staff and that they are receptive to his needs, since pain and depression often accompany xerostomia. The patient must be given detailed counsel on how to maintain good oral health. It is most important that a vigorous regimen of good home care be instituted and properly monitored. Postprandial brushing and flossing is mandatory. Periodontal surgical procedures must be meticulously accomplished in order to ensure that the patient can clean all troublesome areas well.

Sugarless candies and chewing gum are suitable means of stimulating salivation, but the sugar-containing varieties must be avoided at all costs! Lemon juice and glycerine mouthrinses or hydrogen peroxide and warm water mouthrinses aid in maintaining a moist intraoral environment and are helpful in removing food debris and desquamated epithelium from the interdental spaces. Cleansing foods such as juicy fresh fruits are preferred for their ease of ingestion and for stimulation of the oral epithelium. Soft, nonsticky, high-protein foods are also encouraged.

Restorative procedures should be completed as soon as possible. If it is economically feasible, full-coverage restorations should be used in an effort to protect as well as strengthen remaining tooth structure. Because of the poor prognosis of denture patients with xerostomia, it is wise to retain the natural dentition for as long as possible. Such a program must be based upon a recall system that is more frequent than that required for a normal person. Three-month recalls are recommended, as are regularly scheduled fluoride treatments. For patients who must lose their natural teeth, oral lubricants such as glycerine or 2% methylcellulose may offer relative comfort and ease of function with their dentures.

Irradiated patients

Much of the previous information on xerostomia also applies to patients who have received or will receive radiation therapy to the head, neck, or oral cavity. However, there are some additional factors to consider in these patients. Primarily the major concerns involve the increased susceptibility to dental decay, periodontal disease, and *osteoradionecrosis* (osteomyelitis) (Fig. 6-11).

In contradistinction to the other conditions that produce xerostomia, there is usually an opportunity to institute preventive measures prior to the onset of xerostomia. These measures frequently will alleviate the anticipated problems.

In the first place it is mandatory to know the dosage of ionizing radiation that has been used and to determine whether the oral cavity, jaws, and major salivary glands were actually included in the field of radiation.

Although approaches to the dental treatment of preirradiation or postirradiation patients varies somewhat from center to center, the Veterans Administration Hospital at Hines, Illinois, uses the following approach in prevention: Prior to irradiation the patient is instructed in home care. The teeth are meticulously cleaned, and a 0.4% stannous fluoride (SnF_2) gel is applied every 4 hours and particularly at bedtime. For the next 6 days the gel is applied once a day in the clinic. From visits eight to twelve, professional applications are made once every second day; from visits thirteen to twenty, every third day; from visits twenty-one to thirty, weekly professional applications are done; and from visits thirty-one and on, professional applications are made on a bimonthly basis. Recently the Oral Disease Research Laboratory of the Veterans Administration Hospital in Houston reported better anticaries results obtained from the combined sequential use of 0.31% APF and 0.4% stannous fluoride.[3] The APF gel is applied for 2 minutes and is followed by a 2-minute application of stannous fluoride.

Condemned teeth should be extracted at least 1 week prior to commencement of irradiation treatment. A generous alveolectomy is performed so that

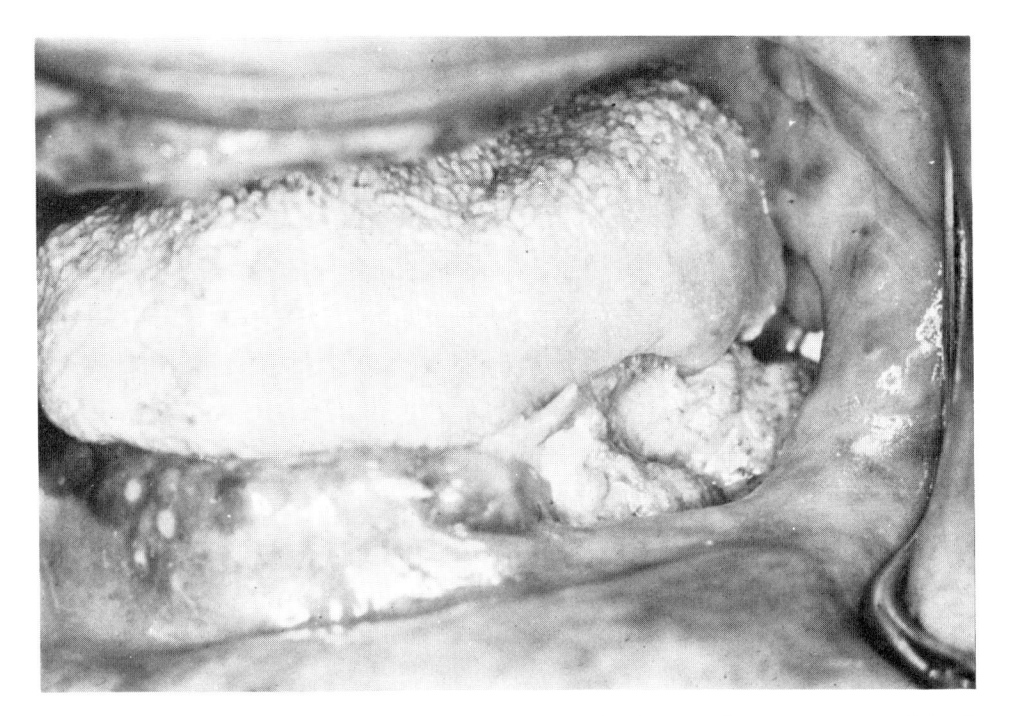

Fig. 6-11. Osteoradionecrosis. Intraoral photograph showing large segment of dead bone in left mandibular alveolus. In addition, patient had sinus tract draining extraorally at inferior border of mandible on left side. Patient had received irradiation 6 years previously for squamous cell carcinoma of floor of mouth.

the mucosa can be carefully closed over the sockets. Some clinicians believe that antibiotic coverage is desirable. Hopefully this approach will prevent the development of an osteoradionecrosis, which tends to develop in these patients because of decreased blood supply of the jawbones and the presence of bacteria.

For patients requiring dentures, it is recommended that at least 1 year should lapse from the time of completion of the radiation therapy. Even then the mucosa must be carefully evaluated for the presence of redness or frank ulceration. If either of these changes are noticed, denture construction must be delayed. However, if the mucosa has a healthy pink color, is free of lesions, and (in the case of male patients) the whiskers show signs of regeneration, the clinician may begin denture construction. When the dentures are delivered, it is important that the patient be instructed to remove the dentures at night in order to rest the mucosa and to reduce the risk of ulceration.

It is critically important to reexamine the denture wearer at frequent intervals in order to detect denture-related ulcerations in their earliest possible stage so that they may be treated and eliminated in short order. Ulcers on the ridges are particularly serious because they permit bacteria access to the underlying susceptible bone, possibly resulting in osteomyelitis. Under such circumstances dentures should be judiciously trimmed and the offending occlusion adjusted, but the denture should be removed until the ulcer has completely healed.

Artificial saliva is being successfully used by some researchers. Workers at the Veterans Administration Hospital in Houston report that a saliva substitute, VA-OraLube, has been developed and is currently being successfully used at that institution.[3-5] It is designed specifically for use in head and neck irradiated patients but is equally effective for xerostomia of any cause.

A painful mucositis often occurs during radiation therapy to the head, neck, and oral cavity. In most cases this stems from temporary decrease in function of the major and minor salivary glands. The duration of this reaction ranges from weeks to months. It is important to continue fluoride applications and meticulous home care practices that were instituted prior to irradiation throughout this susceptible period.

In addition, irradiated patients often will experience recurrent superficial bacterial and mycotic infections, which may compromise the patient's ability to eat comfortably. Routine oral smears performed periodically may prove helpful in identifying subclinical candidiasis. Thus the administration of interceptive antimycotic medication may prevent a serious superinfection. Angular cheilitis and intraoral candidiasis should be treated with nystatin (Mycostatin) ointment or rinses, or vaginal suppositories (100,000 units) dissolved in the mouth.

REFERENCES

1. A Committee Report of the American Heart Association: Prevention of bacterial endocarditis, J.A.D.A. **95:**600-605, 1977.
2. Committee on Prevention of Rheumatic Fever and Bacterial Endocarditis of the American Heart Association: Prevention of bacterial endocarditis, Circulation **56:**139A-143A, 1977.
3. Preventive Dentistry Bulletin, vol. 1, no. 2, Houston, July 1977, Oral Diseases Research Laboratory, Veterans Administration Hospital.
4. Shannon, I. L., McCrary, B. R., and Starcke, E. N.: A saliva substitute for use by xerostomic patients undergoing radiotherapy to the head and neck, Oral Surg. **44:**656-661, 1977.
5. Xerostomia and Sjögren's syndrome: artificial saliva. In McCarthy, P.L., and Shklar, G.: Diseases of the oral mucosa, ed. 2, Philadelphia, Lea & Febiger. In press.

BIBLIOGRAPHY

Batsakis, J. G.: Non-neoplastic lesions of salivary glands. In Tumors of the head and neck, Baltimore, 1974, The Williams & Wilkins Co.

Bickley, H. C.: Practical concepts in human disease, Baltimore, 1974, The Williams & Wilkins Co.

Braunwald, E.: Heart failure. In Wintrobe, M. M., Thorn, G. W., Adams, R. D., Braunwald, E., Isselbacher, K. J., and Petersdorf, R. G., editors: Harrison's principles of internal medicine, ed. 7, New York, 1974, McGraw-Hill Book Co., pp. 1117-1127.

Burchenal, J. H.: Hematologic neoplasms. In Holland, J. F., and Frei III, E.: Cancer medicine, Philadelphia, 1973, Lea & Febiger.

Burket, L. W.: Oral medicine, diagnosis and treatment, ed. 6, Philadelphia, 1971, J. B. Lippincott Co.

Committee on Prevention of Rheumatic Fever and Bacterial Endocarditis: Jones criteria (modified) for guidance in the diagnosis of rheumatic fever, American Heart Association, 1955.

Council on Dental Therapeutics: Accepted dental therapeutics, ed. 37, Chicago, 1975, American Dental Association.

Crouse, V. L.: Diseases that may complicate surgery. In Irby, W. B., editor: Facial trauma and concomitant problems, evaluation and treatment, St. Louis, 1974, The C. V. Mosby Co., pp. 172-181, 186-197.

Daniels, T. E., Silverman, S., Jr., Michalski, J. P., Greenspan, J. S., Sylvester, R. A., and Talal, N.: The oral component of Sjögren's syndrome, Oral Surg. **39:**875-885, 1975.

Disorders of the hematopoetic system. In Wintrobe, M. M., Thorn, G. W., Adams, R. D., Braunwald, E., Isselbacher, K. J., and Petersdorf, R. G., editors: Harrison's principles of internal medicine, ed. 7, New York, 1974, McGraw-Hill Book Co., pp. 1580-1682.

Eisen, H. N.: Cell-mediated hypersensitivity and immunity. In Davis, B. D., Dulbecco, R., Eisen, H. N., Ginsberg, H., Wood, W. B., Jr., and McCarty, M., editors: Microbiology, New York, 1973, Harper & Row, Publishers.

Eisenberg, E., and Bernick, S. M.: Anomalies of the teeth with stains and discolorations, J. Prev. Dent. **2**:7-20, 1975.

Feinstein, A. R.: Rheumatic fever. In Wintrobe, M. M., Thorn, G. W., Adams, R. D., Braunwald, E., Isselbacher, K. J., and Petersdorf, R. G., editors: Harrison's principles of internal medicine, ed. 7, New York, 1974, McGraw-Hill Book Co., pp. 1171-1177.

Friedman, W. F., and Braunwald, E.: Congenital heart disease. In Wintrobe, M. M., Thorn, G. W., Adams, R. D., Braunwald, E., Isselbacher, K. J., and Petersdorf, R. G., editors: Harrison's principles of internal medicine, ed. 7, New York, 1974, McGraw-Hill Book Co., pp. 1154-1170.

Harper, P. L., Jr.: Laboratory values–normal, abnormal, and their significance. In Irby, W. B., editor: Facial trauma and concomitant problems, evaluation and treatment, St. Louis, 1974, The C. V. Mosby Co., pp. 220-232.

Hendrix, T. R.: Diseases of the esophagus. In Wintrobe, M. M., Thorn, G. W., Adams, R. D., Braunwald, E., Isselbacher, K. J., and Petersdorf, R. G., editors: Harrison's principles of internal medicine, ed. 7, New York, 1974, McGraw-Hill Book Co., pp. 1425-1427.

Jacobs, A.: Anemia. In Hardisty, R. M., and Weatherall, D. J., editors: Blood and its disorders, Oxford, Eng., 1974, Blackwell Scientific Publications.

Jones, N. L., and Campbell, E. J. M.: Chronic airway obstruction due to asthma, bronchitis and emphysema. In Wintrobe, M. M., Thorn, G. W., Adams, R. D., Braunwald, E., Isselbacher, K. J., and Petersdorf, R. G., editors: Harrison's principles of internal medicine, ed. 7, New York, 1974, McGraw-Hill Book Co., pp. 1275-1285.

King, D. W., Geller, L. M., Krieger, P., Silva, F., and Lefkowitch, J. H.: A survey of pathology, New York, 1976, Oxford University Press.

Koff, R. S., and Isselbacher, K. J.: Chronic active hepatitis. In Wintrobe, M. M., Thorn, G. W., Adams, R. D., Braunwald, E., Isselbacher, K. J., and Petersdorf, R. G., editors: Harrison's principles of internal medicine, ed. 7, New York, 1974, McGraw-Hill Book Co., pp. 1537-1540.

Leavell, B. S., and Thorup, O. A.: Fundamentals of clinical hematology, ed. 4, Philadelphia, 1976, W. B. Saunders Co., pp. 59-62.

Mason, D. K., and Chisholm, D. M.: Salivary glands in health and disease, Philadelphia, 1975, W. B. Saunders Co.

McCarthy, P. L., and Shklar, G.: Diseases of the oral mucosa, New York, 1964, McGraw-Hill Book Co.

McCarthy, M.: Streptococci. In Davis, B. D., Dulbecco, R., Eisen, H. N., Ginsberg, H., Wood, W. B., Jr., and McCarty, M., editors: Microbiology, New York, 1973, Harper & Row, Publishers.

Norman, P. S.: Asthma, hay fever and other manifestations of allergy. In Wintrobe, M. M., Thorn, G. W., Adams, R. D., Braunwald, E., Isselbacher, K. J., and Petersdorf, R. G., editors: Harrison's principles of internal medicine, ed. 7, New York, 1974, McGraw-Hill Book Co., pp. 368-374.

Pallasch, T.: Chemoprophylaxis of rheumatic fever, rheumatic heart disease and bacterial endocarditis. In Pallasch, T.: Clinical drug therapy in dental practice, Philadelphia, 1973, Lea & Febiger, pp. 124-126.

Peery, T. M., and Miller, F. N.: Pathology, a dynamic introduction to medicine and surgery, ed. 2, Boston, 1971, Little, Brown & Co.

Quie, P. G., and Ayoub, E. M.: Rheumatic fever, Postgrad. Med. **44**:73, 1968.

Robbins, S. L.: Blood and bone marrow. In Pathologic basis of systemic disease, Philadelphia, 1974, W. B. Saunders Co., pp. 699-748.

Robbins, S. L.: Heart. In Pathologic basis of systemic disease, Philadelphia, 1974, W. B. Saunders Co., pp. 639-643.

Robbins, S. L.: Lymph nodes and spleen. In Pathologic basis of systemic disease, Philadelphia, 1974, W. B. Saunders Co., pp. 749-781.

Rosenthal, D. S., and Maloney, W. C.: Hematology for the practicing dentist (Symposium on physical and laboratory diagnosis), Dent. Clin. North Am. **18**:171-186, 1974.

Rushmer, R. F.: Structure and function of the cardiovascular system, Philadelphia, 1972, W. B. Saunders Co., pp. 180-186.

Sambh, M. P.: Mechanisms of hypertension, Proceedings of International Workshop Conference, Los Angeles, 1973 (Excerpta Medica Amsterdam), New York, 1973, American Elsevier Publishing Co., pp. 4-5.

Sapiro, S. M., and Eisenberg, E.: Sjögren's syndrome (sicca complex), Oral Surg. **45:**591-599, 1978.

Shafer, W. G., Hine, M. K., and Levy, B. M.: Xerostomia and diseases of salivary glands. In A textbook of oral pathology, ed. 3, Philadelphia, 1974, W. B. Saunders Co.

Shklar, G., and McCarthy, P. L.: The oral manifestations of systemic disease, Woburn, Mass., 1976, Butterworth (Publishers).

Silen, W.: Peptic ulcer. In Wintrobe, M. M., Thorn, G. W., Adams, R. D., Braunwald, E., Isselbacher, K. J., and Petersdorf, R. G., editors: Harrison's principles of internal medicine, ed. 7, New York, 1974, McGraw-Hill Book Co., pp. 1431-1447.

Tisdale, W. A., LaMont, J. T., and Isselbacher, K. J.: Cirrhosis. In Wintrobe, M. M., Thorn, G. W., Adams, R. D., Braunwald, E., Isselbacher, K. J., and Petersdorf, R. G., editors: Harrison's principles of internal medicine, ed. 7, New York, 1974, McGraw-Hill Book Co., pp. 1540-1551.

Walter, J. B.: An introduction to the principles of disease, Philadelphia, 1977, W. B. Saunders Co., pp. 484-487, 528-542.

7

Behavioral considerations

Richard Adelson

Treatment planning as traditionally taught utilizes the objective analysis of examination data, such as the visual exam, roentgenograms, and study casts, to formulate for the patient the necessary treatment activities and their sequencing.

The treatment for a particular problem is based upon a set of criteria established by the dentist. Utilizing these criteria, the dentist must balance the benefits and costs among the treatment alternatives and decide upon the one with greatest benefit and least cost—the word "cost" implying not only money but future problems, time needed, and impact on the dentition.

This design, however, ignores a very important reality. The patient at some point will accept, reject, or wish to modify the plan presented. His decision will be based on criteria generated by psychologic and sociologic considerations, including his attitudes, expectations, priorities, and past experiences with dentistry.

The criteria used by the patient to balance the benefits and costs may then be different than the dentist's to a greater or lesser degree. It is vital to the successful negotiation of the final treatment plan that the discrepancies between what the dentist believes to be the appropriateness of treatment and what the patient desires be resolved.

The dentist, because of his or her training, recognizes that the oral condition with which the patient presents has multiple causes. In addition to the general susceptibility or resistance to oral disease, there are a host of factors, local and idiopathic, that have contributed to the current condition. There are multiple possibilities for the resolution of these problems, each with their own benefits and deficits. The one factor that remains consistent with all the possible treatment alternatives is the uncertainty of outcome. There is no way to assure patients that their periodontal disease will not continue, that a salvaged tooth will not need root canal treatment, or that the crown will last forever. The dentist recognizes that the treatment performed may not eliminate the problem or be serviceable for a lifetime.

The patient, however, comes to the dentist with a potentially different set of assumptions and expectations. The patient often sees his problem as having a single cause: "It was all my last dentist's fault" or "I have soft teeth." This unicausality regarding the factors that have generated the current condition is carried over into its resolution, which is also seen in terms of a single treatment. It is therefore not unusual for patients to say "Take them all out" or "Make me a bridge that does not come in and out" without recognizing that for each of their current problems there may be a multitude of treatment plans.

The patient, because of his assumptions about the nature of dental treatment, develops expectations regarding the outcome as well. A patient often assumes that once entering into treatment, he can reasonably give all responsibility for treatment to the dentist, and that he need have only an insignificant role in the treatment, such as presenting his mouth at the time appointed. Furthermore, the success of the outcome, because of the mechanical nature of the treatment, will be directly related to the quality of care the dentist provides. Treatment performed by the "good" dentist will fix his problems and can reasonably be expected to last a lifetime.

The result of this discrepancy between the expectations and assumptions of the patient and practitioner has serious implications unless it is explored and resolved. Clearly the patient must expect to become actively involved in the treatment process for it to be successful.

A pragmatic approach to treatment planning recognizes the patient's active role. It requires a practitioner who uses this approach to include as part of the examination the acquisition and interpretation of psychosocial information about the patient. This information will be used to formulate an individualized treatment plan, present the plan to the patient in a manner that will facilitate acceptance, manage the patient's anxieties and fears, and motivate the patient to long-term preventive care.

This chapter will provide the reader with a rationale for the vital importance of the behavioral aspects of treatment planning, a method of acquiring this information from the patient through the dental interview, and a description of how the information collected may be integrated with the other examination data into a treatment plan.

DENTAL INTERVIEW
Purpose and goals

It has been only about 30 years since dentistry recognized the importance of how the patient's medical condition influences dental treatment and the manner in which it is performed. It is now routine for practitioners to take a careful medical history and use this information as an integral part of the treatment plan. Only recently, however, has the profession begun to appreciate that psychologic and sociologic considerations have as great an affect on treatment as medical ones.

Psychosocial considerations relate to a person's expectations, priorities, past experiences, perceived needs, and a variety of socioeconomic factors. As inappropriate as the full-month reconstruction might be for the debilitated geriatric patient, it would be as inconceivable for the patient who places little value on his teeth—who in fact has come to the dental office to have them all extracted and dentures made.

These factors, then, influence the patient's desire for treatment and the value he places on both dental care and his teeth.

The psychosocial information gathered in the dental interview will allow the dentist to reach the following goals:
1. Develop a unique treatment plan for this individual based on psychosocial factors integrated with other examination data
2. Facilitate motivation of the patient toward acceptance of the treatment plan as well as ongoing motivation throughout the care process
3. Appropriately manage the actual delivery of care, especially as it relates to anxiety and pain control.

This information, in order to achieve these goals, must have a factual as well as an attitudinal component. The data collection, to be useful and effective, requires that both components be acquired.

During the process the practitioner also has the opportunity to provide information and to develop rapport with the patient. Although this does not relate primarily to the treatment plan, it has considerable implications for treatment acceptance and the permission to perform that treatment.

The process conveys to the patient (1) that the practitioner is concerned about this patient as a person (the act of sitting down to talk before any treatment is discussed or performed demonstrates this interest); (2) the need to involve the patient in the treatment decision; and (3) that the practitioner is actually interested in the patient's experiences, attitudes, and expectations and will use this information in designing treatment.

The successful interview will obtain valid, reliable, and precise knowledge about the patient and his dental problem and, at the same time, develop a solid interpersonal relationship. The dentist, in this role, can be described as a data gatherer, data processor and analyzer, decision maker, and helper.

The dental interview is conducted as the first contact of the dentist with the new patient and should be the first step in gathering diagnostic data. Unfortunately this sequence is seldom followed. Some dentists routinely have the patient's roentgenograms and study casts taken first before they see the patient. In other offices the interview with the patient takes place after the dentist has examined the patient's mouth. Following are reasons why failure to conduct the interview first will limit the data gathered as well as provide the potential for future patient management problems:
1. Information gathered at the interview session will influence the kind and amount of further data to be collected. For example, it would be valuable to know that a full series of roentgenograms was recently taken and is available before the patient is subjected to additional roentgenograms. Knowledge about particular past dental problems might require special diagnostic procedures, such as occlusal films, temporomandibular joint roentgenograms, or a face-bow mounting of the patient's study casts.
2. Eliciting the patient's anxieties and concerns about the examination and dealing with them beforehand will avoid potentially serious patient management problems. Knowing, for instance, that the patient has a severe gagging problem will allow the dentist to perform helpful procedures beforehand. Concerns expressed about radiation provide an opportunity for the dentist to describe the necessity for the films and the degree of radiation safety that is practiced.

3. It is vital to know the patient's perception of the condition of his own mouth. It is clear that the dentist must present the proposed treatment very differently to the patient who, for example, does not recognize the existence of any periodontal problems as opposed to one who does. The ability to elicit this information will be restricted if the dentist has already examined the patient's oral cavity. In the instance of the practitioner attempting to determine whether the patient recognizes a periodontal problem, the practitioner may find difficulty in getting a response to a question such as "How are your gums?" The patient, knowing that the dentist already has the "correct" answer, will avoid a direct answer or may pose a question such as "How do they look to you?"

Site of the interview

The consideration for the site of the dental interview should include three criteria: first, the location should be a place that will be most conducive to communication; second, it should be a place that makes a statement about a philosophy of the office that relates the treatment of the mouth as part of total health care; and third, it should afford sufficient privacy that patients will have no concern that their conversation will be overheard. It is for these reasons that a consultation room rather than a treatment area should be used for the interview.

In order to facilitate communication, it is important that the environment itself not arouse anxiety. For many patients, concern about treatment can arouse considerable distress. Research has shown that subjects in a dental reception room, awaiting treatment, have difficulty in solving puzzles or even following directions. In addition, they have elevated heart rates, blood pressure, and galvanic skin responses. The anxiety produced by the dental equipment found in the treatment room will clearly impede the flow of information.

The treatment room, in addition, produces patient expectations of dental treatment. Patients seated in a dental chair can reasonably expect care rather than talk. If we would like to encourage active patient involvement, we should provide an environment conducive to generating patient participation.

The consultation room is the place where the physician most often talks to his or her patients. It therefore begins to state nonverbally to the patient the medical rather than the mechanical nature of the treatment. The dentist who wishes to convey to the patient that he or she is, in fact, a physician treating oral disease, healing affected tissues, and preventing the recurrence of the problem, can do this best in the private office consultation room. In order for the dentist to begin reeducating the patient, it requires that he or she be dissociated, when possible, from the dental treatment room, which provides the more mechanical message.

In selecting the interview site, one should also keep in mind the necessity for privacy. The patient will be reticent to discuss matters he would not like overheard and thus may refrain from giving possibly critical information. The patient may conclude that the dentist's lack of concern over his privacy may indicate that personal matters may not be kept confidential.

Furniture arrangements

The arrangement of the furniture within the room and its comfort also provides an opportunity for the dentist to demonstrate his or her willingness to be open. Certain arrangements promote the atmosphere necessary for patients to be able to communicate their feelings. Psychologists have shown increasing interest in the effect of environment upon people's behavior. Research efforts have looked at space and how its use affects the individual. Other work considered seating arrangements that would foster cooperativeness versus competitiveness.

Fig. 7-1 shows three configurations of chairs and desks. Fig. 7-1, A, showing the chairs across from one another with the desk separating them, presents the clearest physical barrier between the two people. The desk location limits the dentist's ability to see and consider the patient's body language and psychologically restricts the free exchange of information. This is the seating arrangement used by people in a competitive situation.

Moving the chair to the side of the desk begins to eliminate the barriers (Fig. 7-1, B). This situation promotes considerably more familiarity, and yet at the same time the corner of the desk maintains a certain distance. This is referred to as the conversing arrangement and can be recognized as the position most often used by junior-level employees in banks and by employment offices.

Fig. 7-1, C, is most ideal for the purpose of the interview. In this situation there is the least amount of physical barrier between dentist and patient. This open environment encourages the patient to express himself both verbally and nonverbally. It permits easy visibility of the patient's body language.

The arrangement of furniture must also be in accordance with the prac-

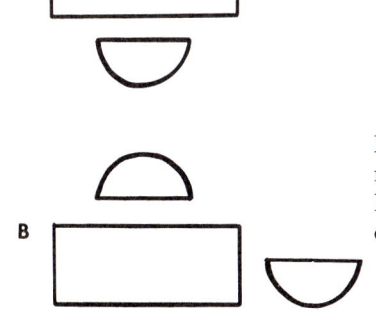

Fig. 7-1. Configurations of chairs and desks. A, Arrangement used by people in a competitive situation. B, Conversing arrangement. C, Ideal arrangement for dental interview.

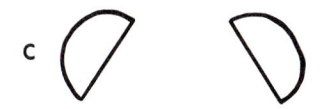

136   Modifying factors in treatment planning

titioner's and patient's personal space. This space describes an invisible envelope that surrounds each of us. Another person entering this space causes a sense of discomfort, anxiety, and need to reestablish the distance. The preferred size of the envelope varies with the situation, the person who enters the space, and the cultural background of the individual. During the interview, especially when utilizing the chair arrangement in Fig. 7-1, *C*, it is important for the dentist to be aware of the danger of encroaching on the patient's personal space. The patient's movement to increase the distance will be obvious if the dentist is sitting too close.

Interview process

The interview process is important, for the greater the skill of the interviewer, the more complete and reliable will be the information upon which he or she bases the diagnosis and treatment plan. This goes beyond the simple acquisition of a factual history. It involves developing an understanding of patients as people—their anxieties, fears, and motivations. In addition, their social history, especially as it relates to their view of the dentist and dental care, is critical to the development of an appropriate treatment plan.

Techniques have been developed by psychologists and others to facilitate communications between the dentist and the patient. All of these techniques tell a patient that the practitioner is

1. Interested in what he has to say
2. Concerned about misunderstanding his meaning
3. Receptive to his expressing himself fully

Setting the stage

Part of establishing the patient's receptiveness to the interview is the manner in which it is begun. The dental interview must get off to a good start. The way in which the interview is presented to the patient will set the tone and improve the effectiveness and efficiency of this initial interaction. It is critical, at the outset, that the patient understands why he is there. The introductory statement is made after the patient is seated in the consultation room. An example of such a statement would be, "Good morning, Miss Jones. Before we examine your mouth, I would like to spend a few minutes with you so that I can learn a little bit more about you." This avoids situations where the patient, who has never been interviewed before and is being exposed to a very different dental care environment, begins saying to herself, "There must be something terribly wrong. Why am I sitting in here?"

Verbal communication

Once the patient understands the reason for the interview, there are a variety of techniques that will help to facilitate the communication between the practitioner and the patient. As was mentioned before, it is important to establish a climate where the patient can express himself fully. Clearly the manner in which questions are phrased on a medical history checklist would be least appropriate. Medical history questionnaires typically ask questions that are answered with a simple "yes" or "no" or with a short statement of fact. These are called closed-ended questions.

Open-ended questions

Open-ended questions ask for information in general terms and cannot be answered with a single word or a simple statement of fact. Questions of this type will tend to generate a greater amount of information and will also provide the practitioner with the patient's feelings or attitudes.

An example of a closed question, one that provides very limited information, would be "Are your teeth sensitive to cold?" If the answer is "yes," then it tells us that the patient has teeth that are sensitive to cold and nothing more. It would now require an additional series of questions in order to determine the parameters of their cold sensitivity as well as to determine whether they are sensitive to hot, pressure, sweets, and so on. Contrast the question "Are your teeth sensitive to cold?" with an open-ended question that, by being of wider scope, generates information more efficiently and thoroughly. A question like "Tell me what makes your teeth hurt" or "Would you describe your teeth sensitivity?" will provide the practitioner much of the necessary information with fewer questions. It will also provide some expression from the patient as to the degree and duration of the pain. Closed-ended questions will be used, but only where there are details that have not been made clear or have been left out.

Silence

Often the patient is prevented from providing complete answers because the practitioner has filled the momentary pause with another question, thus preventing the patient from completing his last thought. In other cases, patients unused to having practitioners who are interested in what they have to say will, initially, often be reluctant to give more than cursory answers. Patients wonder, "Does the doctor really want to hear what I have to say?" or "I wonder if it's really *that* important to the doctor?"

The dentist, by not speaking, provides the patient not only with room to speak, but also with the clear message that he or she would like to hear what the patient has to say. This nonverbal message, silence, is enhanced when the dentist uses other signals such as nodding, leaning forward, and expressions such as "uh-huh" or "go on." All these encourage the patient to continue to elaborate and to explain himself more fully.

Feedback

Feedback is a question or statement that summarizes the practitioner's understanding of what the patient is saying. Essentially it restates in the practitioner's own words what the patient has been conveying to the dentist. It essentially asks the question "Is this what you mean?"

A patient presents a series of problems that he has had with a past dentist. The impression from this listing of problems is the patient's dissatisfaction with the previous dentist. The practitioner asks, "You sound as if you are unhappy with your previous dentist." The patient then has an opportunity to either concur with what the practitioner has just said or possibly say, "Oh, no. I thought he was an excellent dentist. I don't think the problems could have been helped."

The use of feedback ensures that the dentist does, in fact, understand the patient's statement. It also provides an opportunity for the patient to clarify by restating his answer or to agree with the dentist's impression.

The practitioner can use feedback to express how he or she is affected by the patient's statements. An example might be for the dentist to say, in response to a patient's expression of interest in regular checkups and a preventive program, "I'm pleased that you feel so strongly about saving your teeth."

SUPPORT

Expressions of support are responses that show interest, concern, or understanding to patients. This should be typical of all responses, and when nonjudgmental in nature, such expressions produce a climate in which the patient comfortably expresses his feelings. If this is to be achieved, the dentist must withhold responses that reflect his or her own values. If perceived by the patient as an expression of disapproval, it may generate a reluctance to give further information. A patient describes the long period of time that he has been away from dental care. The dentist responds by saying, "I don't think that was too good." The patient may now feel that the dentist would not be understanding of the possible fear, anxiety, or economic problem that has prevented him from seeking care and will be less willing to reveal these reasons.

An important by-product of this nonjudgmental climate is that the patient has an opportunity to reexamine some of his own thoughts about dentistry. The statement that "I don't like my teeth" or "I don't know why I bother to spend any money to try to save them" is the first step by which he can begin to examine those factors that have led to his making that decision and its possible consequences.

The dentist can assist this process by not responding "You shouldn't feel that way." Instead a statement such as "Tell me why you feel that way" sets up an exchange where the patient can reexamine the basis for his attitudes and whether different outcomes under different circumstances are possible.

REFLECTION

Reflection is another method by which the patient is essentially told to continue and elaborate on his previous statement. This is a response that repeats, mirrors, or echoes a portion of what the patient has just said. The patient says, "My last dentist told me that I didn't have to replace the missing tooth." Your reflective statement, which asks for more details, might be "She told you that you didn't need a replacement?" The patient now has been given encouragement to explain this particular incident more fully.

CONFRONTATION

A confrontation response points out, in a nonjudgmental way, an inconsistency in what the patient has been telling the dentist. For example, the patient says that he is concerned about keeping his teeth and yet has not been to the dentist in 6 years. In the confrontation of the patient the dentist may say, "It seems inconsistent that you are concerned about keeping your teeth and yet have not been to the dentist for such a long period of time." This statement assists the patient in clarifying his own feelings about dentistry, for it provides an opportunity to talk about other factors that might have prevented him from seeking dental care. Another form of confrontation is an inconsistency with the current situation. Statements like "You seem angry" or "You seem upset" allow the patient to more accurately get in touch with his feelings. It also gives the practitioner an opportunity to check out his or her own perceptions of what the patient is feeling about a particular event.

Nonverbal communication

Up to this point we have examined ways to receive information from a patient through spoken communication. However, it is important to realize that nonverbal messages that accompany any spoken statement are critical to its meaning. They can also make a statement on their own. One must also bear in mind that in the communication process the practitioner will also be giving information nonverbally to the patient, which will affect to a large extent the quality and quantity of information given by the patient. It is therefore important that practitioners carefully monitor their own nonverbal messages.

Attending to the nonverbal behavior of the patient is important for a number of reasons. It provides an additional source of information that can enhance, clarify, or possibly contradict the patient's spoken statement. The nonverbal message provides an instantaneous response to something just said. The attentive interviewer will note the patient expressing emotions such as interest or hostility before and even without anything being said.

Confronting the patient with what appears to be the interviewer's interpretation of some attitude expressed nonverbally provides an opportunity for patients to clarify their own feelings as well as affirm or correct the practitioner's interpretation. In a case where the patient is describing his past treatment, the practioner notices from body posture, tone, and facial expression a sense of hostility. By saying to the patient "You seem angry when you talk about this" the dentist gives the patient a way of reflecting on his own attitude and possibly reexamining his feelings. It will also, if correct, provide an opening for the patient to more fully describe his feelings.

Many times the inconsistencies are between statements the patient is making and his nonverbal messages. An example would be the patient who describes a situation that appears to have been a considerable problem but whose facial expressions and body attitude do not reflect this. There will be other situations in which a patient describes with great emotion what might appear to be some minor incident. It is at this point that the practitioner can again make note of the inconsistency by saying, "Although you seem to have had a very frightening experience with dentistry, you don't seem very upset" or "That particular incident seems to have upset you greatly."

Attention to nonverbal communication can
1. Improve the accuracy of the message
2. Provide information
3. Provide opportunities for clarification of feelings
4. Build stronger practitioner-patient relationships

Receiving nonverbal communication requires "listening" with the eyes as well as the ears. One should note the following aspects of the patient's behavior:
1. Posture
2. Facial expression

140   *Modifying factors in treatment planning*

3. Position and activity of the hands
4. Position and activity of feet and legs

The combination of the above means of communicating nonverbally will provide information regarding both the patient's involvement in the interview situation and the patient's emotional state. Concerning the patient's interest in the interview, is she sitting forward in her seat or withdrawing? Is she maintaining eye contact or staring off into some corner of the room? Are her hands and feet relatively quiet? Or is she drumming her fingers or tapping her feet? Concerning emotional state, patients can and will express the whole gamut of emotions without words. Affectual states can be classified as anger, sadness, anxiety, and disgust; these are the unpleasant states. Happiness, joy, and excitement are the pleasurable ones. The recognition of the patient's behavior that accompanies these emotions does not require unusual practitioner skills. The practitioner must first be attentive to the messages being sent. With some practice, using his or her imagination, he or she can visualize the facial expression of the person who is anxious and distinguish it from the facial expression of one who is sad. One can readily imagine the angry person's clenched fist and the person who "turns away in disgust."

As important as watching, observing, and noticing the patient's attitudinal state is the need for the practitioner to check out with the patient the accuracy of his or her observations. The practitioner's feedback will be valuable even when he or she has not correctly interpreted the patient's emotions. First, the patient will be given an opportunity to translate his affectual state, which will allow a more valid interpretation of his communication. It also communicates to the patient the practitioner's interest in fully understanding his meaning because of its importance to being able to better design and implement treatment.

DEVELOPING THE TREATMENT PLAN
General areas

This discussion will deal with the specific information that should be collected during the interview and how this data needs to be integrated with the results of the other examination procedures in developing a treatment plan. The interview information will also assist the dentist in motivating the patient toward more complete care and establishing a methodology for the control of pain and anxiety.

The data, both factual and attitudinal, can be broken down into the following six general areas:

1. Patient expectations
2. Past experiences
3. Perceptions of current oral condition
4. Attitudes
5. Economics
6. Family history

The practitioner can be assured of acquiring all the necessary information by using an item checklist. The following example is one that is used at the School of Dental Medicine at the State University of New York at Stony Brook. This list can provide a beginning for a personalized one the reader can develop based on his or her own needs:

1. Reason for visit
   a. Problems
   b. Expectations
2. Why did you come to the dental school for treatment?
3. Past dental history, including attitudes
   a. Last visit
   b. Frequency of visits
   c. Change of dentist (why?)
4. Social and family history
5. Economics
6. Family history of tooth loss, including attitudes toward
   a. Dentures
   b. Missing teeth
   c. Replacements
7. Feelings about mouth
8. Mouth odor
9. Feelings about current dental cosmetics
10. Health attitudes
    a. Perception of personal state of health
    b. Health care in general
11. Attitudes toward preventive dentistry, including current usage
12. Lifestyle

The interviewer should use the checklist as a reminder of data required but not as a list of questions one would find on a yes/no medical history. Questions should be designed to provide the patient with opportunities to freely express her feelings and attitudes. Because of this the interview does not follow a specific format. The questions asked are based upon the answers the patient gives. Transition from one area to another should be based upon the patient's responses. One would want to avoid as much as possible the sense of routinely proceeding through a standard set of questions.

The patient's answers to any of the checklist items can provide data in one or more areas. The interviewer must remain aware of how this information will be used so that he or she can determine how the interview can best be directed. The interview data gathered from the patient will contain two components—one factual, the other attitudinal. It is important to know, on a factual level, that a patient has had a tooth removed, when it occurred, and whether there were complications with the procedure. Equally important is how the patient feels about the missing tooth or how those complications affected this person as far as his attitudes toward this type of care.

PATIENT EXPECTATIONS

The first of the areas on the checklist relates to patient expectations. It is critical that we understand the following in the development of any treatment plan:

1. What problem or reason prompted the patient to seek treatment?
2. What does the patient expect from you as a dentist in terms of the types of care and the manner in which the care would be delivered?
3. What expectations does the patient have as to what dentistry is able to do for him on a long-term basis?

The first question that should be asked in the area of expectations after introducing the patient to the dental interview is "Why are you here?" or "What brought you in?" This question provides a wealth of information. It will immediately identify those problem areas the patient considers important. In addition it supplies the reasons for the visit and thereby some initial idea as to the patient's expectations from the care process. Patients may come to a dental office and respond to this question with, "I haven't been to the dentist for 6 months, have just moved to the area, and would like a checkup." This expression of expectations for treatment is very different from the patient who says, "All I would like is to have this tooth filled."

It is important that the patient's reasons for seeking treatment be written down in his own words.

The problem as stated by the patient, no matter how insignificant it appears in the dentist's estimation of the total dental needs, must be used as the initial problem discussed with the patient.

An example of the need to address the patient's presenting problem is Mrs. M., who came in for treatment because of a "rough spot on the upper left." After a complete examination with full-mouth roentgenograms, considerable decay was found under many of the restorations. The decay was so advanced that some of the involved teeth required root canal treatment. An incipient periodontal problem was also discovered. The rough filling as judged by the dentist was insignificant in comparison to this patient's other needs. After the dentist gave Mrs. M. a detailed description of the required treatment for the restorative, endodontic, and periodontal problems, Mrs. M. asked, "Well, what about that rough area that brought me in?" This is an example of a dentist whose priorities established a treatment plan without the recognition of the patient's expectations and values.

A more appropriate beginning for this presentation to Mrs. M. would have been, "I recognize the rough area that you have in the upper left, and the first thing that we will do when we begin your treatment will be to attend to that. There are, however, some other serious problems that I feel we ought to discuss."

Another question that relates to the patient's expectations is one that asks, "Why did you come to see *me?*" The answer to this question provides important information related not only to the patient's expectations from you as a dentist, but also as some indication of the quality of the referral. Motivating the patient who says "I was looking up a dentist in the phone book and your name starts with 'A'" will be very different from motivating the patient who states that "Mrs. Smith came to you for some extensive dentistry and I feel that I need the same kind of work; she recommended you very highly."

How the next question is built upon the patient's previous comments to provide the flow in the interview could be shown using the above example of the patient referred by Mrs. Smith. The question, "You feel you need the same kind of dentistry that Mrs. Smith had done?" provides a line of questioning that will give a better understanding of this patient's view of her current condition as well as her expectations for treatment.

There is a third area of expectations, and this relates to dentistry in general. These expectations relate to the patient's view of the longevity of his teeth, the ability of dentistry to control disease and maintain aesthetics and function, and the outcomes he can expect from dental science.

The patient's expectations for the type of treatment and the manner in which it will be delivered may be realistic. It is possible, however, that his expectations are unrealistic. The patient may expect dentistry to do the impossible, such as saving teeth with severe periodontal disease or placing fixed bridges in a mouth with extensive tooth loss. On the other hand, patient expectations of treatment may be more pessimistic than necessary. One might hear for example, "Fixing my teeth probably won't help—I'll lose them anyway," when the patient can expect considerable longevity from his teeth. In both cases patients will need to be educated so that their expectations from treatment are reasonable and attainable under the constraints of their oral condition.

PAST EXPERIENCES

The next area relates to the patient's past experiences. This category includes specific experiences related to the dental care he has received and his feelings about such experiences.

Information relating to the patient's past experiences falls into the following categories:

1. Experience with dentists
2. Experience with dentistry
   a. Crown and bridge, endodontics, oral surgery, orthodontics, prosthetics, prevention
   b. Tooth loss
   c. Anxiety and pain control

As with each of the checklist items, patient responses will often provide information and understanding of other items at the same time. While questioning the patient regarding his past dental experience, the interviewer should be aware of the additional data generated regarding the patient's expectations from dentists and dentistry, his perception of his current oral condition, attitudes toward the importance of various aspects of dental care, his economic situation, and his family dental history.

A way to begin exploring the area of the patient's past experience is to ask, "Tell me about your past experiences with dentistry." As was mentioned in the previous discussion regarding the interview process, this would be the time to employ "silence" to allow the patient to provide, in sufficient depth, those personally significant aspects of his past experience.

The interview is then directed toward specific areas that the patient might not have covered. One of these areas is the date of his last dental visit and what was done at that time. If the interval was longer than the usual recall period, the interviewer should try to determine the reason.

Did the patient change dentists often? What are the reasons for the changes? Information about how the patient feels about his previous dentist(s) is also an important consideration. Was this dentist someone he felt extremely confident in, a friend of the family, someone that he loves dearly, or, on the other hand, was it someone with whom he had problems? This information will be vital when the patient interview data is reviewed and the need for future treatment is planned and presented.

It is important to know prior to the time the patient is examined whether he has had any care in one or more of the dental specialty areas. Equally important is whether the treatment was rendered by a generalist or specialist. As with the other items, the patient's experience has a factual component that describes what was done and when and an attitudinal component that contains the patient's feeling about the treatment and the quality of the result.

Examples of questions one might ask to stimulate the attitudinal responses would be "What was it like?" or "How did you feel it worked out?"

This knowledge of the patient's experience and attitudes toward care in the specialty areas will be of great assistance if in the examination process it is determined that he will need treatment of this type. In cases where the patient has had a positive experience in his contacts with dental specialists, there would be little problem should there be a reason for additional care. If, on the other hand, the patient has negative feelings about some types of care, the value of knowing this beforehand is clear. The treatment plan proposed will need to allow for treatment alternatives with the benefits and costs of each. The dentist must also discuss with the patient whether his experience in that single case can be generalized to all other situations.

An example of how the patient's past experience in a specialty area will affect the manner in which recommendations are made would be in the case of a tooth that requires endodontic treatment. It will be dramatically different for the patient who says "I feel lucky to have had the root canal treatment so that I didn't have to lose my tooth" as opposed to the patient who says "Root canal treatment was the most painful thing that has ever happened to me. I would rather have the tooth extracted than to go through that again!"

Other areas of dentistry not usually considered as requiring a specialist, and for which there is a need to explore the patient's past experience, would be prosthetics, crown and bridge, operative dentistry, and prevention. Again the interviewer should be aware of the two components that are required from the patient's answer: the factual component will describe what was done and when; the attitudinal component will describe what the experience was like and the patient's perception of the result.

It is important to review whether the patient has lost any teeth. Since the interview is being conducted prior to the examination of the patient's mouth, this question would not be inappropriate. Certainly the dentist can easily determine the absence of teeth by examining the patient. What is not known is whether the patient is aware of the loss. In the case where the patient does not know or says she does not have any missing teeth when in fact she does, there is increased difficulty in convincing her of the necessity for replacement.

If the patient recognizes that she does have missing teeth, two kinds of further information are required. How does she feel about the missing tooth (teeth)? This will give the practitioner information regarding the patient's desire to have it replaced. A patient may say "It's in the back and nobody can see it and, besides, I can eat everything," or else may be very concerned and specifically request a replacement.

The second area that requires exploration is whether there has been any suggestion for replacement by previous dentists. Patients will reply in various ways, each requiring a different approach and having an effect on the resulting treatment plan. For example, a patient may say that "the dentist suggested a removable bridge, but I can't stand anything that goes in and out of my mouth." It is clear that the decision as to the type of replacement the dentist will suggest may be altered by this response; that is, the dentist may plan for a fixed bridge if at all possible.

Parenthetically, one can easily recognize the importance of knowing if some appliance was made for this patient and currently is not being used. Ignorant of this fact, the dentist may suggest the need for a partial denture, only to be informed that the patient already has one and cannot wear it. This will cause not only embarrassment but loss of credibility as well. Furthermore, it creates a situation where the dentist must first begin to ask questions regarding the reasons for not wearing it after the treatment plan has been finalized.

Questions regarding whether the patient has considered tooth replacement might give some clues to the patient's economic problems either past or current. Patients may talk about their "not being able to afford it" as well as whether their financial picture (sometimes with the assistance of dental insurance) has changed, making complete dentistry currently possible.

One important part of any treatment plan deals with a preventive program. The patient's past experience in this regard will assist not only in developing the treatment plan but also in recognizing the need for motivation and education.

As an example, the frequency of past recall visits will provide the dentist with some indication of the patient's commitment or lack of commitment. What is the patient doing now as far as oral hygiene and was he ever taught? If, for example, the patient has been notably unsuccessful at using dental floss, even with careful instruction, it would clearly be a mistake to attempt to use flossing as the major element of his home care preventive program.

An area to be explored in some depth in the patient's past experience is that of anxiety and pain. The question "What was it like having your dentistry done?" or "How did (do) you feel about going to the dentist?" is a way of getting at this information without prejudging the quality of the patient's experience. By this neutral phrasing the patient is free to honestly describe his previous exposure to dental care. The interviewer's interest is related to experiences that were fearful or anxiety provoking. Was there anything that caused the patient any pain, such as an extraction or root canal? Is the patient afraid of the injection or the noise of the drill? This information will be extremely valuable in planning the case presentation and subsequent treatment.

In this same vein, the interviewer should elicit information regarding the manner in which previous dentists have controlled pain for the patient. The range of answers is so far-reaching that there is almost no way to either categorize or predict them. Patients will describe their fear of the injection as the "worst thing about going to the dentist" and will state that they would prefer to have their dentistry done "without anything rather than have the needle." Other patients who have experienced the pain of dental treatment without a local anesthetic now welcome the injection as a means to painless dentistry.

People will present a similar range of responses to pain control adjuncts such as nitrous oxide, intravenous sedation, and premedication. It is important to know what the patient has had and how he felt about it. To attempt to give a patient one of these analgesics without knowing that he has previously experienced an adverse frightening reaction with it will doom its introduction to failure. It is also useful when designing a pain management strategy for this patient to uncover any preconceived notions he might have about some of the methods that might be used. Patients, because of incomplete or inadequate information, might mistakenly feel that some method may be dangerous, will not work, or that they would not like it. Having this data prior to treatment planning will be invaluable in designing the presentation and managing the patient.

This information will also determine, to some degree, the sequence of treatment. For the patient who is particularly anxious about dental treatment, it would clearly facilitate her future care if treatment began with a simple procedure. In this instance the dentist could demonstrate a painless injection and gentle technique. To begin the treatment of an anxious patient with a lengthy, demanding, and extensive procedure may reinforce the patient's conviction that her anxieties are warranted.

PERCEPTIONS REGARDING ORAL CONDITION

It is important that the practitioner establish a fairly good understanding of what the patient perceives is the condition of his own mouth. The exploration falls generally into four categories:
1. Condition of hard tissue
2. Condition of soft tissue
3. Aesthetic appearance
4. Mouth odor

This discussion on patient perceptions of his oral condition will build on the material already presented on patient expectations and past history. It would not be unusual for the patient to present a clear picture of his view of the relative health and disease status for each of the items without the need for direct questioning.

This data, how the patient perceives the health of his mouth, has implications for motivation and treatment planning. Clearly the need to motivate a patient to accept treatment for a condition he already recognizes as a problem is minimal. Conversely, it does identify those problem areas revealed in the subsequent examination of which the patient is unaware.

Condition of hard tissue. The patient's perceptions of the condition of the hard tissue, including missing teeth, will be revealed with questions like "How do you feel about the condition of your teeth?" It should be determined to what the patient attributes its cause. Does the patient feel his teeth are particularly susceptible to decay? Or does he attribute the breakdown of his teeth to the dentistry he has received? Is he happy with the restorative dentistry he has received? Or are there individual crowns or bridges he feels need to be redone?

Condition of soft tissue. Patient perceptions regarding the health of the soft tissue have even greater importance. The adult patient becomes more susceptible to periodontal disease with increasing age. This is combined with the nature of the disease process, which will allow fairly extensive progression of the destructive process before the patient realizes he has a problem. It is also possible that the patient may have received only the most cursory care for this problem.

The question "Tell me about the condition of your gums" followed, if necessary, by "How about bleeding?" should generate the degree to which the patient perceives the existence of a problem. This data will be correlated, of course, by the oral examination and study of the patient's roentgenograms. As with all the patient's perceptions of his oral health status, the failure to recognize the existence of a problem requires the dentist to take special pains to educate the patient.

Aesthetic appearance. An important factor regarding the proposed treatment that must be explored during the interview process is how the patient views his dental aesthetics and with what degree of concern. This situation is highly individualized, and it would not be unusual for a person to wish to correct even minor irregularities. The opposite case is also found in which even large defects or discolorations are not even noticed by the patient, and where there is no desire to have it modified. A question such as "How do you feel about how your mouth looks?" will provide an opportunity for the patient to describe his own sense of his oral aesthetic appearance.

There is a danger in prejudging aesthetics for another person. A patient, Mrs. Z., was an attractive woman in her mid-thirties who was interviewed at the dental school in Stony Brook. She was outgoing and smiling, so there was no difficulty in noticing the left central with root canal treatment and considerable darkening. The student mentioned its condition to the patient and told her that it could be easily fixed. The patient angrily replied that she did not mind it the way it was and had no intention of changing it. There have been other cases where a patient, who has what appears to the dentist to be perfect aesthetics, complains about not liking how his teeth look.

The resulting treatment plan should reflect both the patient's and dentist's estimation of the need for treatment. It is therefore appropriate for there to be discussion of a treatment plan in which both the dentist's recognition of the potential problems for particular treatment and the patient's desire for modification of his current aesthetic appearance can be met.

Mouth odor. A frequently unexplored area related to the patient's perceptions of his oral health relates to mouth odor. It is a condition that the patient will rarely bring up of his own accord and is often an area that the dentist, in his or her misplaced concern not to embarrass the patient, will not question. In over 100 interviews conducted at the dental school at Stony Brook where a question in this area was included as part of a total dental interview, there were only a few cases where patients were reticent to answer. In the majority of the cases, patients welcomed the opportunity to talk about what they perceived as a problem. The question "Is mouth odor a problem?" asked in the interview before the examination does not imply the interviewer has noticed anything. If the patient notes that a problem exists, the practitioner can then determine whether an oral condition is contributing to the odor. In addition, it will provide for the patient who recognizes a problem with his breath a powerful motivating tool as well as an indication for treatment.

PATIENT ATTITUDES

At this point in the interview the patient's attitude as actually expressed should be fairly clear. It is possible that a more definitive expression of his attitude toward a particular aspect of dental care might be necessary as related to the following items:
1. Tooth loss—dentures
2. Replacements
3. Prevention—oral hygiene
4. Aesthetics or function
5. Dentists and dentistry

The patient's attitudes toward the above areas are important first in terms of gauging the priority that will be placed upon various aspects of dental care. They will be useful for motivating this individual as well as in designing the treatment plan.

The patient's attitudes toward the potential loss of teeth or replacement of missing ones must be accounted for when developing the treatment plan. Although it is difficult to establish the priority the patient places on dentistry, one can assume that, for most people, seeking dental care implies some level of concern regarding preserving their teeth. The reasons are varied but essential in explaining the need for particular dental treatment. Patients are interested in saving their teeth for a wide range of reasons: aesthetics, function, comfort, or the psychologic implications of tooth loss. The interview should provide some feeling for the factors that are most important for an individual. Motivation of this patient regarding dental care is facilitated by demonstrating how treatment can help this person retain or maintain his dental goals.

In the area of replacements, the patient's attitudes or feelings about certain kinds of replacements will be a factor in considering alternative treatment plans. For example, patient concerns about gagging and having something on their palate might be the basis for the dentist to consider a fixed prosthesis as an alternative.

Another aspect of this same issue of the patient's desire to preserve his own teeth is his attitude toward prevention. The question asked might be "How do you presently take care of your teeth?" This will give you some idea of his current oral hygiene activity. Closed-ended questions can then supplement this question to find out if he brushes and flosses and how often. It is also useful to find out if he has ever been taught this method by his previous dentist. This will indicate if there are procedures he has abandoned or techniques he is currently using that were taught in a previous dental office.

There are two areas that already have been discussed but bear repeating. The first area is the patient's attitude toward dentists and dentistry. Some patients view the dentist as a professional who performs valuable services and who is qualified and honest. On the other hand, there are patients who view dentists and dental care with suspicion. A patient might feel, for one reason or another, that he has been mistreated by the dentist or has had treatment performed that was not necessary or of poor quality. In addition, dental experiences of friends and relatives, when related to the patient, also might lead to a situation in which the data being provided by the new practitioner is treated with a high degree of skepticism. The patient becomes convinced that the dentist is determined to perform unnecessary procedures of low quality for high fees. This attitude will be evident by the answers the patient has given regarding his past dental experience and his expectations for care.

When faced with low credibility on the part of the patient, it becomes important for the practitioner to modify, if possible, the treatment plan sequence in the design stage. Although it is important to describe to the patient the entire treatment process, an initial strategy might be for the practiioner to begin with some simple part of the treatment and, once that is completed, proceed with the other more involved parts. This initial treatment of the patient provides an opportunity to improve the patient's confidence in that dentist's ability and recommendations.

ECONOMICS

Two factors, when combined, will determine the willingness of patients to embark upon complete care as defined by the dentist. The first, described before, is the patient's attitude toward preserving his teeth and the methods and system in which dental care is to be delivered. The other factor is the patient's ability and willingness to make the necessary financial investment. It is useful for the dentist to have some advance information regarding the patient's financial ability so as to be able to offer patients installment payment arrangements or alternative treatment plans.

FAMILY DENTAL HISTORY

An additional means of understanding the patient's attitudes toward dental care is through the description of the family experience with dentistry. It should be noted that the patient's feelings need to be ascertained concerning the data collected regarding the patient, siblings, spouse, and children. The patient who states that both his parents have dentures needs to be asked, "How do you feel about that?" Patients have answered, "It was the happiest day in my mother's life. She had suffered so much with her teeth and now she can finally chew" and "The day my father stopped smiling was when he got his dentures." These answers provide another piece of data regarding the individual for whom the dentist will be providing care.

The family dental history is also important for its implications for modification of treatment. The practitioner who is or expects to be treating the whole family will find that the extent of treatment for one member will have impact on the others. Factors such as the time and expense involved, the family configuration, whether the patient lives alone, and constraints on the family economic situation will affect treatment decisions. In addition, it is important to know if there is a family member to care for the patient after an extensive dental procedure.

SUMMARY

The treatment plan for the individual patient as defined here has multiple components including specific intraoral procedures and an educational preventive plan. In addition, the treatment plan should include the manner in which the treatment will be provided, dealing with problems of anxiety and pain control and sequencing of treatment. The information generated from the dental interview will be used in all aspects of this treatment plan. The process of formulating this plan then must take into account the information from the dental interview. The patient's expectations, past experiences, attitudes, economic situation, and family dental history will all play roles in the way the patient makes his treatment decisions. The practitioner using this information can assist the patient in making decisions that are compatible with his dental goals.

BIBLIOGRAPHY

Bernstein, L., and Dana, R. H.: Interviewing and the health professions, New York, 1970, Appleton-Century-Crofts.

Enelow, A. J., and Swisher, S. N.: Interviewing and patient care, New York, 1972, Oxford University Press.

Froelich, R. E., and Bishop, F. M.: Medical interviewing: a programmed manual, St. Louis, 1969, The C. V. Mosby Co.

Froelich, R. E., and Bishop, F. M.: Clinical interviewing skills: a programmed manual for data gathering, evaluation, and patient management, ed. 3, St. Louis, 1977, The C. V. Mosby Co.

Froelich, R. E., Bishop, F. M., and Dworkin, S. F.: Communication in the dental office: a programmed manual for the dental professional, St. Louis, 1976, The C. V. Mosby Co.

Hall, E. T.: The silent language, Garden City, N. Y., 1973, Anchor Press.

Jackson, E.: Establishing rapport. I. Verbal interaction, J. Oral Med. **30:**105, 1975.

Jackson, E.: Managing dental fears: a tentative code of practice, J. Oral Med. **29:**96, 1974.

Jackson, E., and Mealiea, W. L.: Stress management and personal satisfaction in dental practice, Dent. Clin. North Am. **21:**559, 1977.

Kross, L. A.: Body language, Dent. Econ., July 1977, p. 62.

Robinson, H. B.: Listening to your patients: therapy for them—and you, Dent. Surv., Oct. 1977, p. 8.

8

Preventive and prognostic considerations

Milton Arnold

Prevention is one of the major aspects to consider in tailoring a treatment plan to the needs of the individual patient. Although preventive aspects are multiple and varied, they may be categorized into two major groups: (1) those that serve as a prognostic index guiding the dentist in the choice of treatment and (2) specific aspects of prevention woven throughout the treatment plan.

GUIDANCE AND PROGNOSTIC INDEX

Preventive and prognostic considerations are frequently utilized by dental clinicians but often in a subconscious manner. Unfortunately these concepts are seldom formally discussed or written about, possibly because they seem so simple and so obvious. However, these very helpful and practical guides need to be set forth in as clear a manner as possible. The considerations in this group are subdivided into two categories: (1) current preventive measures evident at the initial visit and (2) evaluation of home care improvement.

Current preventive measures evident at initial visit

The level of the current status of preventive measures practiced by the patient are readily evident after the history and clinical examination have been completed. On one end of the spectrum is the patient with the clean mouth, current low caries activity, and healthy periodontium. Let us say that the patient is now drinking fluoridated water, has practiced excellent home care for some years, and is restricting sucrose consumption. Barring the existence of other contraindicating factors such as certain systemic diseases, financial hardships, or untoward oral conditions, the treatment plan should be designed with the thought in mind that the work done will be successfully maintained for *many* years to come. Thus the excellent prognostic index for this patient would favor cast restorations, possibly extensive reconstruction, and perhaps adult orthodontics if the oral conditions suggest the need.

152 Modifying factors in treatment planning

The patient presenting with poor oral hygiene, broken-down teeth, moderate to advanced periodontitis, and high sucrose intake occupies the other end of the spectrum. To immediately decide on a final treatment plan for this individual, which consists of complex periodontal, restorative, reconstructive, and perhaps orthodontic work, is absolute folly. The current prognostic index is much too poor indeed!

Evaluation of home care improvement

If the patient and the dentist desire to conserve the teeth in the case just discussed, then it becomes necessary to determine first whether such a plan is feasible. If the patient demonstrates that he can institute and continue a satisfactory home care program, then an extensive plan to conserve the teeth may be workable. If he is unable to institute and continue such a program, then such a plan is not suitable. Thus the first step is to test the patient on this very point.

The patient should be carefully instructed in the importance as well as all the details of a successful home care program: flossing, brushing, other cleaning aids, disclosing agents, and reduction of sucrose consumption. The patient's efforts are monitored frequently, and necessary points are reinforced. At the end of the 6 month test period his efforts should be finally evaluated. If he has shown that he has continued to maintain a successful home care program, the prognostic index has vastly improved, and a treatment plan containing complex extensive measures may be designed and the work commenced. On the other hand, if he fails this test, the prognostic index remains poor, and extensive and expensive dental procedures are not warranted.

It is also during this observation period that an effort is made to arrest the major destructive processes in a rapid but conservative way to prevent further pathologic changes (see Chapter 10). Accordingly, minimal procedures such as scaling and moderate curettage, in addition to the home care instruction, as well as quadrant excavations of deep carious lesions, especially of potentially critical abutment teeth, should be done. Provisional dressings should be selected that will minimize possible discomfort and be durable enough to last for the required time interval. It may also be desirable to replace missing teeth with transitional appliances for aesthetic as well as functional reasons.

SPECIFIC ASPECTS OF PREVENTION WOVEN THROUGHOUT THE TREATMENT PLAN

In planning treatment, the incorporation of preventive features in order to maximize the prognosis represents the practice of dentistry at its best. In this aspect, prevention can be thought of as taking place on three levels:
1. Primary prevention: steps taken to ensure that disease does not occur.
2. Secondary prevention: detection of incipient disease and halting its progression by simple repair or remedial measures.
3. Tertiary prevention: treatment of well-established disease in order to minimize or eliminate the gross destructive effects, to restore healthy function, and to resist further attacks by the disease process.[10]

Primary level of prevention

SYSTEMIC DISEASE

While the dentist's main focus is on the prevention of oral diseases, he or she also is concerned with the prevention of systemic diseases. Accordingly, the dentist might rearrange, modify, or even eliminate some aspect of dental treatment to prevent systemic problems.[13,30,33] Conceivably the altered treatment plan will favorably affect the prognosis of the systemic disease.[42]

Engaging the patient's physician as an ally in the preventive aspects is not only wise but necessary. He or she will supply the detailed information that will make the preventive procedures rational and the planning realistic. Furthermore the dentist must be concerned with prophylactically protecting himself or herself, as well as other patients, from the possibility of serious infectious disease such as syphilis and hepatitis B.[40] Medical considerations in treatment planning are discussed in Chapters 5 and 6.

The dentist has the responsibility to acquaint himself or herself with the latest available information on primary preventive procedures. He or she may be called on to advise the community or to personally apply this knowledge during treatment planning sessions in his or her office. These procedures may encompass every phase of dentistry as well as some of medicine, and may start from the time the patient first comes into the office.

DISEASES OF THE ORAL MUCOUS MEMBRANES AND JAWS

Preventive aspects of the practice of dentistry at the primary level would include the prevention of diseases of the oral mucosa and jaws. For example, patients are advised not to use tobacco and to minimize the consumption of alcohol in order to decrease the risk of developing cancer of the oral cavity or indeed cancer of the other organs. The oral cavity, jaws, and neck should be examined periodically in order to detect oral lesions in their earliest stages so that they may be successfully treated and hence prevented from developing into larger, more destructive, and possibly life-threatening lesions.

Some primary preventive procedures may unwittingly cause harm. This was brought out recently in a letter to the editor of the *Journal of the American Dental Association* criticizing a report of a screening for oral cancer in a community.[18,38] A group of 1769 individuals were examined, and 108 were referred to their dentists for further evaluation. It was pointed out that the likelihood of oral cancer appearing in our population in 1977 is one in 9000. If the group screened was a random sample, the probability is less than one in five that someone who would develop oral cancer was even evaluated at that screening. Nevertheless, 108 were screened positive. Not only do these false-positives cause needless mental anguish, no matter what assurances are pressed on these people, but they also tend to discredit the screening. The writers add, "We know of no proof that there is improved survivorship of subjects with oral cancer detected at a screening over these diagnosed without a screening procedure."

DENTAL CARIES AND PERIODONTAL DISEASE

As the guardian of the structures inside the oral cavity, dentistry has the responsibility of dealing with the two major oral diseases: caries and periodontal disease. Caries has been one of the more prevalent diseases of our civilization for the past 400 to 500 years.[19] It continues to exert a health and economic impact of epidemic proportions.[4] Periodontal disease has also been characterized as a major health problem in the nation and in the world, and is said to be responsible for more loss of teeth than any other single cause.[28]

Interestingly, both diseases have a common pathogenic locus: dental plaque, a sticky, tenacious mat of mixed microorganisms and other ingredients on the tooth. The progression of both diseases depends on other factors besides plaque. It has been said that we know how to prevent caries, at least in theory, and that we have known for a long time that periodontal disease is largely preventable. Both diseases can thus be discussed in light of the first stage of prevention.

It may surprise recent dental graduates and present students to learn that the concept of prevention is not something that came into existence with the incorporation of the American Society of Preventive Dentistry in 1968. Giovanni of Arcoli (1412-1484) in his *Practica*, published in Venice in 1483, presented what has been called a "decalogue of dental hygiene" that presents ten rules for preventing dental problems,[9] some of which include the following:

1. Sweet and viscous food, such as dried figs, preserves made with honey, and so on, must not be eaten.
2. The teeth must be cleaned at once after every meal from the particles of food left in them; and for this purpose must be used thin pieces of wood. . . . Care must be taken not to injure the gums. . . .
3. After this, it is necessary to rinse the mouth. . . .
4. The teeth must be rubbed with suitable dentifrice before going to bed. . . .

It is fair to say that dentists, at least for the past hundred years, have been aware of the harmful potential of sweets and debris to the teeth. While prevention was probably not the organized and formal type of presentation it is today, in most offices it was taught, and information was passed along to the patient.

We will first discuss prevention of both these diseases in light of our present knowledge in terms of the primary level. Since these diseases are responsible for most of our problems, we will attempt to show how they are dealt with in the varying disciplines of dentistry where preventive principles or concepts are incorporated in the treatment planning on the second and third levels of prevention in order to obtain a better prognosis.

It is important to note that while many of the rehabilitative ideas that are practiced and taught are based on solid evidence, there are still many that are the unproved fruits of someone's clinical experiences. Some of these have been passed down through lectures, and others have found their way into books and then recopied and repeated as "gospel." As we discuss treatment planning, we will attempt to pinpoint them. Their validity may have a bearing on prevention and, consequently, prognosis.

Dental caries. Dental caries is an infectious disease characterized by a series of complex chemical reactions that result initially in the destruction of the enamel and ultimately of the entire tooth. This destruction results from acids that are formed by oral bacteria that metabolize fermentable carbohydrate.[19]

Four factors have been listed as being involved in the initiation of dental caries. Each factor is a necessary but insufficient condition to initiate the lesion. As a result, caries has been characterized as being multifactorial. It has led to some interesting observations such as freedom from caries in individuals who do not brush their teeth or in gnotobiotic (germ-free) animals on a highly cariogenic diet. But most important, it has pointed the way for primary preventive procedures.

The susceptible tooth. The first factor, the susceptible tooth, is related mainly to the ability of the enamel to resist dissolution by acids. This is determined to a great extent by the amount of *fluoride* that has been taken up by the hydroxyapatite crystals in the enamel to become hydroxyfluoroapatite. This can take place systemically during the development of the clinical crowns of the teeth from birth until about age 13 when the third-molar crowns are completed. (Evidence that prenatal exposure to fluoride protects deciduous teeth is conflicting.[16,36]) Fluoride ions can also be taken up topically, to a lesser extent, even long after the tooth has erupted. To what extent other factors determine resistance is problematic. Here we might consider genetic and congenital influences on tooth development, where the actual formation, fissure defects, and so on, are the factors. Other regulatory mechanisms, such as antibacterial properties and buffering capacity of the saliva and its quantity, may be hereditary and affect the overall susceptibility, but are not part of tooth structure.

In treatment planning on a community level we can use *communal fluoridation* in primary prevention. The safest, most efficient, and economical means for providing partial protection against dental caries is the ingestion of natural drinking water containing 1 to 2.5 ppm of fluoride from infancy to about age 13. Numerous studies have repeatedly demonstrated that this procedure reduces the prevalence of dental caries about 50% to 60%.[25] If the communal water supply does not provide the optimal level, adding fluoride to bring the level to 1 ppm will provide the benefits, which are mainly systemic, on the preerupted teeth.

The use of *fluoride tablets* is an alternate means of providing systemic fluoride to unerupted teeth when the water supply is lacking fluoride. In these cases the dentist must take into account the age of the patient, the fluorine content of the drinking water, and the ion concentration available from each tablet. Tables are available that take all these factors into account.[37] The major problem here is the failure of even the most conscientious parents to follow through after a while. The amount of caries reduction that can be expected from the daily ingestion of fluoride tablets ranges from 20% to 50%.[16]

Application of fluoride topically is another means of making enamel more resistant to the acids that initiate caries. While neutral sodium fluoride as a 2% solution has been used successfully, better results are obtained with an 8% to 10% stannous fluoride solution. Acidulated phosphate-fluoride (APF) solution or gel, which provides a 1.23% fluoride ion concentration, yields the best results. The benefits from these three methods are 30% to 40% less decay.[16] Prior to topical application, it is recommended that a thorough prophylaxis be given to remove all deposits. Etching with a 0.5% phosphoric acid solution has also been incorporated in some techniques. The APF gel has also been applied inside plastic trays with good effects. A 4-minute treatment semiannually is the optimal way to use this modality. A recent study used APF tablets, having children swallow them after chewing in order to obtain both a preeruptive (systemic) and posteruptive (topical) benefit.[8] The preeruptive benefit was 41.9% to 50% reduction in decay, while the posteruptive benefit was 26% reduction in decay.

It has been suggested that *fluoride dentifrices and rinses*, such as a stannous fluoride or sodium monofluorophosphate dentifrice, be used daily in conjunction with other topical application for an additional benefit (20% to 30%). Daily mouth rinsing with a 0.02% fluoride solution (0.1% of fluoride if used weekly) or supervised brushing with a fluoride prophylactic paste as seldom as one to five times a year will also provide benefits. Reports have ranged from 11% less DMFS to 80% caries reduction.[19,27]

The use of *pit and fissure sealants* is still another means of providing the tooth with resistance to caries on the occlusal surfaces. Various studies have indicated caries reduction from 55% to 99%.[2,14,17] Even when the sealant was not retained there still was an effect. There is some question, however, as to whether covering incipient caries will retard or prevent the progress of decay.

Plaque. The second factor that has been implicated in the initiation of caries is the plaque attached to the tooth. Plaque is essentially a mixed mat of microorganisms and other ingredients. Both the saliva and the gingival fluid supply a mucoid type of protein, called glycoprotein, that forms a tenacious pellicle on the tooth. This pellicle attracts and anchors organisms. As the bacteria grow and divide, they produce an extracellular sticky gel called dextran, which not only reinforces the attachment, but attracts other bacterial forms that then become part of a complex flora-plaque maturation. A milligram net weight of plaque may contain 200 to 500 million microorganisms, while a similar amount of saliva contains less than 1% of this number.[24]

The reason plaque itself is so deleterious is that by clinging to the tooth it is able to maintain the end products of bacterial metabolism in intimate contact with enamel long enough for demineralization to take place. It even does this on smooth surfaces that normally would not be expected to maintain anything in position for any length of time. Another consequence of the stabilization of plaque is that when the aerobic bacteria use up the available oxygen, the anaerobic bacteria can start proliferating because of the lack of oxygen. This condition would not happen if the aerobic microorganisms were shifted around during mastication, so that oxygen would not be depleted in a confined area.[23]

Bacterial activity in plaque. The third factor in the initiation of dental caries is bacterial activity in plaque. After the bacteria have colonized, they act on the available carbohydrate, which is usually sucrose, to form dextrans which are polysaccharides. Dextrans, usually formed by *Streptococcus mutans*, are extremely adhesive. They help gather other microorganisms, which then metabolize the fermentable carbohydrates (mainly sucrose) to form acids, particularly lactic, and to a lesser extent acetic, propionic, pyruvic, and probably fumaric. These acids first dissolve the inorganic component of the enamel. The organic matrix is subsequently destroyed mechanically or enzymatically.[19]

The primary preventive measures for the elimination of plaque and the bacterial activity in plaque are designed to keep the plaque from forming in the first place and, if it does form, to remove it as rapidly as possible. The prime instrument for this task is the toothbrush. Since plaque optically blends with tooth structure, it is wise to use a disclosing solution to aid in its visualization. The technique used, type of brush, and thoroughness of the method employed are all important.

The toothbrush will not reach all areas, particularly the interproximals and under the gingivae. Here dental floss and the rubber tip will be invaluable aids. Floss threaders will help under solder joints and pontics. It has been estimated that it should take approximately 5 to 7 seconds to clean each tooth and 7 minutes for the entire dentition.[20]

A thorough cleaning should last about a day. Cleaning after meals may not do more good than before, and possibly less, because the plaque has to be present to capture the fermentable carbohydrate. However, most people feel more comfortable removing food and debris after meals and before going to bed. The major problem is motivation. Clinical experience shows that it is very difficult to change people's habits regardless of their intelligence and education, the amount of money they have spent on their teeth, or the amount of instruction or reinforcement they have received.

Craig and Montague found in a family oral health survey that more than 40% admitted that instruction had not changed their habits.[5] It is probable that an equal amount were ashamed to admit this. Schulman found that there was general agreement that no education or motivational technique has consistently been associated with long-term success in causing patients to maintain hygiene![31] Fear of losing teeth usually does not motivate for long.

In a letter to the editor of the *Journal of the American Dental Association*, James Bouman, the representative of Blue Cross in Wisconsin writes, "The sad fact is that the task of motivating the dental patient to learn a whole new approach to maintaining his/her own oral health is probably effective (meaning a permanent behavior change) with no more than 20% of the patients who are exposed to the information."[1]

Concerning children, the critical factor in success was whether their mothers were willing and able to help them during their school years. Linn found that even when mothers were involved in an oral hygiene program, they rarely checked the thoroughness of brushing.[21] In spite of their indoctrination, the parents seldom used disclosing tablets and gave sugar-containing snacks with little concern. Eighty-six percent of these mothers had at least graduated from high school.

Much has been written about motivating the dental patient. The area that needs investigation and documentation is "habit formation." Is there a critical age for establishing behavior? How can old habits best be changed?

Other means of dealing with plaque have been considered.[24] These have included antibacterial or antibiotic agents aimed at preventing proliferation of bacteria. The antibacterial agent that has shown most promise has been chlorhexidine gluconate. While it has inhibited plaque formation, it has caused desquamation of the mucosa, stain on restorations, and bladder cancer in laboratory animals. It has been known that antibiotics such as penicillin produce marked reduction in caries. The problem, however, is the possibility of creating resistant organisms and sensitization that would limit the effectiveness of the antibiotic in a serious medical situation.

Enzymatic as well as nonenzymatic mucolytic agents have been studied in attempts to disperse the gellike matrix that holds plaque together. For example, dextranase has been very effective in animal studies because of its effect on dextran. It is not as effective in humans where other polymers, in addition to dextran, are present. Mixed results have been found with mucolytic agents such as ascutal T (Ascoxal), a mixture of ascorbic acid, percarbonate, and copper sulphate.

Carbohydrate ingestion.[10] The final method in caries prevention concentrates on the fourth factor: carbohydrate ingestion into the plaque. One of the most effective means of altering plaque accumulation and cariogenicity is by the restriction of sucrose intake.[24] Sucrose plays the major role in caries production except in "baby bottle" and "milk bottle" syndrome, where lactose plays a part.

Sucrose and lactose are disaccharides. The monosaccharides, such as fructose and glucose, are less cariogenic, and even less so are the alcohol hexoses, mannitol and sorbitol. Starch, a polysaccharide, is low in cariogenicity. Xylitol, an alcohol derived from the wood sugar pentose, xylose, was shown to produce a significant reduction in plaque when substituted for sucrose in a recent study with dental students.[24] Unfortunately a recent report has indicated that xylitol may be carcinogenic in high doses.

The key to the dietary control of caries lies in limitation of sucrose ingestion. This can be accomplished by elimination of certain sugar-containing foods, restriction of sugar to mealtimes, or the substitution of mannitol, xylitol, starch, or an artificial sweetener when feasible. The roadblock again is habit.

Most people are unaware of the extent of their sucrose intake. A small bar of chocolate may supply 7 teaspoons of sugar, while a serving of apple pie may give 12 teaspoons.[7] Manufacturers of breakfast cereals have been adding various forms of phosphate to modify the caries potential of their sweetened products.

Some rather innocuous-appearing foods and beverages have a low pH in addition to a substantial sucrose content. For example, clear tea has a pH of 5.8, but with lemon, 3.4; apples, 3.3; grapes, 2.8; grapefruit juice, 3.2; and cola, 2.3. Even when the sugar has been eliminated, as it is in the low-calorie drinks, the acidity is still present.[3]

Dentists have been attempting to inform the public about the role of sugar. They have recommended the substitution of noncariogenic snacks such as nuts, pretzels, celery, radishes, carrots, popcorn, and so on. Some have talked about the protective role of protein and fat while wondering if the urea formed in the saliva, from protein, is a major substrate of plaque, and if the fat forms an oily film on the teeth. Clearly, much is known about the role of nutrition in caries production, but a great deal more still has to be learned.[35]

The dentist has a means of monitoring his or her patients as to whether they are following their dietary recommendations. The Snyder test, which is correlated with a quantity of acid-forming bacteria in the saliva, gives a colorimetric picture of the activity. Presumably, if all caries are taken care of and the diet is low in carbohydrate, there would be no color change. The amount of change within a measured time interval gives a measure of the caries potential of a mouth.

Primary preventive procedures need to be tailored to the individual needs of the patient. Needless to say, it is ridiculous to run patients with caries-free dentition and healthy periodontium through a rigid preventive program. On the other hand, certain patients have problems that have a known potential for increasing caries activity. An example would be the patient who has received irradiation to the head and surrounding structures as treatment for a malignancy. Here the increased caries results from the poor oral hygiene of the debilitated patient as well as the change in the quantity and quality of the saliva. The saliva becomes viscous and has a lower pH than normal, while the quantity is so sparse that its ability to counteract the effects of the bacteria is lost.[29] Another example is the patient suffering from Sjögren's syndrome where the xerostomia has a similar effect. Obviously, patients with these predisposing problems require special attention. All our knowledge should go into planning a program for prevention.

The dentist has an even greater responsibility to the patients he or she is treating so as not to iatrogenically set the stage for caries because of the quality of his or her dentistry. Examples of dental treatment that might present problems are filling overhangs, open contacts, unfavorable contours of crowns and bridges, poorly adapted orthodontic appliances, ill-fitting prosthetic appliances, and unpolished surfaces, especially approximating noncarious areas. Further discussion is detailed under the disciplines responsible for the treatment.

Periodontal disease. Periodontal disease, the inflammation and destruction of the supporting tissues of the teeth, may start in childhood, where about 9% of children between ages 11 and 15 are affected. This incidence increases with age so that 10% to 29% of those between ages 19 and 25 have it and from age 45, about 98% of the American population is affected.[11] The initial inflammatory response, characterized by reddening and swelling as well as easy bleeding of the gingivae, is reversible and is called gingivitis. The more advanced stage, periodontitis, is characterized by periodontal pockets and the loss of alveolar bone, which is irreversible.[12]

Gingivitis, a fairly universal condition, is amenable to primary preventive procedures. To the extent that it can be prevented, periodontitis can be eliminated too. Microbial plaque lying close to the patient's gingival tissue is the primary etiologic factor initiating gingival inflammation. In contrast to caries, which is multifactorial in its initiation, gingivitis has only one necessary requirement—the bacteria in the plaque.

This dental plaque is a little different from the plaque involved with caries. It is the early plaque that harbors the colonies of gram-positive streptococci and lactobacilli that produce the largest amount of acid, which is responsible for caries. As the plaque continues to mature and gathers in different types of microorganisms, it changes. In areas opposite the salivary glands and in subgingival areas where the crevicular fluid is rich in calcium and phosphate, the plaque can become mineralized to form calculus. It is this mature form of plaque and calculus that is responsible for periodontal disease.

The bacteria, many of which are now gram negative, do not invade the gingiva. Instead, endotoxins, which are part of the cell membrane, are potent inflammatory agents. The gingivae react with vasodilation, edema, massive accumulation of inflammatory cells, and frequently hemorrhagic necrosis.[34]

The primary preventive measure is plaque removal (same as for caries) before it elaborates its inflammatory products. Prevention involves the use of the toothbrush, dentifrice, dental floss, interproximal cleaners, and floss threaders where necessary. According to Loe, complete removal of plaque *once* every second day is compatible with the maintenance of gingival health.[22] Recently there was a report on an alexidine mouthwash for dental plaque and gingivitis.[39] It is shown to be safe and effective, but it has the drawback of staining the teeth and anterior restorations brown.

Plaque removal encounters the same problems discussed in caries control—motivation and thoroughness. Forrest[10] echoes what many writers and lecturers have said, "If it were possible to initiate a perfect and rigid plaque control then the vast majority of our patients would never have gingivitis or, later periodontal disease."

Those of us who have indoctrinated patients and have observed them diligently apply themselves to home care procedures will appreciate the frustration they feel when they develop problems in spite of their efforts. Golomb, a periodontist and the editor of the *New York Journal of Dentistry*, writes, "Meticulous cleansing, the do-it-yourself branch of dentistry, neither solves nor prevents all dental difficulties. To lull the public into assuming that it does (or most of the time, anyway) can be no service to the patient or profession."[15] On the other hand, we see other patients who ignore our warnings and seem to have no apparent effects of gingivitis or periodontitis when they do not brush regularly, carefully, or at all.

There are other considerations that deserve attention in the prevention of gingivitis and periodontal disease on the primary level. These are factors that predispose to plaque accumulation and so require attentiveness to either prevent their occurrence or, if that is not possible, to mitigate their effects through an increased diligence in plaque removal. These factors include the following:
1. Iatrogenic: overextended, unpolished, deficient, or undercontoured restorations
2. Developmental: nonocclusion or poor tooth form or tooth position
3. Systemic: debilitating disease (Parkinson's disease or stroke)
4. Habits: diet, unilateral mastication, indolent mastication

Secondary level of prevention

At the secondary level of prevention, incipient disease is already present. Thus the clinician must detect its presence and do simple repairs or undertake remedial measures in order to prevent its advance. Efforts in this category include treatment of incipient caries, gingivitis, early periodontal disease, and the correction of faulty restorations.

DENTAL CARIES

The carious lesion that starts insidiously and has the potential for rapid growth requires prompt attention. The detection of the initial lesion and halting its progression by simple repair or remedial measures is the essence of secondary prevention.

Unfortunately, incipient caries is frequently difficult to diagnose on the two most vulnerable surfaces of the teeth: the occlusal and interproximal surfaces. The criterion on the occlusal surface is the "sticky" explorer. However, since pits and fissures that tend to catch the explorer are commonplace, the dentist is frequently faced with a dilemma. Similarly, while a slight radiolucency is the criterion for initial decay at the contact point, this roentgenographic darkening may also be anatomic or hypoplastic in nature or even an artifact.

About 50 years ago, Hyatt proposed a solution to the problem of the occlusal "lesion." He suggested the "prophylactic odontotomy," which involved the operative removal of all pits and fissures and filling them with amalgam. The rationale for this treatment was that these areas would decay anyway and that it was more efficient to fill them while they were small. This idea, as well as variations of it, have persisted to this day.

The incipient interproximal lesion does not lend itself to prophylactic odontotomy because it would involve the removal of a great deal of tooth structure. Accordingly, if this radiolucency does not appear to extend into dentin in good quality roentgenograms using magnification, continued observation is the treatment indicated. Nevertheless, other considerations such as past dental history, age, oral hygiene practices, and frequency of dental examinations might cause the clinician to place a class 2 restoration in some cases.

Currently a greater emphasis is being placed on patient responsibility. This has resulted in a modification of certain secondary preventive procedures. For example, there has been an increasing tendency to abandon G. V. Black's extension for prevention principles in cavity preparation in lieu of conservation of tooth structure. It is thought to be unnecessary to extend a preparation into a self-cleansing area; it is now sufficient to bring it to a "cleansable" area. This concept has been abetted by the many studies that have shown that the gingival sulcus is in no way sterile. Since restorative materials, no matter how well polished, retain plaque to a greater extent than natural tooth structure, the gingival margins should be above the gingival crest when feasible.[41]

The following considerations, observed during the completing of routine restorative dentistry, help to ensure the arrest of dental disease, effect the prognosis, and qualify as secondary preventive procedures.

1. Rubber dam or cotton rolls should be used for better visibility, elimination of moisture, and safety.
2. Water should be utilized with high-speed instrumentation, making sure that it strikes the bur for proper cooling effect.
3. Since at least 50% of restorations fail because of poor cavity preparation, careful attention must be given to removal of unsupported enamel, adequate retention, and depth. (However, the limit should be 1 mm maximum into dentin, if possible.)

4. Because the odontoblasts react to the cutting of their Tomes' fibers, more care must be given to restricting the area covered by the preparation. (There is a relation between sensitivity and number of tubules cut.)
5. Desiccation also has a deleterious effect on the odontoblasts. The use of long, steady blasts of air should be avoided. Instead the tooth should be dried with cotton or air used only for short periods.
6. Silicates, cold cure acrylics, and composites cause destruction of odontoblasts; therefore bases should be accurately placed so that as much dentin is covered as is possible.
7. High-contact (high surface tension) cavity liners (e.g., Copalite) prevent marginal leakage under amalgams.[43]
8. Low-contact (low surface tension) cavity liners (e.g., S.S. White) provide better pulp protection under amalgam.[43] They can be used in shallow preparations.
9. Composites last about twice as long as silicates, but they tend to wear. Eugenol and varnish affect them; calcium hydroxide does not. They are best placed with a special syringe to avoid air bubbles.
10. Avoid the use of sterilizing agents in the cavity. No medication will selectively kill bacteria without harming the odontoblasts.

Gingivitis

Gingivitis is the initial stage in periodontal disease. It is possible, in early cases, to return the gingiva to its original state with the institution of secondary preventive procedures. Frequently, in more advanced cases of gingivitis, we must be content with preventing its progression to a more advanced periodontal condition, thus accepting the irreversible recession or other damage that has already occurred.

As was described earlier, the simplest method of treating gingivitis is to institute a rigid regimen of toothbrushing and plaque removal. Hopefully this can be done by the patient after proper instruction. In those instances where the patient has lost control of his arms or has poor coordination, the electric toothbrush can be of great help.

The dentist's responsibility involves the correction, where feasible, of faulty dentistry. This may include every aspect of restorative measures from the polishing of a restoration to the rehabilitation of an entire occlusion. The objective is the elimination of plaque-accumulating areas by promoting normal bilateral function with restorations that themselves do not encourage the retention of plaque and are capable of being cleaned by ordinary procedures.

Where development of tooth alignment and irregular arch form produced areas that cannot be properly cleaned, corrective procedures should be undertaken. These might range from special plaque removal instruction to restorative changes or even orthodontia.

Periodontal disease

While gingivitis is the first stage in periodontal disease, periodontitis is its successor in its progression, and 90% of the time both are present. Periodontitis is characterized by the formation of periodontal pockets and the loss of alveolar bone underlying the inflamed gingiva. In contrast to gingivitis, where bacterial plaque is the prime etiologic agent, periodontitis can be considered multifactorial in origin.

Periodontitis can be thought of as the product of a number of varying factors, both qualitative and quantitative, acting in concert. The net effect of any one factor, for example, food impaction, may range from no apparent consequence to a severe bony defect, depending on other influences. It seems as if the product must exceed a threshold in order to produce a clinical manifestation of periodontitis.

These factors can be grouped under two major categories: *local* and *systemic*. Each factor must also be rated for its intensity and frequency of action.

1. Local factors
   a. Dysfunctional factors[26]
      (1) Overfunction (e.g., excess stress on teeth during mastication)
      (2) Underfunction (e.g., too little stress, that is, nonocclusion)
      (3) Habits (e.g., unilateral mastication)
   b. Irritational factors
      (1) Abnormal anatomy (e.g., inadequate proximal contact)
      (2) Deposits on teeth (e.g., calculus)
      (3) Nondetergent diet (e.g., soft foods)
      (4) Food impaction (e.g., plunger cusps)
      (5) Mechanical irritants (e.g., overhang)
      (6) Chemical irritants (e.g., alcohol)
      (7) Atmospheric irritants (e.g., mouth breathing)
      (8) Improper toothbrushing
      (9) Improper orthodontic procedure
2. Systemic factors
   a. Nutrition
   b. Debilitating diseases
   c. Blood dyscrasias
   d. Endocrine dysfunction
   e. Pregnancy
   f. Allergies and drug reactions
   g. Metallic poisoning
   h. Radiation
   i. Psychosomatic factors

Each of the above factors must be considered as a potential contributor to the disease known as periodontitis. This disease is curable to the extent that the factors involved in the etiology can be eliminated or controlled. The key to this is establishing a proper diagnosis. Thus it is mandatory not only to recognize the condition, but also to identify the factors operating to create the problem. This must be coupled with a proper treatment plan designed to remove the etiologic agents, minimize or eliminate the destructive effects, restore healthy function, and increase the resistance to further attacks of the disease process. By definition the level of severity of periodontal disease that is treatable under secondary level measures would involve those cases with no bone loss and with gingival pockets only. Therapeutic measures utilized at this level would be polishing, scaling, root planing, and curettage. It must be recognized that in periodontitis it may not be possible to restore the periodontium to its predisease state.

Tertiary level of prevention

In the tertiary level of prevention the dentist attempts to deal with gross destructive effects and restore function in a way that will prevent further attacks. Basically treatment is either periodontal and instructional or restorative. *Prevention and prognosis are to a great extent related to pinpointing the etiologic factors, eliminating or controlling them, and the quality of the therapy for removing the effects.*

PERIODONTAL THERAPY

Treatment of advanced periodontitis is the essence of tertiary prevention. The objectives of periodontal treatment in this tertiary stage are no different than they are in the secondary—to arrest the disease process and to restore the periodontium to a state of health. The difference is that the disease has progressed so that a true periodontal pocket is now present, instead of a simulated one caused by inflamed gingiva. In addition, there is a loss of alveolar bone. At the present level of our knowledge, we cannot expect to return the tissues damaged by periodontitis to their original state. The functional impairment depends on how far the disease had progressed when treatment was commenced. The greater the tissue loss, the more severe the functional problem.

The periodontal pocket is a deep sulcus produced by the migration of the epithelial attachment in an apical direction. Now plaque can form at the base of the pocket where it is inaccessible to the patient. In dealing with this problem the clinician usually divides the treatment into two phases. The first phase is conservative and includes scaling, root planing, patient instruction, and motivation for home care. It is during this stage that the dentist removes hopeless teeth and attempts to eliminate or control the other etiologic factors.

A reevaluation of the patient takes place after the completion of the first phase. If pockets still remain and adequate plaque removal is impossible, the second or surgical phase is instituted. This includes procedures such as deep curettage, gingivectomy, gingivoplasty, mucogingival surgery, ostectomy, and osteoplasty. The first three procedures are designed to eliminate the gingival pockets through reattachment of the epithelium or by removing the tissue. Mucogingival surgery corrects nonpocket deformities such as high muscle attachments that tend to pull the gingiva in an apical direction. Ostectomy and osteoplasty are performed for infrabony pockets and other osseous deformities, such as exostoses, to facilitate plaque removal by the patient.[6]

In assessing the foregoing treatment for periodontitis, it is important to keep in mind that, while we are treating periodontal disease, we are attempting to prevent further destruction. Nevertheless, surgical procedures carry with them certain hazards that have prognostic implications. The guiding principle should be to "exhaust all conservative means before attempting gross tissue removal."

Even though gingival surgery has advanced to the point where its results are predictable, at least more so than osseous surgery, there are problems that

affect the prognosis. Recession or loss of gingival tissue is the biggest concern and may lead to several problems:
1. Root sensitivity is a frequent aftermath. Sensitivity to thermal, tactile, and sweet stimuli are the usual complaints. This complaint may be so severe that treated teeth will have to be extracted.
2. Aesthetic concerns result from exposure of the margins of crowns and the increase in length of the clinical crowns.
3. Root caries are the consequence of nonprotected dentin exposed to the oral environment in a vulnerable position.
4. Pulpal pathology may occur as a hyperemia because of the constant insult of hot, cold, and other stimuli.
5. Gingival sensitivity may result when alveolar mucosa is left to serve as marginal gingiva.
6. Increased mobility may be evident postsurgically for approximately 1 year.[32]

Other aspects of periodontal therapy and prognosis, which are beyond the scope of this chapter, would include occlusal correction and the use of night guard appliances.

Following are additional factors influencing prognosis:
1. Degree of patient cooperation obtainable.
2. Extension of the pocket. Miller claimed that bifurcation and trifurcation involvement and pockets that extend to the apex rendered the prognosis hopeless.[26] In recent years, surgical techniques and endodontic therapy and implants, as well as restorative techniques combined with periodontal treatment, permit the conservation of *some* of these teeth.
3. Alveolar bone support. Miller felt that at least one-half root support should be present for a good prognosis. In addition, the bone should be evenly distributed and dense. Experiences involving periods of observation combined with other therapy have led to a reexamination of this thesis.
4. Mobility. Teeth that can move more than one millimeter in every direction are questionable. Still, if occlusion is an important factor, mobility may be reduced remarkably after occlusal correction. Teeth that can be depressed in their sockets are deemed hopeless. However, in many cases reasonably priced splinting with provisional techniques, such as wires, A splints, and acid-etch composites, may be used. This approach enables the clinician to observe the progress of the case during an evaluation period before making a final decision on the rehabilitation phase of the treatment plan.
5. Number of teeth remaining.
6. Distribution of remaining teeth.
7. Service required of teeth to be saved.
8. Age. Older patients with the same amount of bone as younger individuals have a more favorable prognosis. There are periodontists who teach that there should be no bone loss with aging.
9. Presence of systemic disease.
10. Probability of successfully removing causative factors.

Preventive and prognostic aspects of operative dentistry

Successful application of primary preventive procedures for caries should obviate the need for operative dentistry, at least as far as it is causally related to caries. However, utopia has not been attained, so operative dentistry continues to form a large part of clinical dentistry. This discipline is responsible for the repair of all lesions of the clinical crowns of the teeth, regardless of their cause.

The greatest challenge that operative dentistry faces is the treatment of well-established caries in attempts to restore function in a *lasting* manner. Such efforts define the tertiary level of preventive dentistry and would include the following procedures:

1. Mass excavation of caries and temporization for rapid control of this destructive process.
2. Pulp extirpation and root canal therapy for acute infections and pain control as well as for chronic infections.
3. Direct pulp capping with calcium hydroxide for pulp exposures that are asymptomatic.
4. Placement of zinc oxide eugenol dressing for nonexposed sensitivity.
5. Removal of most of the decay and placement of a sealing restoration over it. The cavity is reentered in 6 months, the remainder of the decay is removed, and the permanent restoration is placed. This technique may be used for deep cavities.
6. Indirect pulp capping (coiffage indirect, coiffage neutral). This is basically the same procedure described in 5, except that the permanent restoration is placed right away.
7. Caries control measures.
8. Permanent restorations placed. Casting should be used and thin cusps protected where possible in order to minimize the possibility of fractures.
9. Proper seating and cementation of cast restorations.

Preventive and prognostic aspects of fixed partial prosthesis

Preventive aspects of fixed partial prosthesis start with the diagnosis. It is generally agreed that if there is a choice between a fixed and removable prosthesis, everything else being equal, the fixed appliance would be selected on the basis of comfort, tooth stability, and kindness to tissues. Yet there are times when it is difficult to make a decision. The reasons for indecision include number and position of abutments, their bone support, the caries index, the patient's finances, and the quality of home care.

Fixed partial prostheses, as well as supplying missing teeth, splint teeth together. Thus if the plan and design are correct, weaker teeth that have lost some bone support will be stabilized. This prevents further breakdown because a tooth that has class 2 mobility is more vulnerable to traumatic occlusion than one with class 1 mobility. The benefits may be multiple: aesthetic in supplying the missing tooth; functional in increasing masticatory efficiency by reestablishing bilateral mastication, restoring and maintaining lost contacts and thus preventing food impaction, extrusion, and drifting; and periodontal stabilization. In addition, these fixed appliances provide a measure of caries control and prevention. Not only are existing caries on the abutment teeth cared for, but there is a likelihood that new caries will be prevented as a result of the crowns and the improved chewing ability. All these attractive benefits help to ensure a satisfactory psychological attitude on the part of the patient.

Treatment planning, based on a thorough diagnosis, takes into account all modifying factors. The potential abutments are studied individually. Their relation to the other teeth in the arch as well as to the opposing arch is evaluated to determine if a fixed prosthesis is even feasible. Without detailing the criteria, there are a number of minimum requirements that must be met. As a result, some teeth are considered hopeless, while others are deemed very satisfactory. The problem is with teeth that fall into an intermediate category where there may be disagreement about prognosis. Unfortunately there are no definitive guidelines in many of these cases. The individual dentist must make a decision based on his or her own limited experience, a lecturer's personal opinion, or a book that may well be perpetuating a myth.

In some situations certain problems can be anticipated and the following specific modifications made in the design of a fixed prosthesis in order to improve the outcome.

1. A posterior cantilever bridge supplying a molar might require three abutments and a pontic half the mesiodistal and one-third the buccolingual width of the tooth it replaces. A cantilever supplying a first premolar (not to involve the canine for aesthetic reasons) might have a canine-shaped pontic supported by the second premolar and first molar.
2. In a long span, many posterior bridge problems could be prevented by narrowing the pontics to one-third instead of the usual two-thirds buccolingual width.
3. If we want to connect a posterior fixed bridge made of gold to an anterior fixed bridge made of porcelain baked to precious metal, we can use a precision attachment, placing the female keyway on the distal end of the canine crown and the male key on the mesial key of the first premolar crown. The forces of occlusion will tend to seat the parts. In contrast, putting the female end on the posterior section would have the opposite effect. An additional benefit may accrue if the posterior abutment should be lost. The attachment on the canine could be useful for the design of the removable partial denture.
4. In those instances where a tooth is to serve as an abutment, but it is anticipated that in the future the tooth may be needed as an abutment for a bridge adjacent to the one we are making, we can make a coping first and then cement an individual crown over it temporarily. In the event that its services are needed, the single crown is simply removed and incorporated into the new bridge and is cemented over the coping.
5. A tilted tooth, which might become exposed during the preparation to parallel it, can be prepared for a nonparallel coping to cover the whole tooth, and the coping can be partially prepared parallel to the anterior preparations. The final crown is cemented over it and is referred to as a "telescoped" crown.

Modifying factors in treatment planning

Preventive and prognostic aspects of removable partial prosthesis

Removable partial prosthesis is usually completely involved with prevention on the tertiary level—the treatment of well-established disease in order to minimize or eliminate the gross destructive effects to restore healthy function and to resist further attacks by the disease process. This is true to the extent that we consider the state of partial edentulousness a disease state. Our concern here is the preservation of the remaining teeth and the ridges. Since much of the alveolar bone is lost with the teeth, the ridges may be mostly composed of basal bone.

Usually there are several teeth missing, and those present are located in a manner that is not conducive to fixed partial prosthesis. In many cases the edentulous span is long. Frequently the case has a free end saddle, that is, there are no teeth at one end of this span. The prosthesis depends not only on the teeth but also on the edentulous ridges for support.

Concern with the following considerations will promote a better prognosis in removable prosthodontic treatment.
1. Careful treatment planning and denture design.
2. Careful evaluation of teeth to be conserved (Questionable teeth should usually be extracted.)
3. Institution and maintenance of good home care
4. Proper preparation of the mouth to receive the denture
5. Use of temporary or provisional dentures where indicated

Importance of prognostic considerations

It is particularly important that the patient be as completely informed about the prognosis of the proposed treatment plan as possible. In practical terms this means that the dentist should give the patient an idea of how long the contemplated work should last. This involves discussing the chances of success as well as the risks involved in specific avenues of treatment. In many instances the seasoned dentist is able to give the patient an accurate estimate of success rate. For instance, it is known that approximately 95% of teeth treated by conventional endodontics respond satisfactorily. In contrast, it is very difficult and often impossible to accurately predict the degree of success to expect in advanced periodontal cases that require complex reconstructive treatment. The dentist hopes that such treatment will be successful. In such cases it is vitally important to explain to the patient that we cannot predict how the tissues will respond to treatment and that there is a chance that the treatment will not be successful. Advising a patient about the prognosis is necessary for two reasons: (1) it will enable the patient to make an intelligent choice in the light of all the facts; and (2) if the treatment does fail, then the patient will have been prepared for this possibility and will more readily accept it.

Unfortunately there may be great disagreement as to what constitutes success in treatment. What represents success to the dentist may be interpreted as failure by the patient. Therefore, before treatment commences, the discussion concerning prognosis should clearly define to the patient what the dentist feels constitutes success in that particular case.

REFERENCES

1. Bouman, J.: Letter to the editor, J.A.D.A. **93**:515, 1976.
2. Buonocore, M. G.: Caries prevention in pits and fissures sealing with an adhesive resin polymerized by ultraviolet light: a two-year study of a single adhesive application, J.A.D.A. **82**:1090, 1971.
3. Bridges, M. A., and Mattice, M. R.: Yearbook of dentistry, Chicago, 1951, Yearbook Publishers, p. 408.
4. Carlos, J. P.: Caries research: the current status, J.A.D.A. (special issue) **87**:998, 1973.
5. Craig, T. J., and Montague, J. L.: Family oral health survey, J.A.D.A. **92**:326, 1976.
6. Deasey, M. J., Vogel, R. I., Schubach, P., and Simon, B. I.: Periodontal therapy, principles of pocket elimination, J.A.D.A. **92**:1173, 1976.
7. Doyle, W. A.: Utilization of dietary counseling in a private office, Dent. Clin. North Am., July 1965, p. 517.
8. Driscoll, W. S., Heifetz, S. B., Korts, D. C., Meyers, R. J., and Horowitz, H. S.: Effect of acidulated phosphate fluoride chewable tablets in children: results after 55 months, J.A.D.A. **94**:537, 1977.
9. Foley, G. P.: Foley's footnotes, J.A.D.A. **92**:408, 1976.
10. Forrest, J. O.: Preventive dentistry, Bristol, Eng., 1976, John Wright & Sons, pp. 8, 49.
11. Galagan, D. J.: Dental health and the need for prevention. In Curators symposium on applied preventive dentistry, Columbia, Mo., 1964, University of Missouri.
12. Genco, R. J.: Periodontal disease as a plaque disease. In Preventive dentistry, New York, 1972, Medcom, p. 16.
13. Glasser, S. P.: The problems of patients with cardiovascular disease undergoing dental treatment, J.A.D.A. **94**:1158, 1977.
14. Going, R. E., Conti, A. J., Haugh, L. D., and Grainger, D. A.: Two-year clinical evaluation of a pit and fissure sealant. Part II. Caries initiation and progression, J.A.D.A. **92**:578, 1976.
15. Golomb, I.: Editorial, N.J. Dent., Dec. 1976.
16. Horowitz, H. S.: Research on clinical and public health applications, J.A.D.A. (special issue) **87**:1013, 1973.
17. Horowitz, H. S., Heifetz, S. B., and McCune, R. J.: The effectiveness of an adhesive sealant in preventing occlusal caries, findings after two years in Kalispell, Montana, J.A.D.A. **89**:885, 1974.
18. Kamen, A., Schreer, S. B., and Schmee, J.: Letter to the editor, J.A.D.A. **94**:799, 1977.
19. Katz, S., McDonald, J. L., and Stookey, G. K.: Preventive dentistry in action, Upper Montclair, N.J., 1972, D.C.P. Publishing, p. 236.
20. Less, W.: Mechanics of teaching plaque control, Dent. Clin. North Am. **16**:653, 1972.
21. Linn, E. L.: Mothers' involvement in oral hygiene program, J.A.D.A. **92**:398, 1976.
22. Loe, H.: Plaque control in periodontal disease, J.A.D.A. (special issue) **87**:1034, 1973.
23. Mandel, I. D.: Bacterial plaque defined. In Preventive dentistry, New York, 1972, Medcom, p. 13.
24. Mandel, I. D.: New approaches to plaque prevention, Dent. Clin. North Am. **16**:661, 1972.
25. McClure, F. J.: Water fluoridation—the search and the victory, Bethesda, Md., 1970, U.S. Dept. of Health, Education, and Welfare, National Institute for Dental Research.
26. Miller, S. C.: Textbook of periodontia, ed. 3, Philadelphia, 1950, The Blakiston Co., p. 70.
27. Report of Council on Dental Therapeutics, J.A.D.A. **91**:1250, 1975.
28. Rizzo, A. A.: Periodontal research introductory remarks, J.A.D.A. (special issue) **87**:1019, 1973.
29. Rubin, R. L., and Doku, H. C.: Therapeutic radiology—the modalities and their effects on oral tissues, J.A.D.A. **92**:731, 1976.
30. Santinga, J. T., Fekety, R. F., Jr., Bottomley, W. K., Else, B., and Willis III, P. W.: Antibiotic prophylaxis for endocarditis in patients with a prosthetic heart valve, J.A.D.A. **93**:1001, 1976.
31. Schulman, J. Clinical evaluation of the phase-contrast microscope as a motivational aid in oral hygiene, J.A.D.A. **92**:759, 1976.
32. Selipsky, H.: Osseous surgery—how much need we compromise? Dent. Clin. North Am. **20**:105, 1976.
33. Simon, A. B., Linde, B., Bonnette, G. H., and Schlentz, R. J.: The individual with a pacemaker in the dental environment, J.A.D.A. **91**:1224, 1975.

34. Snyderman, R.: Immunological mechanism of periodontal tissue destuction, J.A.D.A. (special issue) **87:**1020, 1973.
35. Stanton, G.: Three approaches to diet therapy. In Preventive dentisty, New York, 1972, Medcom, p. 44.
36. Statements of general policy or interpretation: oral prenatal drugs containing fluoride for human use, Washington, D.C., *Federal Register*, 1966, U.S. Food and Drug Administration.
37. Stookey, G. K., and Katz, S.: Using fluorides for preventing dental caries Dent. Clin. North Am. **16:**681, 1972.
38. Tomme, C.: Military civilian groups cooperate in oral cancer screening project, J.A.D.A. **94:**499, 1977.
39. Weatherford III, T. W., Finn, S. B., and Jamison, H. C.: Effects of an alexidine mouthwash on dental plaque and gingivitis in humans over a six-month period, J.A.D.A. **94:**528, 1977.
40. Weil, R. B., and Bernstein, B.: Viral hepatitis: its importance to dentists, N. Y. State Dent. J. **41:**467, 1975.
41. Welk, D. A., and Laswell, H. R.: Designing cavity preparations, Dent. Clin. North Am. **20:**231, 1976.
42. Workshop on relative analgesia, J.A.A.S. **15:**14, 1977.
43. Younis, O.: Permeability and wetting properties of four cavity liners, J.A.D.A. **94:**690, 1977.

BIBLIOGRAPHY

Arnold, M.: Case history, Oral Med. News., April 1974.
Caputo, A. A., and Standlee, J. P.: Pins and posts—why, when and how, Dent. Clin. North Am. **20:**299, 1976.
Eames, W. B.: A clinical view of dental amalgam, Dent. Clin. North Am. **20:**385, 1976.
Gratzinger, M.: The use of removable orthodontic plate appliances in the management of chronic periodontal disease, Dent. Clin. North Am. **3:**403, 1959.
Handelman, S. L., Buonocore, M. G., and Heseck, D. J.: A preliminary report on the effect of a fissure sealant on bacteria in dental caries, J. Prosthet. Dent., **27:**390-392, 1972.
Kaufman, E. G., and Papirno, R.: Stress concentration in full crowns, N.Y. State Dent. J. **29:**370, 1963.
Langeland, K.: Prevention of pulpal damage, Dent. Clin. North Am. **16:**709, 1972.
Lau, V.M.S.: The reinforcement of endodontically treated teeth, Dent. Clin. North Am. **20:**313, 1976.
Lefkowitz, W.: The treatment of carious teeth, Dent. Clin. North Am. **4:**629, 1960.
Lerman, M. D.: Hydrostatis appliance therapy of the myofascial (TMJ) pain dysfunction syndrome (abstracted from IADR program and abstracts), March 1970.
Miller, E. L.: Planning partial denture construction, Dent. Clin. North Am. **17:**571, 1973.
Morse, D. R., Seltzer, S., and Sinai, I.: Endodontic classification, J.A.D.A. **94:**685, 1977.
Powers, J. M., Farah, J. W., and Craig, R. G.: Modulus of elasticity and strength properties of dental cements, J.A.D.A. **92:**588, 1976.
Shore, N. A.: Occlusal equilibration and temporomandibular joint dysfunction, Philadelphia, J. B. Lippincott Co.
Silvestri, A. R., Cohen, S. N., and Wetz, J. H.: Character and frequency of discomfort immediately following restorative procedures, J.A.D.A. **95:**85, 1977.
Simring, M., and Posteraro, A. F.: Hazards and shortcomings of splinting, N.Y. State Dent. J. **30:**19, 1964.
Sullivan, H. C., and Dragoo, M. R.: Regenerative techniques in periodontal therapy, Dent. Clin. North Am. **20:**131, 1976.

9

Additional considerations

David M. Dickey

In almost any field of knowledge that has been divided into categories, there are exceptions or matters of interest that do not really fit under major headings. We are constantly faced with exceptions. The area of treatment planning illustrates this point. While the chapter topics in this book have been very thoughtfully chosen and developed, there are a few additional points to consider, and an attempt will be made to deal with them; hence the title of this chapter.

OPERATOR EXPERIENCE AND COMPETENCE

While in school the dental student functions in a more or less protected environment. Any mistakes in patient management or treatment are minimized by the fact that he or she is under the supervision of qualified faculty members. The danger of exercising bad judgment is minimized for the same reason. Soon after the state board examinations have been passed and the D.D.S. is added, the picture changes. The new dentist is solely responsible for each decision made and each treatment rendered. Happily, the vast majority of dentists can and do cope successfully with this situation. They are able to provide first-class dental care within their framework of knowledge and experience.

The experienced practitioner who has managed cases of increasing difficulty over a sufficient period of time can no doubt formulate an appropriate treatment plan for a relatively difficult full-mouth rehabilitation and carry it out successfully. The novice dentist probably should approach that difficult case with caution, and consider the merits of referral to a specialist if this form of treatment seems to be what the patient truly needs. Remember, the spirit may be willing when the flesh is still weak. Every dentist has had case failures at some time and to some degree. The trick is to avoid openly inviting them.

This admonition is in no way intended to undermine a feeling of self-confidence. Most dentists have a fine education and are well qualified when they begin their careers. This is simply a plea to temper enthusiasm with some practicality and reality. Perhaps it could be stated more succinctly: Not every dentist is capable of effectively carrying out everything that his dental license says he is allowed to do. Name your game, but know your limits.

OPERATOR AND PATIENT TIME

We have all heard the phrase "time is money." Time and motion studies are now an accepted routine in many phases of human activity. In the dental profession, experts in practice management have made us well aware that the dentist's time must be carefully planned in order to achieve financial success. The practitioner must also keep in mind that there is only so much time available in each day.

The patient's time availability must also be considered. His time may be every bit as valuable to him, and treatment plans must sometimes be adjusted accordingly. Sometimes treatment can be successfully carried out over extended periods of time when the patient's time is limited. However, it would be foolhardy to embark on a difficult full-mouth reconstruction case requiring multiple lengthy appointments when the patient states that he can make it to your office only from 1 to 2 PM on Wednesdays, providing his employer does not schedule a business meeting at that time.

It would seem, then, that in formulating a treatment plan the dentist must determine first of all if it can be accommodated within his or her schedule. Then the dentist must consider the patient's time availability in the same light in order to arrive at a workable agreement. In most cases, patients can make special arrangements for appointment time when they have been informed what their dental needs are. When they are resistant to such arrangements, or simply cannot make them, they must be made to understand that their treatment will be of a limited maintenance type, and not the ideal kind that the dentist would like to provide. This may be agreed to in writing if the dentist so desires.

In some cases the busy dentist will be literally unable to accommodate a treatment plan that will best suit the patient because of previous commitments. If this happens, it is of course appropriate to refer the patient to a dentist who can arrange the needed time rather than to offer the patient less than he deserves.

Every dentist will at one time or another confront the patient who is leaving town in 2 weeks, or is in town visiting her daughter for a week, and wants her neglected oral cavity restored in that available time. This section will be ended without further comment.

DENTAL LABORATORY AND SPECIALIST AVAILABILITY

Dental laboratory service is available to every practicing dentist, no matter how remote the office location might be. The mail is full of circulars and pamphlets advertising every imaginable technical procedure within the realm of dental laboratory service. However, there are definite limitations to this widespread availability.

If a treatment plan calls for a considerable amount of laboratory service, the dentist must proceed very carefully if he or she is in a "mail-order" situation. How long will the mailing process take both ways? How much time does the laboratory require for a given procedure? In what sequence must the treatment plan be carried out, and how many separate mailings will be required? Allowance must be made for delays in the postal service and delays in laboratory work time (even though the advertisement said they would complete a bridge in 2 days after receipt). Heaven forbid that the laboratory will complain that the dental impressions are unsatisfactory and send them back, but it does happen. Also, there may be occasional mishandling of material by the laboratory, which is another delay.

After projecting your treatment plan schedule to allow for all these contingencies, the dentist should tell the patient how long his dental treatment will take. If he accepts the dentist's plan and has time to wait, there should be no problem. In fact, if some of the potential delays do not materialize and the work is completed ahead of schedule, he will be delighted. On the other hand, even though they have delayed needed dental care for long periods, many patients become quite impatient about having their work completed once they have committed themselves to the dentist's care. Failure to inform such patients of possible delays in the course of treatment imposes a considerable strain on the dentist-patient relationship.

In most cases, local laboratory service is available, and this is by far is the best arrangement. The delay and cost of mailing parcels are eliminated, and the dentist and laboratory technician may more conveniently talk on the telephone or even have personal visits for consultation on a case. Even though written instructions and recommendations should always accompany a case to the laboratory, additional interchange of ideas is often beneficial.

Even when local laboratory dental service is available, there may be cause for further consideration. If there is only one laboratory in the community, is the dentist satisfied with the service received from it? Does this laboratory deliver good dentures, but is inadequate in the crown-and-bridge department? If there are several laboratories and the dentist has determined that one is better than the others, how busy is that one? Can the needed services be expected within a reasonable time? These are all considerations that each individual operator must take into account when determining what dental services can be offered and in what time frame.

The availability of dental specialists is another consideration in treatment planning for the general dentist. How much of a problem this presents again depends in part on the dentist's location, but it also depends on how "general" the general dentist is. If the dentist has been well grounded and is considered proficient in such areas as periodontal treatment, endodontics, removal of impacted third molars, and so on, this consideration may have limited importance. It is difficult to conceive, however, that any general dental practice can exist as an island. Both the dental patient and the dental profession can be better served if the dentist has the wisdom to know when to refer.

Fortunately for all concerned, dental specialty practices are far more widespread than they were even 5 or 10 years ago. This fact, coupled with the easy availability of transporation to most people, means that the majority of dental patients can reach the services of a specialist with little difficulty if their dentist feels that this step is indicated. Again, this plan of action must be incorporated into the treatment plan, and the patient should understand why it is necessary.

MANUAL DEXTERITY OF THE PATIENT

Various patient afflictions may necessitate a modification of thinking in formulating a treatment plan. Among these are muscular disorders, some types of paralysis, epilepsy, and disorders associated with mental retardation. Many forms of dental treatment are based on the assumption that the patients have adequate physical and mental control to provide oral hygiene preventive and maintenance measures for themselves. A mentally retarded patient may not remember or be able to use dental floss or brush the teeth daily (unless he has special care and supervision). Also it may be dangerous for the epileptic patient to wear a removable appliance because of imminent seizures. These patients should at least receive interim treatment. As described by Clark,[2] this is "the phase of dental care planned to interrupt the oral disease process." (Sommers and Ebinger refer to this stage as "stabilization" in Chapter 10.) Some cases of this type may force the dentist to resort to plans involving minimal maintenance and no replacements or removal of otherwise usable teeth. Although this may seem distasteful to the dentist who wants to provide first-class dental care, it will often be the kindest and most beneficial treatment for that patient.

In reflecting on "exceptions to the rule," I am reminded of a 40-year-old woman with scleroderma who is currently being treated at our dental school. Because this is a chronic condition of 18 years duration, there is considerable circumoral constriction, and the patient's hands are fixed in a partially flexed position. The chief complaint originally was dental pain caused by dental caries and moderately severe periodontitis. This was an interdisciplinary case, and members of all potentially involved departments were consulted.

In the opinion of the Department of Periodontics the prognosis of periodontal treatment for this patient would be quite limited in the posterior portion of the mouth. Oral hygiene would present a problem. Extractions could be accomplished and complete dentures constructed if this became the choice, although the patient was unhappy at the thought of this alternative. Interestingly enough, during the gathering of data-base information, it was learned that one of the woman's main activities is presenting puppet shows for children's groups in various churches. She is able to handle this activity in spite of the condition of her hands. In addition, she has a strong religious faith, which she feels has carried her through many difficulties.

Since most of the more severely involved teeth were in the lower posterior arches, it was suggested that these be removed and a minimum preparation lower partial denture be constructed. The remaining operative dentistry could then be accomplished with only moderate difficulty. It was also suggested by our prosthodontist that a hand holder might be fabricated for the patient on an electric toothbrush. This would be done by molding the holder directly to the patient's hand with self-curing acrylic. With this unique instrument the patient would hopefully be able to provide the home care treatment necessary to maintain her remaining teeth and periodontium in an acceptable condition.

It is likely that this plan of treatment will be successful for this patient for a considerable time. The example illustrates the importance of gathering all pertinent data and understanding the background and attitudes of patients.

PLANNING TREATMENT FOR THE ELDERLY PATIENT

One very important segment of our population is a group referred to as the elderly. In dentistry and medicine we call them geriatric patients. The system of retirement in business and government in this country seems to have designated 65 as the age beyond which an individual becomes elderly. According to Cameron,[1] "census figures for 1970 indicate that there are now 20 million persons age 65 and over, or 10 percent of the entire population." Cameron also states that by the year 2000 the number of Americans age 65 and over will probably increase by about 50% for a total of 30 million, and with breakthroughs in the control of heart disease and cancer, and the trend to earlier retirement, an individual may live 30 or more years in retirement.[1]

For most of us the term "elderly" is synonymous with nursing homes, debility, and in-house care. On the contrary, however, only 5% of geriatric patients are nursing home residents. The remainder are either actively caring for themselves or are being cared for by relatives.

Personality and intelligence are remarkably stable in the advanced years. Elderly people would like to talk to someone about the problems they confront with aging, but younger people have a natural aversion to this kind of discussion. As a result, many old persons become withdrawn and resentful and are considered by others to be senile. The same "others" are likely to think that many personal needs, including professional help, are no longer as important to these individuals as they once were, and as a result these needs are pushed to the background. This is obviously an undesirable and unfair situation. One can only hope that the prediction of Mitchell, Standish, and Fast[4] will indeed be realized: "Gerodontics someday in the future may reach the proportions of the practice of pedodontics at present."

Most senior citizens live on limited retirement incomes or are dependent on relatives. Still they frequently desire adequate dental care and feel entitled to it. As they become older and less active, the pleasures of visiting with family and friends and enjoying good food become more and more important to them.

Treatment planning must be approached with special attention in the case of the geriatric patient. While prognosis is an important consideration, it should not necessarily be the all-important one. The ideal treatment must often give way to more practical application. For example, minimum preparation partial dentures may make more sense than intricately designed cast-abutment crowns. If a patient has been happy with his complete dentures for many years, but they are simply worn out, it may be desirable to fabricate duplicate dentures instead of requiring the patient to adjust to completely new dentures.

The oral soft tissue examination is particularly important in the geriatric patient. Since a high percentage of the intraoral malignancies that are discovered occur in patients of middle age and beyond, judicious employment of tissue biopsy becomes an important factor. It has already been mentioned that time is money, and this is true. It is also true that the moral satisfaction derived from serving the public well should be part of the income of every practicing dentist. No other segment of the public is more deserving of this service than those we call the elderly.

SUMMARY

Most of the situations that might arise to challenge the art and science of treatment planning have been or will be dealt with in this book. However, unusual circumstances can still offer surprises, and no one volume can anticipate all of these. The dentist should remain sensitive to the different and unusual and maintain flexibility in developing expertise in treatment planning. To be less than idealistic does not necessarily mean abandonment of basic ideals and principles. Kerr, Ash, and Millard[3] put it this way: "One should keep in mind that alternate treatment plans are not poorer forms of dental treatment, but rather forms of treatment that come as close to the ideal as possible." To show compassion and empathy for the patient, and to be realistic with oneself as well as the patient, will only enhance the dentist's chances for a successful end result.

REFERENCES

1. Cameron, M. J.: Views of aging, Ann Arbor, Mich. 1976, Institute of Gerontology.
2. Clark, J. W.: Clinical dentistry, vol. 1, Hagerstown, Md., 1976, Harper & Row, Publishers.
3. Kerr, D. A., Ash, M. M., and Millard, D. H.: Oral diagnosis, ed. 4, St. Louis, 1974, The C. V. Mosby Co.
4. Mitchell, D. T., Standish, S. M., and Fast, T. B.: Oral diagnosis/oral medicine, ed. 2, Philadelphia, 1974, Lea & Febiger.

PART III

Sequencing, classification, case analysis, and case treatment planning

10

Sequence of treatment and flexibility

Earl E. Sommers
John C. Ebinger

The order in which the treatment plan is completed is an important factor in resolving and managing a patient's disease complex. The sequence in which care is rendered can be the difference between case success or failure, even though the choice and execution of treatment is performed correctly. Therefore the dentist must possess expertise in sequencing treatment.

Patient care that is not completed in the correct sequence can result in one or more of several undesirable situations:

1. Threat to the total health and life of the patient. A situation that can serve as an example is the patient with a damaged heart valve who requires periodontal surgery. Improper management of the heart condition prior to proceeding with the surgery may lead to additional irreversible valvular damage. The damage to the valve may be sufficient to decrease cardiac output, which is a life-threatening situation.
2. Unnecessary discomfort to the patient. Consider a patient with temporomandibular joint pain resulting from an arthritic condition who requires extensive crown and bridge procedures. If the temporomandibular joint problem is not resolved first, the patient will be subjected to prolonged joint pain. The pain from the arthritic condition will be aggravated by the extended periods of mouth opening during the crown and bridge procedure. In addition, the final occlusal relationship will be designed to the specifications of inflamed joints and will change after the joint heals, leaving an unacceptable attempt at rehabilitation.
3. Irreversible destruction of tissue. Consider the patient with a deep carious lesion that is sequenced to be treated following months of periodontal therapy. The carious lesion may expose the pulp and produce irreversible destruction of the pulp prior to completion of the periodontal therapy. Should root canal therapy not be possible, the only

option for treatment of the tooth would be extraction. In this case the loss of the tooth would be a direct result of incorrect sequencing.

4. Failure of treatment. A common example of failure of treatment because of improper sequencing is the placement of a crown restoration on a tooth prior to treating a severe periodontal condition. Should the periodontal therapy prove to be unsuccessful and the tooth need to be removed, then of course the crown is also lost.

5. Lost time for the dentist and patient. Inefficient use of time will occur when all appropriate procedures are not sequenced for the same appointment. An example is the time lost from the dentist placing three simple restorations in the same quadrant on three separate appointments. A much wiser use of time would be to complete all three in one appointment.

6. Financial loss for both dentist and patient. Inefficient use of time becomes a financial loss for the dentist because of the continuous cost of operating a business. The dentist's financial loss is often passed on to the patient in the form of higher fees for the same service. In addition, if patients spend unnecessary time in the dental office, this may mean decreased income because of time off from their employment. The inefficiency and ineffectiveness that result from improper sequencing of patient care create a great deal of frustration and dissatisfaction for the dentist. In addition, the patient's image of the inefficient dentist will be lowered because of the wasteful management of the patient's time and money.

In this chapter, two general goals will be discussed that must be considered while sequencing the care of patients. The first goal is to establish the most ideal sequence to effectively and efficiently restore health and function. This sequence will be called the "biologically ideal" sequence. The second goal is that the sequence must be compatible with the patient's wishes, financial capabilities, and time constraints without jeopardizing the health of the patient (Fig. 10-1).

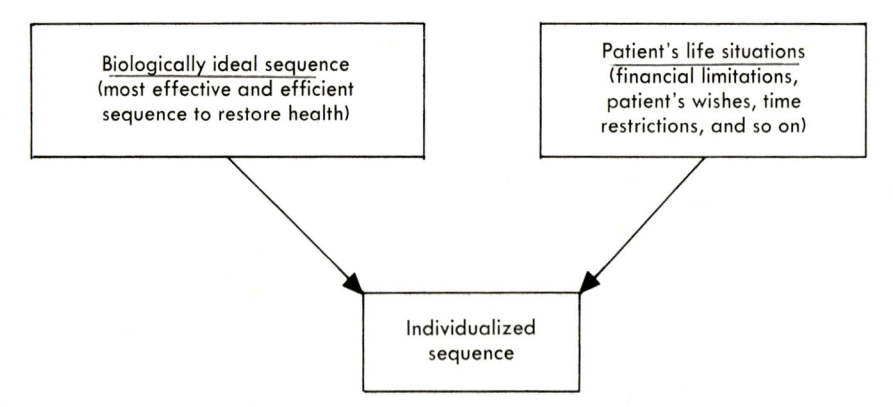

Fig. 10-1. Both sequencing goals (the biologically ideal sequence and the sequence compatible with the patient's life situations) must be carefully considered and the most acceptable sequence for each patient established without jeopardizing the patient's health. A compromise between these two goals is often necessary in order to arrive at an acceptable sequence.

The biologically ideal sequence is the most effective order to follow in efficiently completing a plan for treatment that will restore oral health and function. Essentially, it is the best sequence of treatment to manage the oral and related systemic problems resulting from a pathophysiologic process. This sequence is established without the influence of the patient's wishes, financial capabilities, and time constraints or other modifying factors. More than one sequence may be equally efficient and effective in restoring health and function for a patient. Therefore more than one possible sequence may be biologically ideal. For example, a patient may have several carious lesions of equal severity that require amalgam restorations. In this case all restorations within the same quadrant should be completed at the same appointment for maximum convenience and efficiency. However, it may not make any difference which quadrant is done first. Therefore more than one ideal sequence is possible for this patient.

In order to accomplish the first goal stated above, four general criteria have been established. These criteria state that the sequence of the plan must (1) reflect the relative urgency of each component of the plan, (2) establish an acceptable technical interrelationship of the components, (3) establish convenience for completion of the plan, and (4) enable the dentist to be efficient in completing the plan. These criteria will be discussed in detail later in this chapter.

The second goal mentioned above is to establish a sequence that is compatible with each patient's life situations. As with other health professionals, the dentist comes into contact with many different types of people, each with different life situations. With respect to this great variety of life situations, the dentist must sequence therapy that not only is biologically acceptable but also is suitable for the life situation of each individual. Life situations that may require flexibility of the biologically ideal sequence include patient's wishes, time restrictions, financial limitations, and physical and mental disabilities. Flexibility in this chapter will refer to the ability to make alterations of the biologically ideal sequence that are necessary to accommodate the life situations of the patient without significantly compromising the patient's care. For example, consider the patients whose employment involves direct contact with the public. These patients may have a specific request related to missing, fractured, or discolored anterior teeth. They will often request to have problems such as these resolved first in the sequence. The same patients may have very urgent systemic or dental disease problems that should be managed first or their health will be seriously compromised. The dentist must explain the consequences of treating the aesthetic problem first, and the patient must assume the responsibility for the consequences or the dentist should not treat the patient.

Upon careful consideration of the goals and criteria, three major categories of sequencing may be established. The first, *stabilization*, can be defined as the prevention and elimination of disease. The second, *maintenance and monitoring*, includes periodic evaluation of health and completion of those procedures required to maintain health. The third, *rehabilitation*, is the restoration of normal aesthetics and function. The major part of this chapter will deal with the categorization of the diagnostic, treatment, and management procedures in dentistry according to these three major categories and their subcategories.

CRITERIA FOR THE SEQUENCE

In order to establish the biologically ideal sequence to restore health and function, certain general criteria must be met. These criteria are as follows:

1. The sequence must reflect the relative urgency of each component of the plan for treatment. Urgency is the most important consideration when sequencing those procedures employed to control disease. A systemic problem such as cancer of the vocal cords requires treatment before definitive pocket elimination by periodontal surgery because the latter is less threatening to the health of the patient. Also, a patient with a painful acute pulpitis and an asymptomatic, nonhemorrhagic gastric ulcer should usually receive treatment for the pulpitis before the ulcer. The gastric ulcer is not likely to be an immediate problem, and the patient needs relief from the dental pain. Another important example is treating active caries before fabricating a posterior gold bridge. In this instance the procedures required to manage problems of active disease are more urgent than the management of non-disease-control problems.

2. The sequence must establish an acceptable technical interrelationship among components of the plan. The procedures of the plan must be sequenced so each will technically complement the others, resulting in more efficient and effective care. For example, prophylaxis should proceed application of fluoride because more fluoride can penetrate the tooth when the surface is clean. Also, the root canal should be completed on a tooth before a permanent restoration is placed. If the restoration was placed before the root canal was completed, the access for the root canal would need to be prepared through the restoration, which would weaken it. Another example is that a major occlusal adjustment should be completed before permanent restorations are placed. If a restoration is inserted in a tooth that has a major occlusal prematurity prior to the adjustment, a large portion of the restoration may need to be altered during removal of the prematurity. The result may be that the restoration that was designed for the tooth prior to the modification of the occlusal contours of the tooth may be structurally weakened and need to be replaced.

3. The sequence must establish convenience for the completion of the treatment plan. After the criteria of urgency and technical interrelationship of procedures have been satisfied, the various procedures must be sequenced in an order that will provide the least amount of interruptions to the patient's lifestyle and still allow the dentist to accomplish the therapy in an efficient manner. For example, if more than one amalgam restoration is needed in the same quadrant, it is convenient to sequence all the restorations to be done at the same appointment. However, the dentist must be certain the relative urgency of all caries to be restored for the patient is approximately equal before considering the most convenient sequence to restore the teeth. Another example is if one tooth needs to be extracted and others require periodontal therapy,

it is convenient to remove the tooth first to provide easy access to the adjacent teeth for completion of the periodontal curettage and root planing.
4. The sequence must enable the dentist to be efficient in completing the plan for treatment. The sequence of the plan must enable the dentist to efficiently resolve the patient's problems. However, the efficiency criterion can only be considered after the relative urgency and technical interrelationship criteria have been met. For example, the dentist can be more efficient at completing the restorations outlined in the plan if the periodontium is healthy and does not bleed. Hemorrhage into the preparation from inflamed gingiva makes the placement of a well-sealed restoration difficult. Therefore periodontal therapy to decrease gingival bleeding should be sequenced prior to restorations for nonthreatening caries.

The above guidelines will be described further in the following discussion.

SEQUENTIAL CATEGORIES OF TREATMENT

All of the components of the treatment plan, including diagnostic procedures, treatment procedures, and management, can be placed in one of three categories. These categories represent three separate phases of treatment, and each has a different goal, as outlined below.
1. Stabilization (disease control)
   a. Primary care (control of life- or health-threatening disease)
      (1) Emergency care
         (a) Life-threatening emergencies
         (b) Oral emergencies
      (2) Urgent care
         (a) Management of health-threatening systemic conditions
         (b) Management of threatening oral conditions
         (c) Temporary management of major aesthetic concerns and major functional conditions
   b. Secondary care (control of nonthreatening disease)
      (1) Prevention
      (2) Management of nonthreatening oral disease
      (3) Provisional aesthetic and functional management
      (4) Interim evaluation of therapy and nonthreatening conditions
2. Maintenance and monitoring
3. Rehabilitation
   a. Sequencing rehabilitation procedures
      (1) Establishment of sound supporting structure
      (2) Permanent aesthetic and functional management

Stabilization may be defined as that phase of patient care which includes those procedures required to eliminate, control, and prevent all forms of active disease. In essence, stabilization is the control of disease. The goal for this phase of treatment is to *establish* both oral and systemic *health*.

Maintenance and monitoring begins once stabilization is completed. During this phase of care the systemic and oral health is evaluated and those procedures necessary to maintain the desired level of health are performed. The goal is to *maintain health*.

Rehabilitation may be defined as that phase of patient care which includes those procedures required to restore normal aesthetics and function to areas destroyed by disease or modified by developmental disorders. The goal is to *reestablish normal aesthetics and function in a healthy patient*.

In a plan for patient care these major categories are always performed in a specific order. *Stabilization* is always the first phase of therapy. The dentist must recognize that the procedures in this category are his or her primary responsibility as a health professional. The control of disease (stabilization) is the only phase of patient care that should be viewed with *intense urgency* because it is concerned with halting the destruction from each active disease process. The clinician must design the treatment plan and sequence in a manner that will enable the patient to be stabilized in a rapid and inexpensive manner. *Maintenance and monitoring* begins once the stabilization phase is completed. This is an essential phase of care in which the clinician has the opportunity to monitor each patient's natural host resistance and willingness to maintain his or her health. The patients who are unable to maintain oral health should not be allowed to begin the rehabilitation phase of care because the costly, time-consuming procedures required to restore aesthetics and function will fail because of the ongoing disease processes. *Rehabilitation* is always the last category of care to be performed. The procedures in this category are *elective* and should only be completed for those patients who can demonstrate long-term ability to *maintain* health.

The above sequence of categories should be considered inflexible in order to provide the optimum in oral health care. The interrelationship of these categories is summarized in Fig. 10-2.

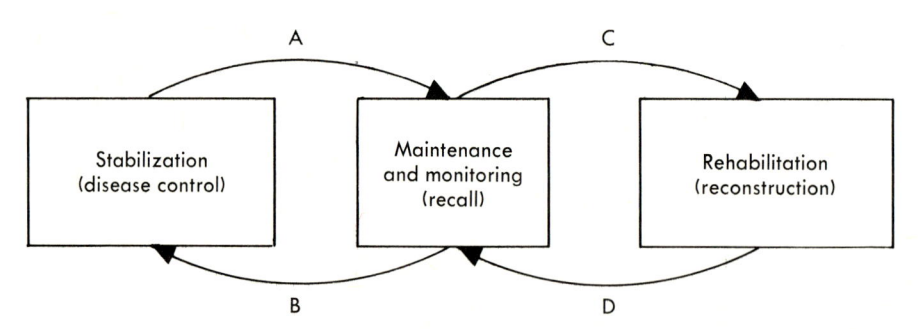

Fig. 10-2. A, Following completion of all procedures in original treatment plan for elimination of disease (stabilization phase), patient is recalled for maintenance procedures and continued monitoring of old and new problems (maintenance and monitoring phase). B, If additional disease is detected at any recall appointment, patient is cycled back into stabilization phase of treatment and then returns to recall phase again, A, for maintenance and monitoring when treatment is completed. C, If patient requires rehabilitation (reconstruction of lost structures), this treatment is completed after patient's mouth has been maintained essentially disease free for one or more years. D, Once rehabilitation phase is completed, patient is continued on periodic recall schedule.

Upon application of the previously described criteria (urgency, interrelationship of procedures, convenience, and efficiency) to each problem or procedure in the major categories of sequencing, a more specific order for care can be established. The remaining portion of this chapter will be devoted to the discussion of the specific sequencing of procedures within each major category. In this discussion each subcategory will be defined, examples of procedures will be given, the rationale for the order will be discussed, and the possibilities for flexibility in the sequence will be considered.

Stabilization

Stabilization may be divided into two arbitrary subcategories—primary care and secondary care. The purpose of making this division is to help establish levels of urgency for the control of disease. In essence, primary care should include those procedures required to control life and health-threatening disease, and secondary care should include the procedures necessary to control nonthreatening disease. Threatening disease may be defined as those problems that, if left unmanaged, may within 4 months cause significant irreversible tissue destruction, pain, infection, or threaten the patient's overall health. Nonthreatening disease may be defined as those problems that should *not* result in the same consequences within 4 months.

PRIMARY CARE

Primary care may be defined as the diagnosis and initial management of threatening disease. In addition, the initial management of urgent aesthetic and functional concerns should be included under this phase of care. Primary care includes those procedures necessary to diagnose and provide initial management of life- and health-threatening problems. It is the most urgent phase of stabilization.

Primary care can be subdivided for the purpose of establishing levels of urgency into emergency care and urgent care.

Emergency care. This phase of primary care refers to the diagnosis and initial management of systemic and oral conditions that are life-threatening or are producing severe pain. In terms of urgency, emergency care takes priority over all other care. The procedures that fall under emergency care are those that should be completed within approximately 24 hours from the time the patient presents to the dentist with a threatening problem.

The procedures and types of problems that should be managed under the emergency phase of primary care may be divided into life-threatening and oral emergencies.

Life-threatening emergencies. Examples of life-threatening emergencies include angina pectoris, thyroid storm, myocardial infarction, anaphylaxis, diabetic coma, and epileptic seizure. The diagnosis and management of each of these problems require the utmost urgency because each can result in loss of the patient's life. The rationale for the need to manage these problems first is obvious. The health professional's primary objective must be to maintain life.

Oral emergencies. Oral emergencies are the diagnosis and management of serious infection, severe pain, and trauma of the oral cavity and surrounding

structures. Following are examples of oral emergencies and their treatment:
1. Drug therapy for a severe infection of a salivary gland
2. Pulpal extirpation for a painful pulpitis
3. Periodontal curettage for a lateral periodontal abscess
4. Extraction of a fractured, painful tooth that has a poor prognosis
5. Reduction of a fracture of the mandible

The problems listed above are potentially life-threatening or are producing severe pain, but do not require the same urgency for care as the life-threatening problems such as myocardial infarction and thyroid storm.

Emergency problems and their management are usually not included in the dental plan for treatment and therefore are not actually sequenced at the time the plan is developed. This is because emergency problems require immediate diagnosis and treatment because of the potential threat to the life of the patient or other serious consequences.

Urgent care. Urgent care may be defined as the diagnosis and management of health-threatening systemic and oral conditions, major aesthetic concerns, and functional conditions. The conditions that should be managed in this phase of primary care require care within approximately 4 months from the time the patient presents to the dentist. Three categories of urgent care may be defined, based on the most important criterion for stabilization—urgency. These are discussed in their order of priority.

Management of health-threatening systemic conditions. The clinician's first responsibility, following emergency care, is to perform the necessary procedures or take the steps required to diagnose or manage health-threatening systemic problems. It should be obvious that such systemic conditions require immediate attention following emergency care because (1) management of the patient's general health usually takes priority over oral problems, (2) treatment of the oral conditions may complicate an existing systemic condition (surgical and emotional stress with dental treatment may precipitate a heart attack in a patient with uncontrolled hypertension), and (3) treatment of oral problems may fail if the systemic problem is not resolved or managed first (periodontal disease is nearly impossible to control in patients with uncontrolled diabetes).

The types of systemic problems that should be managed under this category of primary care are those that are not immediately life-threatening, but could jeopardize the patient's overall health or life in the near future. Examples of such problems are anemia, hepatitis, venereal disease, mild hypertension, and mild hypothyroidism.

Management of threatening oral conditions. Threatening oral conditions should include those oral and paraoral problems that do not require emergency care but should be managed within 4 months. Following are examples of threatening oral conditions:
1. Deep asymptomatic carious lesion approximating the pulp
2. Asymptomatic nonvital teeth
3. Chronic stomatitis
4. Enlarged pericoronal radiolucency around an impacted tooth
5. Bony radiolucencies
6. Neoplasms

The management of these oral conditions usually takes priority over all aesthetic and functional concerns and nonthreatening conditions.

Temporary management of major aesthetic concerns and major functional conditions. The types of aesthetic problems that should be temporarily managed under urgent care are those that cause the patient a great deal of embarrassment, are of concern to the patient for a special social event, or require correction for the patient who must create a good aesthetic impression in his employment. The types of functional conditions that should be temporarily managed in this phase of primary care are those that prevent acceptable speech or mastication.

There is essentially no situation in which any of the procedures of a treatment plan should precede the emergency phase of care. Emergency care requires intense urgency. Within the emergency care phase, systemic problems require management prior to oral problems. Within the urgent phase of primary care, systemic problems usually take priority over oral problems, and oral problems usually take priority over aesthetic and functional conditions. However, some flexibility does exist, again depending upon the relative urgency of the problems. Management of oral problems, whether aesthetic or functional, may proceed or be managed concurrently with a systemic problem if (1) management of the oral problems does not delay necessary management of the systemic problem, (2) management of the oral problems does not complicate the systemic problem, or (3) treatment of the oral problems will not fail if the systemic problem is not resolved first.

SECONDARY CARE

Secondary care may be defined as the management of nonthreatening oral disease and provisional management of nonurgent aesthetic and functional conditions. It also includes interim evaluation of therapy and nonthreatening conditions.

After the dentist has properly sequenced the treatment for the primary care category of problems, he or she must establish a sequence for those procedures required to manage or eliminate the less urgent, chronic intraoral diseases. The secondary care phase of treatment usually involves procedures that require the least amount of time and money for the patient and yet allow the dentist to control or eliminate active disease.

This subcategory is usually the most time-consuming portion of the treatment plan. The majority of dental man-hours are spent attempting to resolve these problems. This phase of therapy can have limitless variations because the profile of asymptomatic intraoral disease varies significantly from one patient to the next. Consequently, establishing hard guidelines for sequencing the individual procedures in this category is difficult. All four criteria (urgency, interrelationships of procedures, convenience, and efficiency) discussed earlier in this chapter should be applied and serve as helpful guidelines for this subcategory.

The procedures required to manage secondary care problems can be divided into four subcategories. These are prioritized below.

Prevention. Prevention includes those procedures required to prevent further destruction of tissue. Preventive procedures should not only be sequenced within the secondary care phase but may also be utilized in any of the three major categories (stabilization, maintenance and monitoring, rehabilitation) as determined by the nature of the problem to be prevented. Following are examples of preventive procedures:

1. Home care instructions to decrease plaque levels
2. Pit and fissure sealants following prophylaxis
3. Counseling the patient for a smoking habit, bruxism, or clenching of teeth, and so on
4. Fluoride treatment following prophylaxis
5. Nutritional counseling

Management of nonthreatening oral disease. This subcategory is usually the most time-consuming of all phases of patient care. The most common and prevalent chronic diseases, caries and periodontal disease, are managed under this phase, in addition to other conditions related to the periodontium and dentition and other chronic oral problems. Following are examples of these problems and procedures:

1. Oral surgery for extraction of teeth with a poor prognosis
2. Management of soft tissue disease such as mucoceles and immune sialosis
3. Temporomandibular joint therapy to include construction of nightguards and administration of antiinflammatory drugs for arthritis of the joints
4. Endodontic treatment for asymptomatic nonvital teeth
5. Prophylaxis, curettage, root planing, removal of restoration overhangs, and minor periodontal surgery for periodontal diseases
6. Occlusal adjustment for significant balancing interference
7. Caries control by use of materials such as amalgam and composite resin

The above examples are arranged in the approximate order in which they should usually be completed. The application of the criteria to this sequence is discussed below.

1. Urgency. Extraction of teeth with a poor prognosis, management of nonvital pulps, management of temporomandibular joint arthritis, and management of immune sialosis should usually be completed before the other problems listed above because any of these problems could result in serious infections and severe pain. Therefore management of this type of problem will usually take precedence over other nonthreatening problems.

2. Interrelationship of procedures. Application of this criterion to the above sequence is demonstrated in the following two examples. First, periodontal therapy was sequenced before the restorations partly because it is much easier to construct well-sealed restorations without gingival hemorrhage resulting from the periodontal disease. Second, the occlusal adjustment was completed before the restorations were placed so that the new restorations could be carved to the correct occlusion.

3. Convenience and efficiency. The teeth with the poor prognosis were removed prior to periodontal therapy. When these teeth are not present, the dentist can more conveniently and efficiently perform the periodontal therapy on the teeth adjacent to the extracted tooth site.

Many exceptions can be cited in which the above general sequencing is not appropriate. For example, consider the following situations:

1. If a patient has numerous failing restorations with large overhangs that prohibit the patient from cleaning these areas, it would be logical to restore the teeth that have overhangs before performing root planing.
2. Consider a patient who has bone loss throughout the mouth and who requires root canal therapy. If the prognosis for the periodontal treatment is questionable, and if there is a possibility that the tooth requiring endodontic therapy is not successful, then the periodontal therapy should be rendered before the root canal is completed.

In sequencing each case, the dentist must apply the criteria and develop the most efficient and effective sequence that will manage the patient's multiple problems.

Provisional aesthetic and functional management. The aesthetic and functional problems that should be managed in the secondary care category of care are those required to establish acceptable aesthetics and function for an extended period of time. The appliances or restorations selected to manage these problems should be those that are the least expensive and that require the least possible amount of time to complete. Even though the restorations and appliances are temporary, they should be designed to be functional for an adequate period of time for the patient to establish and maintain his mouth in a disease-free state. Following are examples of these problems and procedures:

1. Acrylic temporary crown or bleaching for a discolored central incisor
2. Minor tooth movement to correct a single anterior tooth crossbite
3. Fabrication of a temporary partial denture to replace missing posterior teeth where supereruption of the teeth opposing the edentulous space may occur

The dentist must be cautious in utilizing temporary prosthetic appliances because these appliances often create an unhygienic environment that makes it difficult to maintain a disease-free state.

Interim evaluation of therapy and nonthreatening conditions. Because the time needed for the completion of secondary care may be rather lengthy, the evaluation of prior therapy and nonthreatening conditions may need to occur during this category of care. An example of interim therapy evaluation is a 6-week check after nonsurgical periodontal therapy by selected pocket probing, determining plaque levels, and evaluating general tissue health. An example of monitoring nonthreatening conditions is retaking roentgenograms of a bony radiolucency 1 month after it was detected in order to determine if the lesion has changed.

The conditions or therapy to be evaluated during secondary care will not be sequenced according to the four criteria for sequencing, but will be sequenced according to the time interval required for proper monitoring of the treatment or problem. Once the secondary care phase of therapy is completed, the periodic evaluation of therapy and nonthreatening problems will occur during the maintenance and monitoring category of care.

Maintenance and monitoring

Maintenance and monitoring is the second major category of care. As previously described, it is the periodic evaluation of systemic and oral health and the completion of those procedures required to continue the desired level of health.

Following the completion of stabilization, the patient is placed on a systematic recall schedule, which will enable the clinician to evaluate the following:

1. The patient's ability to control disease
2. The effectiveness of the stabilization therapy
3. The prognosis of questionable teeth
4. Problems that only need to be monitored
5. New problems

In addition, the dentist will perform those procedures necessary to *maintain* the desired level of health to include:

1. Prevention procedures such as prophylaxis and topical fluorides, pit and fissure sealants, and so on
2. Oral hygiene reviews

The time intervals and procedures required will vary with the patient's individual needs and abilities to remain stable. For instance, some elderly patients with extensive periodontal defects may require monthly root planing to resist continued periodontal destruction. The usual time lapse between recall appointments is 6 months to 1 year for those patients without special considerations.

For patients who desire rehabilitation therapy, the evaluation period gives the clinician an opportunity to evaluate the long-term ability to remain healthy. There are three reasons why these procedures must only be performed in healthy mouths.

1. The cost and time involved in these procedures can be enormous. Many patients would not be able to afford stabilization if rehabilitation procedures were incorporated into the stabilization phase of therapy.
2. Rehabilitation procedures will fail in unhealthy mouths. These procedures demonstrate their superior characteristics only in healthy mouths.
3. Many rehabilitation procedures add to the difficulty of maintaining oral health. For example, appliances such as the hardware required for orthodontics or large fixed bridges render home care much more difficult to perform.

Sequencing rehabilitation procedures

It is often difficult to establish stringent guidelines for sequencing rehabilitation procedures because there are so many different situations encountered. However, in the majority of cases those procedures required to establish sound supporting structures for the dentition should be completed first and the replacement of tooth structure and teeth should then be completed.

Establishment of sound supporting structures. The establishment of sound support for the dentition is a very important step in the rehabilitation phase. Sound supporting structures are essential to permit success of the remaining procedures under the rehabilitation phase of care. Following is a prioritized list of procedures required to establish sound supporting structures prior to proceeding to aesthetic and functional management.

1. Oral surgery for extraction of third molars and those teeth that did not

respond adequately to the disease control procedures during stabilization.
2. Orthodontics and orthognathic surgery to correctly align the teeth so that masticatory forces are directed parallel to the long axis of teeth. Orthodontics has been sequenced before surgical periodontics because many periodontists prefer to sequence tooth movement before definitive pocket elimination. In some cases osseous defects can be resolved by orthodontics.
3. Surgical periodontics for definitive pocket elimination should be completed prior to replacement of teeth because it is much easier to recontour bone and manage tissue flaps without a complicated prosthesis in the way.
4. Endodontics for those teeth requiring extensive reduction in preparation for crowns, which will encroach upon the pulp. In addition, teeth with insufficient tooth structure remaining to adequately retain a crown will require endodontics so a post can be inserted into the root canal to create the needed retention.

Permanent aesthetic and functional management. Once a sound base has been established, the replacement of tooth structure and teeth may begin. The occlusion must be properly established and stabilized before any permanent restorative procedures are initiated. All single tooth permanent restorations such as full gold crowns, onlays, and porcelain veneer crowns should be completed before replacement of teeth is initiated. The last rehabilitative procedures are those necessary for the replacement of teeth. These procedures include permanent bridges and removable partial dentures.

The main criteria that affect rehabilitation are interrelationship of procedures, convenience, and efficiency. Urgency should never be a consideration because the health of the patient is not dependent on rehabilitation therapy.

11

The simple case

Norman K. Wood
Sol Goldman

In Chapter 4 we have categorized dental cases under the following headings: the simple case, the tooth replacement case, the difficult case, and the transitional case. Early classification of all adult patients along these lines is beneficial because each category of patient represents an entirely different set of problems and thus requires different considerations in treatment planning. This chapter will be devoted to patients in the first category—the simple case.

In order to placate the esoteric academician who declares that there is no such thing as a simple case, it is necessary to explain at the outset that the term simple case in the present context is used in a relative manner only.

WHAT REPRESENTS A SIMPLE CASE?

While admitting that definitions of a simple case will vary considerably from dental practitioner to dental practitioner, depending on their several abilities and points of view, we will lay down some guidelines that should be useful at least as a starting point. First, it must be recognized that a case may be deemed to be simple or complex depending on findings from the various sections of the patient's workup. First let's discuss the clinical findings that delineate the simple case.

Clinical findings

After having gained some clinical experience, it is relatively easy for the dentist to detect those cases whose clinical findings, dictate that the case will be either a tooth replacement case, a difficult case, or a transitional case. These cases are then quickly excluded from further consideration as simple cases, which leaves the adult patient who has a full complement of teeth (except possibly for the third molars) and whose periodontal condition has not progressed far enough to warrant surgical intervention or to cause loss of teeth. The patient's occlusion is judged to be functionally adequate and the aesthetic appearance is generally satisfactory. Caries has not progressed to the point that it is impossible to restore teeth using conventional means. Possibly one or two teeth may need to be crowned. Endodontic treatment may be required on an anterior tooth or two. However, if a nonvital tooth has several canals or other conditions that will render endodontic treatment difficult or questionable, then final decisions on treatment of the whole case will become suddenly more complex. On the other hand, if conditions are ideal, a three-unit bridge might not disqualify the case from being considered a simple case.

Some clinical conditions render simple dental procedures difficult to perform. For instance, frequently the scarring of the lips in scleroderma patients will produce a reduced oral opening. In addition, the tense lip, cheek, and tongue muscles of the nervous patient continually fight against the dentist's fingers and instruments, thus making simple procedures difficult to perform.

Medical considerations

The presence of significant systemic diseases may very well complicate the seemingly simple case and cause its recategorization into the complex or difficult class. For example, patients with a history of myocardial infarction, congestive heart failure, open heart surgery, severe diabetes, hemostatic problems, or prolonged cortisone therapy require physician consultations, careful evaluations, and frequently modification of plans for treatment. Such considerations are detailed in Chapters 5 and 6.

Psychological considerations

The simplest dental procedures may be impossible to implement because of the presence of frank mental illness that renders the patient unable to cooperate. Patient attitudes, although not as dramatic as mental illnesses, also frequently play a deciding role in categorization of cases. Some patients will desire to have all their teeth extracted instead of undergoing treatment to have them restored. Others will prove to be completely retractable to the dentist's efforts to instill a desire to improve their oral hygiene. If such attitudes prevail, then the simple case ceases to be one.

Other considerations

The simplest case (dentally speaking) will rapidly deteriorate into a complex situation if the patient does not possess the financial resources necessary to make satisfactory arrangements for payment of fees. Likewise the situation is complicated if the patient is so busy that he fails to promptly present for his appointments or else fails to appear altogether. Busy executives, physicians, and dentists, as well as individuals who attempt to maintain two or more jobs, often are found in this category.

Case 1. THE SIMPLE CASE

Chief complaint

Mrs. D. is a 43-year-old woman who presents for a periodic dental examination.

Medical history

Mrs. D. enjoys remarkably good health. She currently has no significant symptoms or illnesses that she is aware of. She was hospitalized three times for normal deliveries of her three children. Her only other hospitalization was for an appendectomy 15 years ago.

Social and family history

Mrs. D. denies taking drugs of any kind and does not use alcohol or tobacco. She is not aware of any disease being prevalent in her family.

Past dental history

Mrs. D. has been visiting a dentist regularly since early childhood, except she has missed the last 2 years because of the family's move to South America. Her teeth erupted into satisfactory position both functionally and aesthetically, so orthodontic work was not required. During adolescence she experienced quite a few cavities and received fillings for them, but since then has only required a few fillings placed. Eight years ago she had the upper left second molar (tooth 15) removed because of a pulpitis that developed after a rather deep filling was placed. Unfortunately, endodontic treatment was not feasible because of a rather severe dilaceration of one of the roots. A three-unit bridge was constructed to replace tooth 15.

At about age 30 she began to experience gum problems. At age 37 she underwent periodontal surgery on all posterior quadrants and since has tried to improve her home care. She arranges to have her teeth cleaned and scaled professionally every 6 months.

Attitudinal considerations

Mrs. D. is a happily married housewife who is active in one or two selected religious and community projects. Her husband is an officer at a bank and draws an annual wage of $30,000. The D.'s have three children. The oldest daughter is 24 years old and happily married. The son is 20 years of age and attends the state university. The youngest daughter is 17 years old and a senior in high school. All members of the family are happy and seemingly well adjusted. The importance of good dental care has been stressed in the family, and Mrs. D. has attempted to maintain a semblance of oral hygiene. Now she is quite concerned about her worsening periodontal problem and is anxious for professional advice on how to improve her oral hygiene as well as for treatments to improve the condition of her gingiva.

Clinical findings

The clinical examination of her neck, face, and oral cavity revealed no soft tissue or bony lesions except for a benign hyperplastic node in the left submandibular area and a periodontal condition. Jaw excursions were found to be within normal limits, and no joint noises or muscle or joint pain were elicited during the jaw movements. The saliva appeared to be normal in both quality and quantity.

Mild to moderate periodontal disease was found to be generalized (Fig. 11-1). Bone loss was basically horizontal in nature and slightly more advanced in the posterior regions (Fig. 11-2). None of the teeth were mobile, but 2 to 3 mm gingival pockets were present around the posterior teeth and a 4 mm pocket was present at the distal surface of tooth 14.

All teeth were present except for tooth 15. A three-unit bridge utilizing full gold crowns as abutments is in position replacing tooth 15 (Fig. 11-1). The bridge appeared adequate, and recurrent decay was not detected around these crowns.

New or recurrent decay was found in teeth 2, 3, 5, 6, 7, 8, 13, 19, 20, 28, 29, 30, and 32. Caries on teeth 2 and 3 appear quite deep roentgenographically (Fig. 11-2).

An occlusal analysis revealed a class 1 occlusion with excellent cuspal relationships in the usual jaw excursions. Prematurities were minimal. The clinical findings are charted in Fig. 11-3.

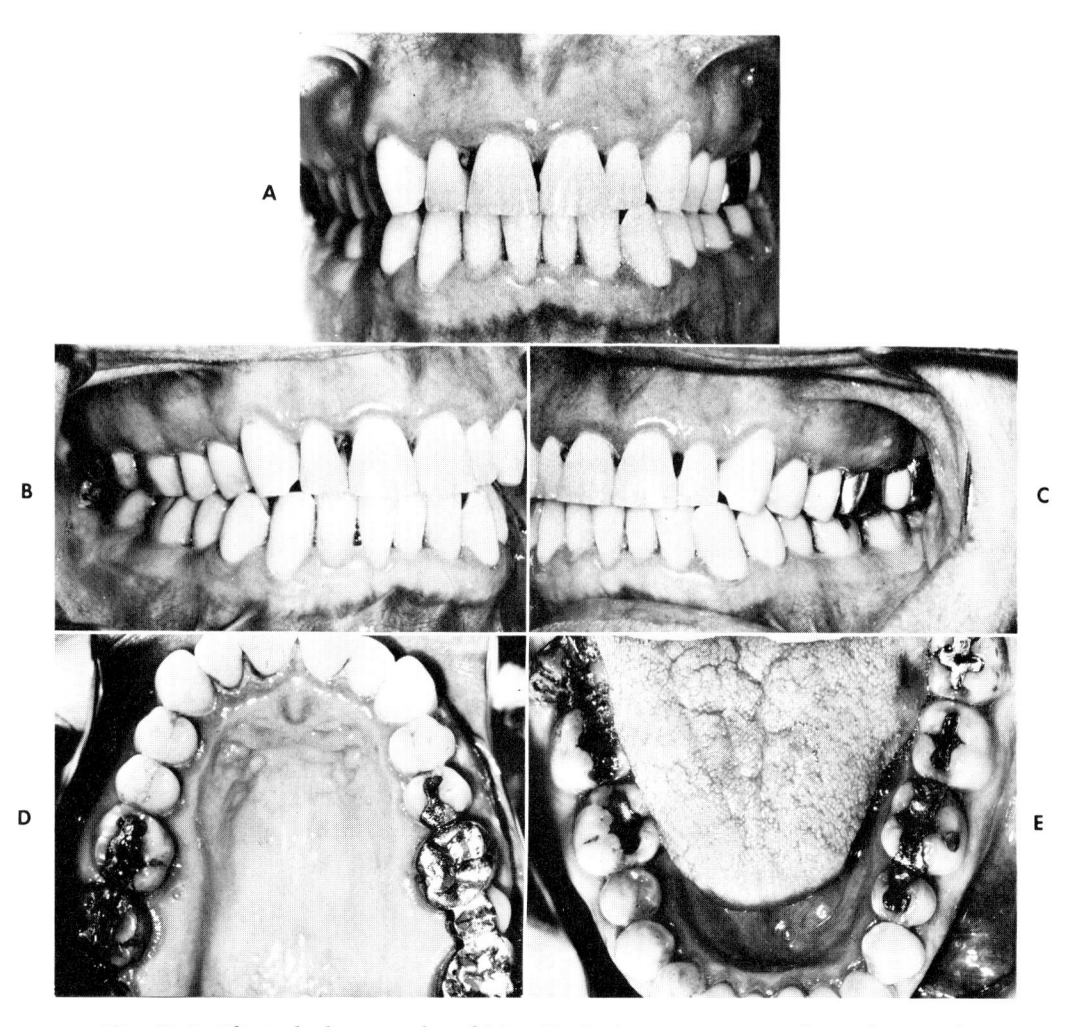

Fig. 11-1. Clinical photographs of Mrs. D. **A**, Anterior view with teeth in occlusion. **B**, View of right side. **C**, View of left side. **D**, Occlusal view of maxillary arch. **E**, Occlusal view of mandibular arch.

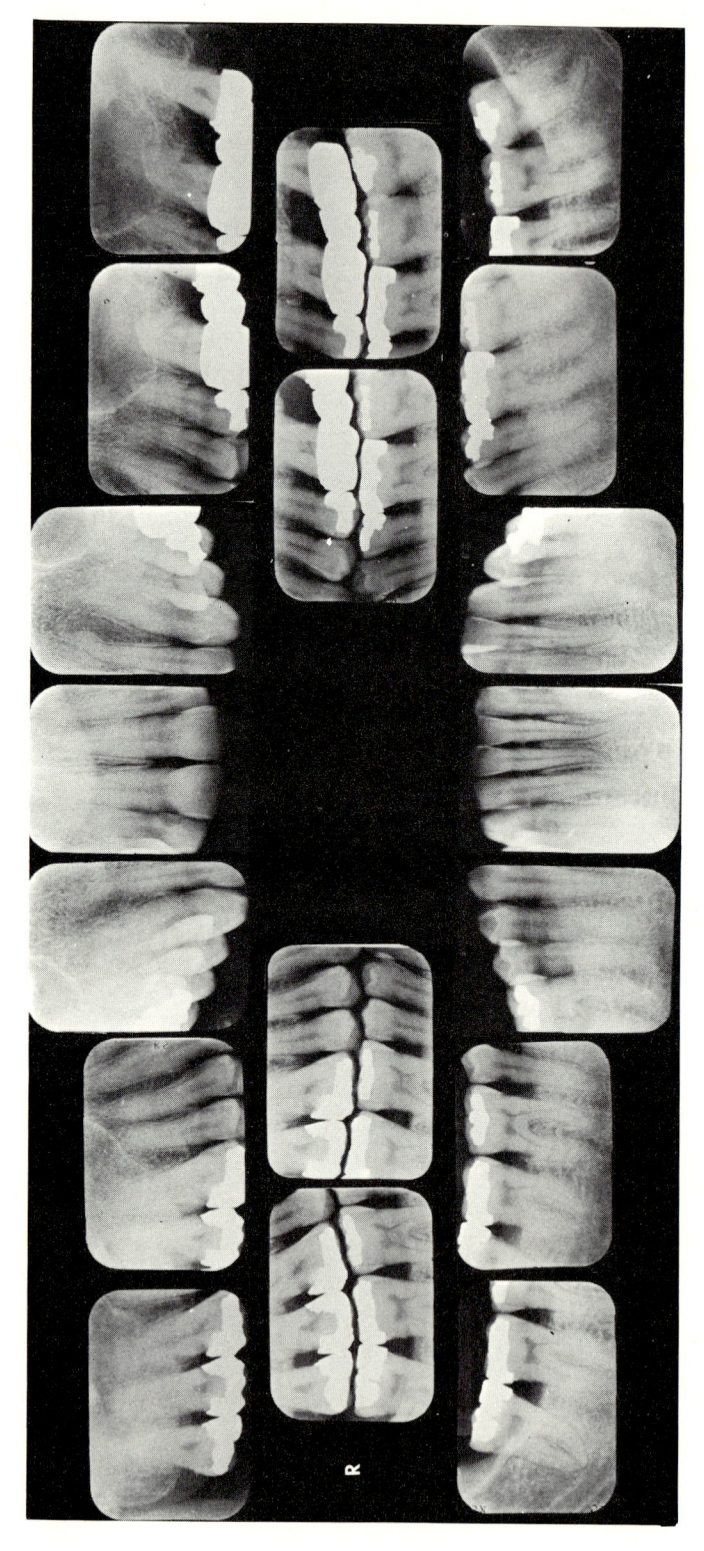

196 *Sequencing, classification, case analysis, and case treatment planning*

Fig. 11-2. Full-mouth roentgenograms of Mrs. D.

The simple case 197

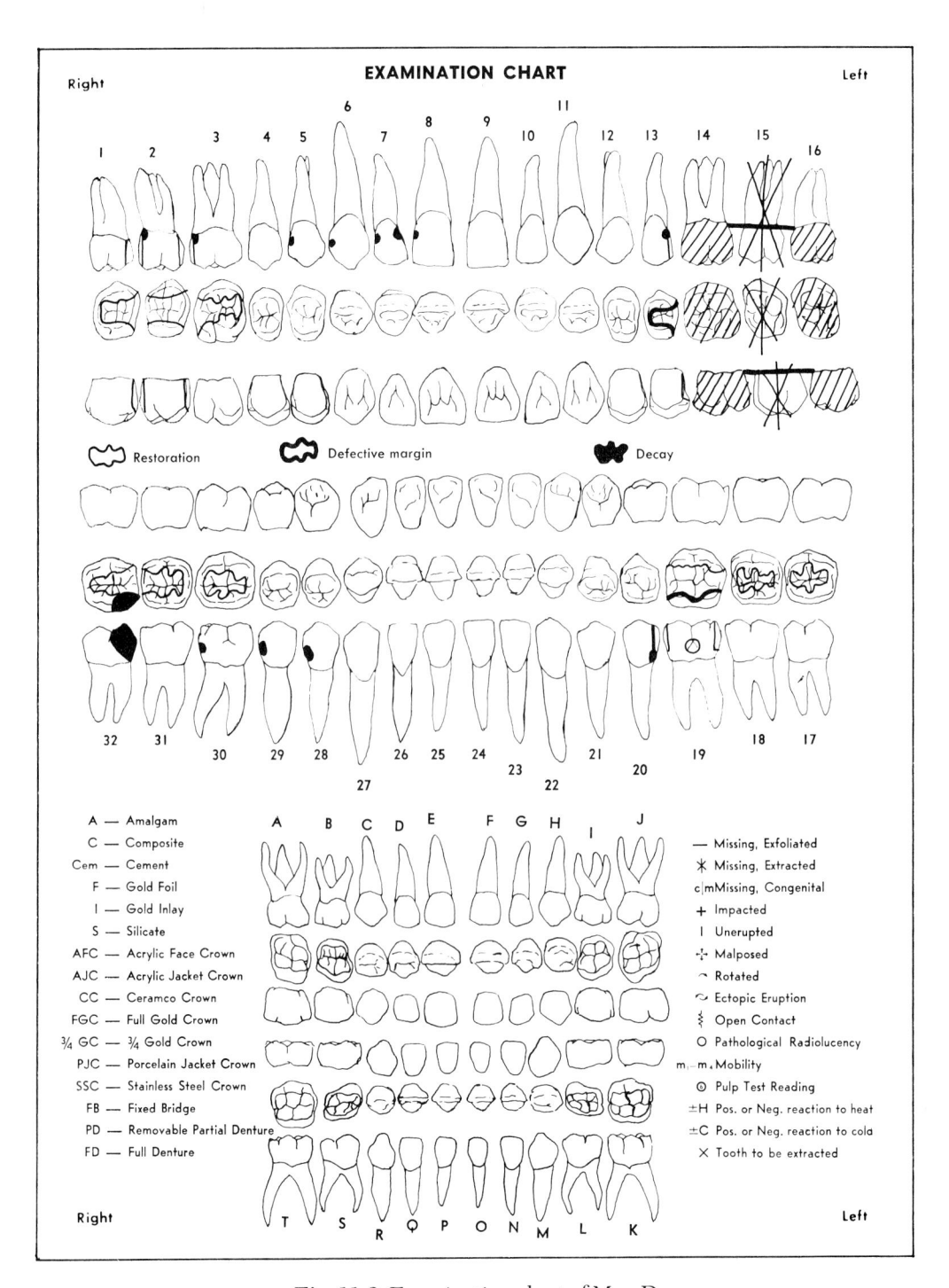

Fig. 11-3. Examination chart of Mrs. D.

Diagnostic summary

1. Mild to moderate periodontitis
2. Twelve carious teeth requiring restorations (Caries is deep in teeth 2 and 3.)

Prognosis

Prognosis is moderately good to good, depending on Mrs. D.'s degree of success regarding home care.

Treatment plan

Summary

1. Home care instruction and reinforcement
2. Periodontal therapy
3. Restoration of the 12 carious teeth
4. Periodic reexamination (maintenance and monitoring)

Rationale

The treatment approach to most simple cases is usually straightforward and the options so limited that a discussion is unwarranted. In discussing details of the treatment plan, we will follow the outline presented in Chapter 10 for sequencing of treatment.

Sequencing

STABILIZATION: PRIMARY CARE. Because no systemic or oral emergencies are present in this case, urgent care is the first category to require attention. There are no known threatening systemic conditions, and so we move directly to consideration of urgent care for the management of threatening oral conditions. In this case the deep carious lesions in teeth 2 and 3 represent threatening oral conditions and need urgent care. The MOD and DO amalgam fillings should be removed in these teeth along with the recurrent decay, preferably under a rubber dam. If a small pulpal exposure is experienced, the pulp should be capped with calcium hydroxide, which in turn should be covered with I.R.M. cement. The cavity should then be filled totally with a temporary cement or a permanent amalgam restoration. If an acute pulpitis ensues, a vital extirpation should be done as soon as possible.

STABILIZATION: SECONDARY CARE. Prevention at the secondary level (see Chapter 7) is the next step to program into the treatment plan. The following procedures are indicated in this order:

1. Detailed home care instruction, including follow-up evaluation and reinforcement (The patient is to be given special instructions concerning floss, needles, and the importance of flossing carefully around the bridge.)
2. Prophylaxis followed by fluoride treatments
3. Dietary analysis and counseling

Management of nonthreatening oral disease will involve minor occlusal adjustment through selected grinding, extensive therapeutic root planing, and restorative dentistry. All the teeth will require extensive therapeutic root planing with special attention given to the deeper pockets around the bridge abutment of tooth 14. This phase of treatment should be completed prior to the restorative procedures for at least two reasons: (1) it will be easier to visualize the interproximal seat areas after the swollen gingiva has regressed to normal size, and (2) the likelihood of gingival bleeding into the cavity will be greatly reduced.

As a general rule, when all emergency and urgent caries are cared for, the remaining restorative procedures should be done by quadrant. In Mrs. D.'s case the distal caries in tooth 29 is by far the deepest cavity remaining. Thus the right lower quadrant should be done first. This would include DO amalgams in teeth 28, 29, and 30, as well as a rather large MOD amalgam in tooth 32. Arbitrarily, the DO amalgam on tooth 13, the MOD amalgam on tooth 19, and the DO amalgam on tooth 20 could be completed during one appointment. During the last restorative appointment, composites on teeth 7 and 8 (mesial and distal on tooth 7 and distal on tooth 8) are to be placed. Finally, all the amalgam restorations should be finished and polished at least 24 hours after their insertion.

MAINTENANCE AND MONITORING. Mrs. D. should now be placed on a 3-month systematic recall schedule, particularly to evaluate her home care program. The periodontal condition on tooth 14 should be carefully checked, as should also questionable teeth 2 and 3, which have been pulp-capped. If these are asymptomatic and Mrs. D. is maintaining good oral hygiene, she should be placed on a 6-month recall schedule.

REHABILITATION PHASE. If during the next 6-month period Mrs. D. has demonstrated that she has brought her periodontal disease and caries activity under control, consideration might be given to placing an MOD gold overlay on tooth 32 because of the large size of the amalgam. Also, if root canal therapy has been done on teeth 2 and 3 previously, consideration should be given to placing gold overlay restorations on these teeth in order to protect these pulpless teeth from fracture.

12

The interdisciplinary tooth replacement case

Charles H. Boozer
Ronald A. Barrett
James W. McGuiness
Norman K. Wood

Tooth replacement cases represent a very significant percentage of the general practitioner's patients. These cases are much more complex than the simple case and are often downright perplexing because there are frequently several modes of treatment possible. The different modes of treatment include the fixed bridge, the removable partial denture, and the full denture. Several questions must be addressed: Is the edentulous space adequate for a tooth replacement? Are the abutment teeth adequate to support the tooth replacement? What is the patient's attitude toward the replacement? Does the patient's oral hygiene and dental IQ indicate a continuing satisfactory treatment result?

It is especially important in tooth replacement cases to follow the sequencing order detailed in Chapter 10. Following this outline, disease control (stabilization) must be attained prior to initiating extensive rehabilitative treatment. If disease control can be established, then the patient enters the maintenance and monitoring stage in which the dentist continues to evaluate his or her oral hygiene efforts as well as the tissue reaction to treatment. If the patient passes this inspection, then the rehabilitative phase may be commenced. However, if the patient fails to maintain good oral hygiene, he must be rerouted through the disease control stage. If the patient again fails to maintain satisfactory hygiene, the extensive costly rehabilitative work is not commenced.

Routine examination includes panorex, full-mouth roentgenograms, serology, hematology, urinalysis, serum biochemistry, health questionnaire, narrative medical and dental history, vital signs, examination of head and neck, soft tissue, periodontium, occlusion, and teeth. Only those findings pertinent to the case are described. The following tooth replacement cases are presented for the purpose of illustrating the extent and degree of oral disease and the decisions and measures necessary to restore function and aesthetics.

Case 1. UTILIZATION OF FIXED BRIDGES

Chief complaint

Miss W., a 35-year-old woman, presents saying, "I need some teeth replaced."

History of present illness

Miss W. has received minimal sporadic dental care over the past few years. Treatment included extractions, restorations, and occasional prophylaxis.

Past medical history

The patient states that she is in good health and has no serious illnesses. Responses to the health questionnaire revealed no significant findings except the continual use of oral contraceptives of 10 years duration. Routine laboratory tests revealed an elevated, 2-hour, postprandial serum glucose level of 145 mg/100 ml, which would be suggestive of a diabetic condition. The laboratory results were transmitted to her physician, who confirmed the presence of mild diabetes by a more definitive analysis. Treatment instituted at this time was diet, weight reduction, and discontinued use of oral contraceptives.

Social and family history

Miss W. is a single white female who denies the use of tobacco and drugs. She admits to being an occasional social drinker. The patient is a schoolteacher who supported her mother until her mother died several months ago.

The patient states that her father died of a heart attack 9 years ago. Her mother died of complications resulting from diabetes and heart disease.

Past dental history

Significant findings in her dental history were mentioned above in the history of present illness.

Attitudinal considerations

Miss W. is an intelligent woman who is quite interested in her appearance and well-being. She dresses well, and her finances are quite adequate. Besides earning a reasonably good salary, she has inherited a substantial amount of money from her mother's estate just recently. Although she has never received oral hygiene instruction, her home care is moderately good. At this time she is quite interested in maintaining her teeth and requests that she be given detailed professional oral hygiene instruction.

Clinical findings

Extraoral examination revealed no significant findings. Intraoral soft tissue examination revealed mandibular lingual tori; all other areas were within normal limits (Fig. 12-1). The gingiva was found to be red, slightly edematous, and to bleed upon manipulation. Pseudopockets were found in several areas because of the edematous condition. Minimal calculus and slight staining were evident in the mandibular anterior region.

Examination of the occlusion revealed that tooth 1 was displaced buccally and extruded. Teeth 18 and 31 were supraerupted, tooth 29 was rotated 90°, and clearance was minimal in the right tuberosity area. Roentgenographically, several proximal carious lesions and defective restorations were observed. Bone trabeculation was normal (Fig. 12-1). The intraoral findings are illustrated in Fig. 12-2.

Diagnostic summary

1. Mild diabetes controlled without medication
2. Gingivitis
3. Missing teeth 2, 3, 13, 14, and 16
4. Supraerupted teeth 18 and 31

Prognosis

1. Diabetes—good
2. Gingivitis—good
3. Rehabilitation—good except for tooth 18

Treatment plan
Rationale

The treatment plan decisions in this case are rather straightforward without many realistic options. It might be wise to maintain tooth 18 by attempting occlusal reduction of the crown after doing endodontics, but its rather severe degree of supraeruption makes this rather difficult. Also, the tooth at present does not have an antagonist. However, if it could be retained, it might become useful in the future as a posterior abutment.

Sequencing

1. Oral hygiene instruction, scaling, and prophylaxis combined with medical correction and supervision of the diabetic condition should return the gingiva to health.
2. Extraction of tooth 18 because of extrusion and lack of an antagonist.
3. Surgically increase clinical crown on tooth 1 in combination with a tuberosity reduction.
4. Root canal therapy on tooth 1 because of extrusion and for the purpose of obtaining pulpal clearance for preparations.
5. Routine single-tooth restorations as indicated (e.g., tooth 31—crown).
6. Fixed prosthetic replacement for missing teeth 3 and 14.

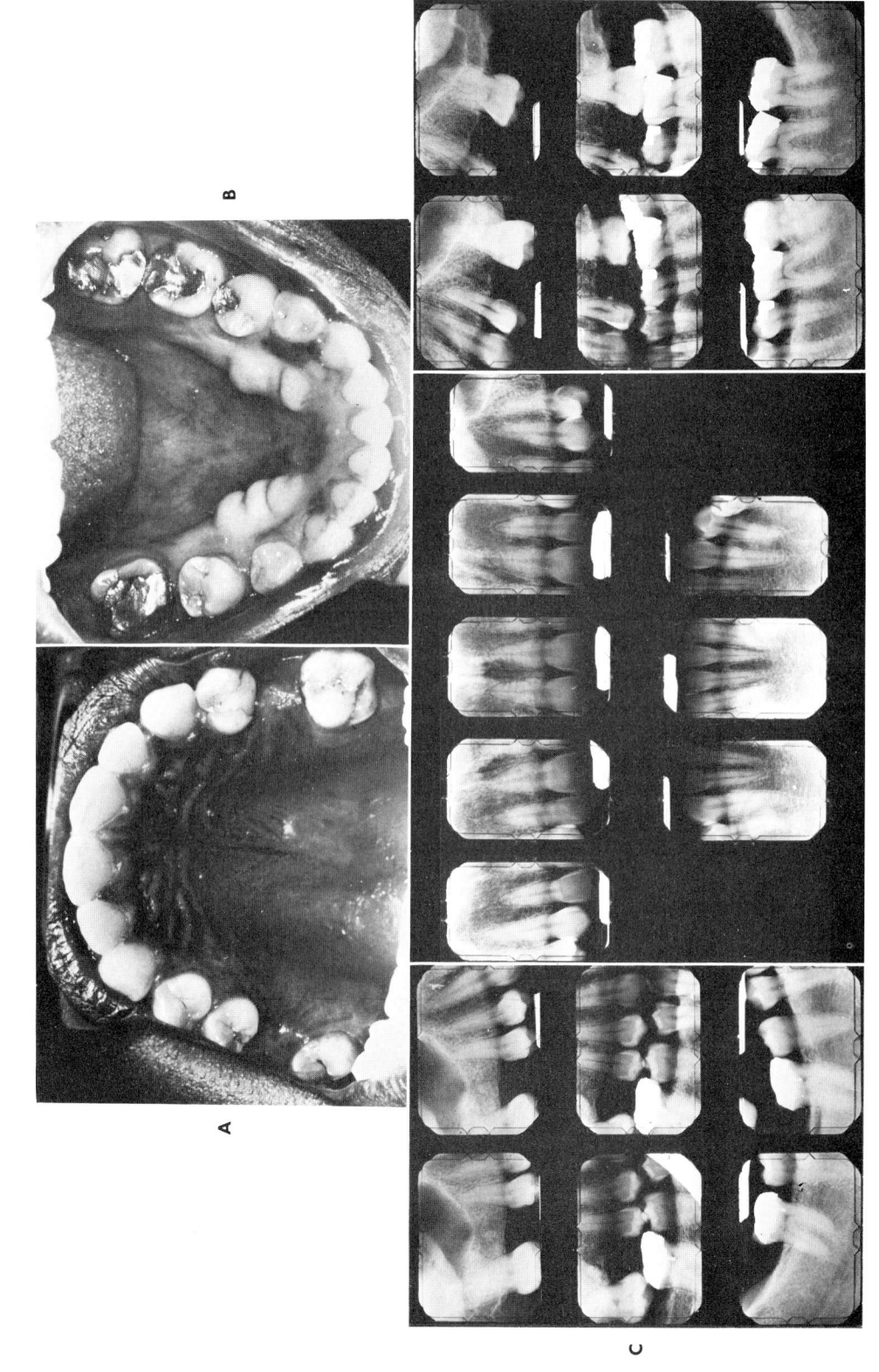

The interdisciplinary tooth replacement case 203

Fig. 12-1. Case 1. Fixed-bridge case. **A**, Occlusal view of maxillary arch. **B**, Occlusal view of mandibular arch. **C**, Full-mouth roentgenograms.

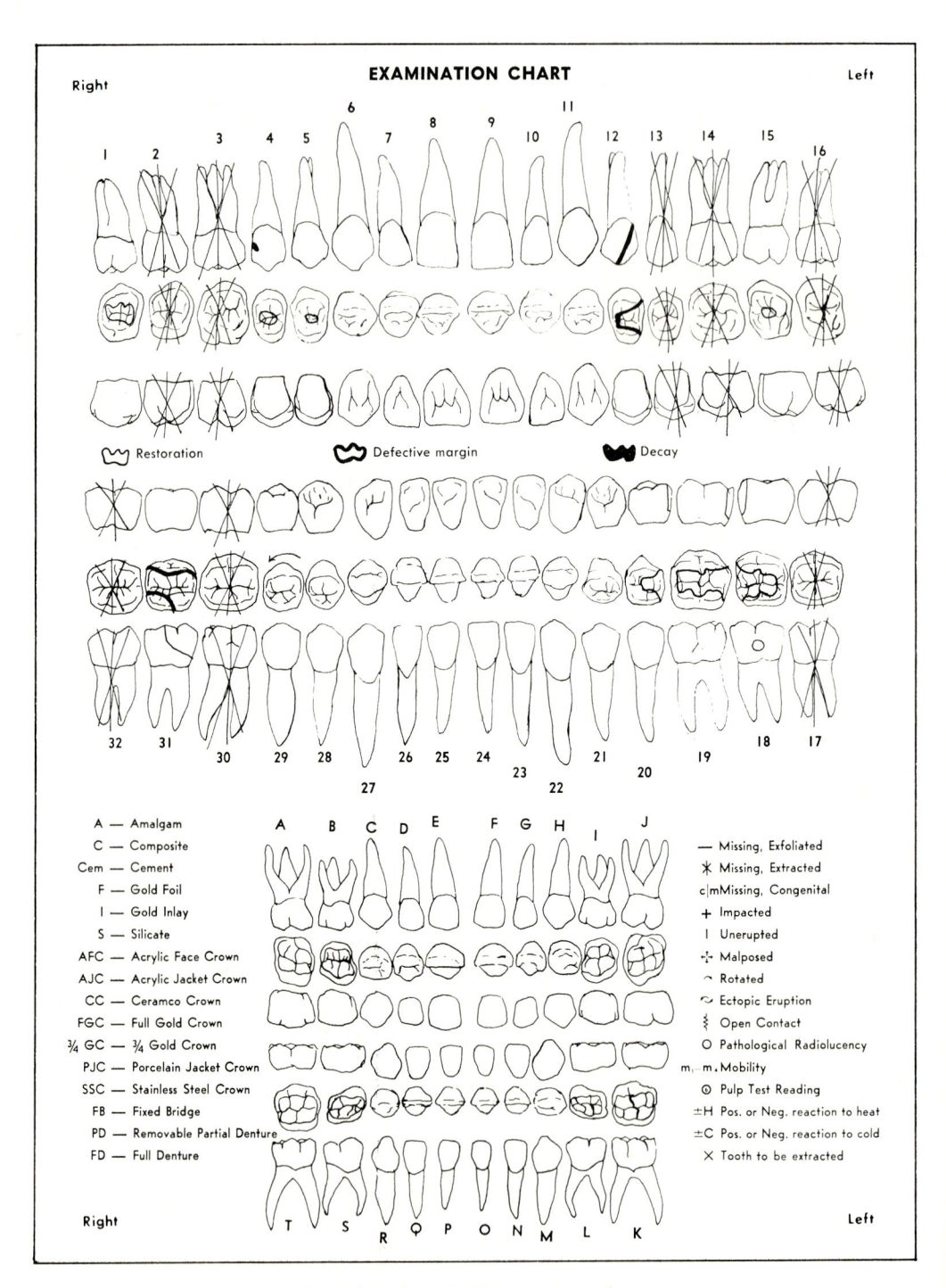

204 *Sequencing, classification, case analysis, and case treatment planning*

Fig. 12-2. Case 1. Examination chart.

Case 2. UTILIZATION OF PARTIAL DENTURES

Chief complaint

Mr. T., a 49-year-old man, presents to have his teeth "all fixed up because some of them were getting loose and sometimes hurt."

History of present illness

Mr. T. has been aware for some time that he has periodontal disease and knows that if he does not attend to the problem he will eventually lose all of his teeth. More recently, however, the upper left canine and an upper left molar have been giving him considerable pain.

Past medical history

Mr. T. states that he currently enjoys good health, has no systemic diseases, and is unaware of any symptoms that would suggest their presence. He was hospitalized only once following an automobile accident in 1942 and then only for observation. He admits to having had mumps and chickenpox as a child. He is not taking any medication at present. He visits his physician yearly for a regular examination.

Social and family history

Mr. T. states that his grandfather died of diabetes and that his father is currently being treated for this disease. He denies knowledge of any other inheritable diseases in the family tree. He has never been in close contact with a person who had hepatitis and has never contracted a venereal disease.

Mr. T. admits to smoking about one-half pack of cigarettes per day but does not use alcoholic beverages at all.

Past dental history

Mr. T. received regular dental care as a child and teenager. Unfortunately he had a relatively high caries rate and usually required a considerable number of fillings at an early age. Mr. T. used to brush very vigorously with a hard brush in a horizontal direction and produced some deep abrasive lesions at the gingival margins of several teeth. However, he was properly instructed on brushing technique and subsequently discontinued the destructive horizontal stroke and also changed to a softer brush. In his early thirties, when he was concentrating on his career development, there was a space of 2 years when he failed to present for his periodic examination appointments. The next time he presented the dentist found that decay was so deep on tooth 31 that the tooth had to be extracted. Also, it was noted that gum disease was present, and since that time he has been undergoing treatment for his periodontal disease. He became so discouraged because of failure of treatment and high cost that 5 years ago he discontinued regular dental care and requested dental care only when he needed teeth extracted. Tooth 32 was the last one extracted.

Attitudinal considerations

Mr. T. was taught by his parents to appreciate his teeth. However, he became discouraged over the years because of the continued decline of his dentition and also because of the high cost of dental care. Recently, Mr. T's financial position has improved remarkably because his two children are now self-supporting and also because he has gained an excellent promotion at work and thus has experienced a handsome raise in salary. Because Mr. T. begins work at 6 AM, he is available for dental appointments at 3 PM on most weekdays. He is now very interested in making a new beginning as far as his teeth are concerned and promises to follow home care instructions *to the letter.*

Clinical findings

The findings during the face and neck portion of the examination were basically within normal limits. A firm, freely movable, enlarged "node" was found in the right submandibular region (working diagnosis was "benign lymphoid hyperplasia").

The oral soft tissue examination (gingiva excluded) also revealed findings that were within normal limits. A moderate degree of leukoedema was observed on the buccal mucosa bilaterally.

Surprisingly, inflammation of the gingiva, although generalized, was only moderate in degree (Figs. 12-3 and 12-4). Bogginess and recession was particularly evident in the anterior region. Pocket depths of 6 to 8 mm were pres-

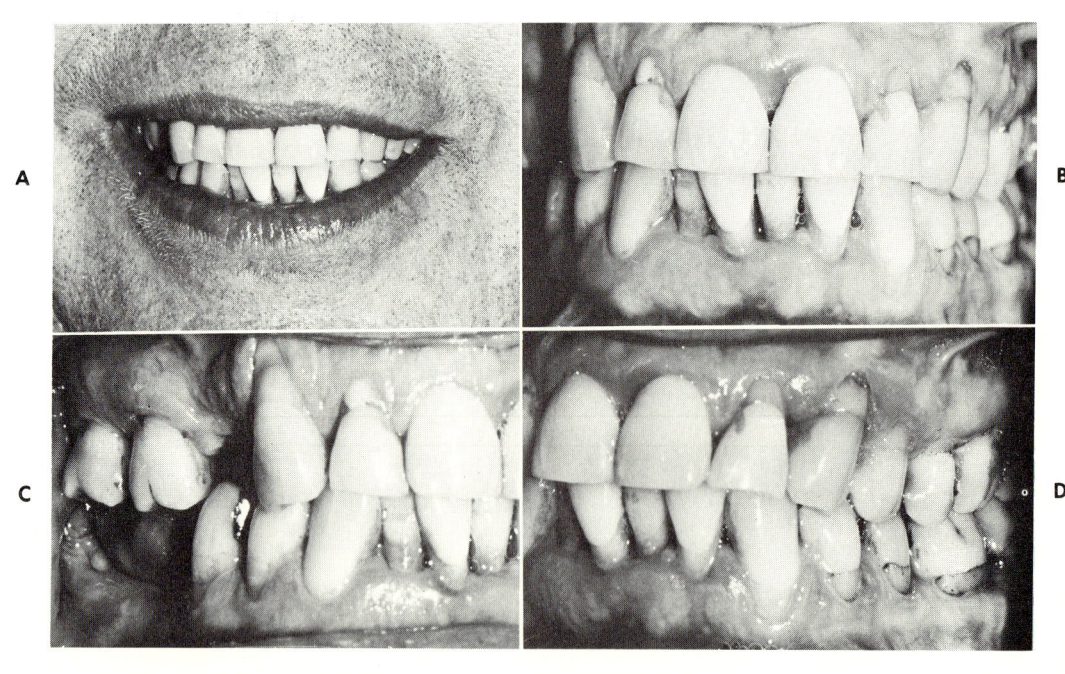

Fig. 12-3. Case 2. Partial denture case. **A,** Appearance of teeth with patient smiling. **B,** Anterior view with teeth in occlusion. **C,** View of right side. **D,** View of left side.

ent around the four mandibular incisors and the maxillary left molars. A 5 mm pocket was identified at the mesial surface of tooth 18. Pockets of 2 to 3 mm could be probed around the remainder of the teeth. Teeth 15, 16, 23, 24, 25, and 26 were very mobile. Abundant subgingival calculus could be visualized roentgenographically on all teeth (Fig. 12-5).

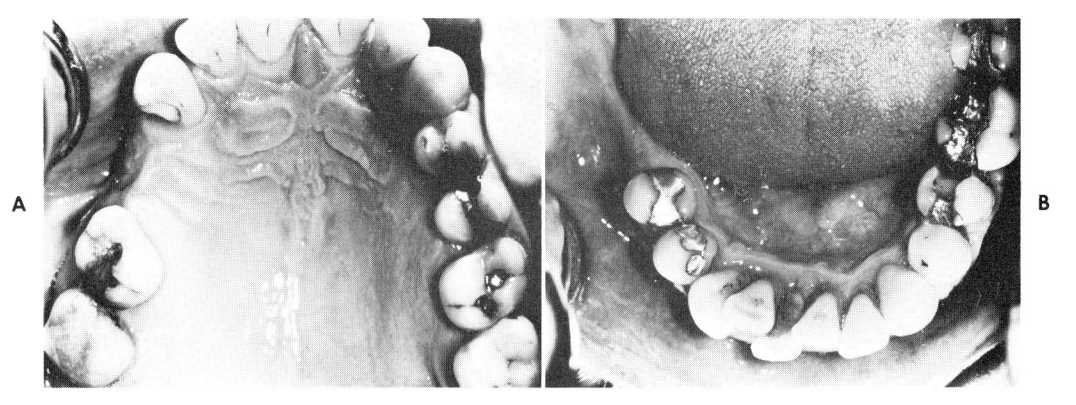

Fig. 12-4. Case 2. **A**, Occlusal view of maxillary arch. **B**, Occlusal view of mandibular arch.

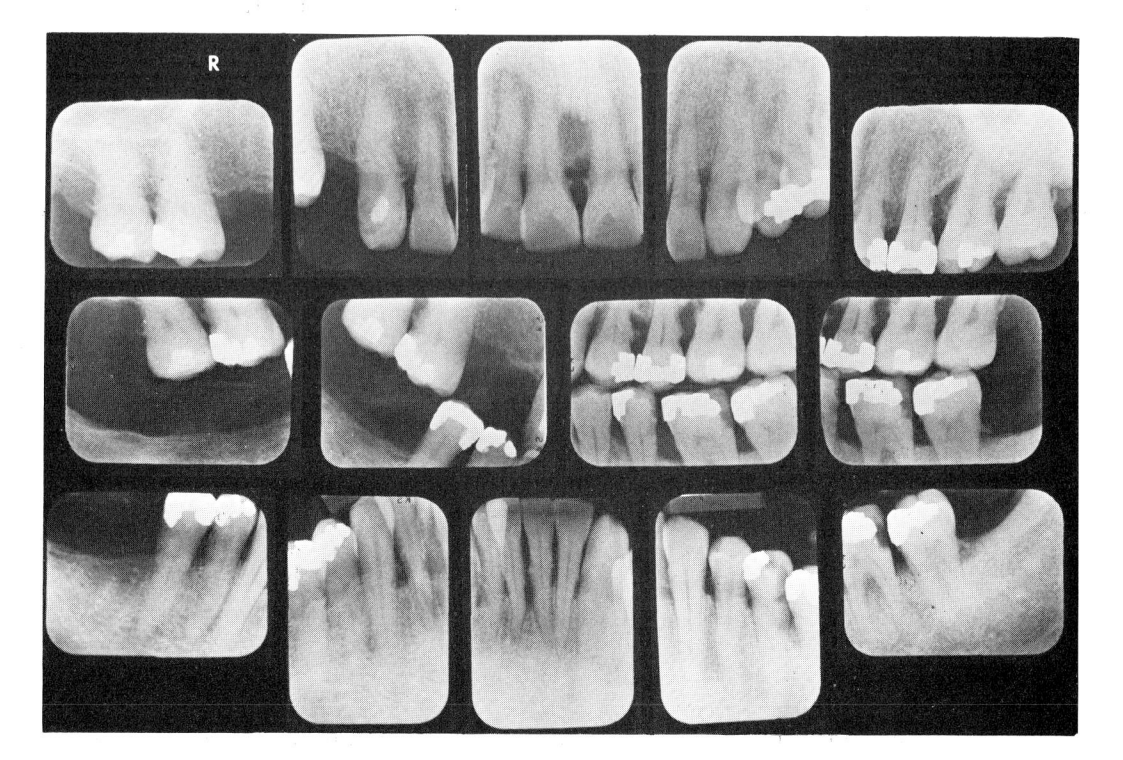

Fig. 12-5. Case 2. Full-mouth roentgenograms.

Present restorations in the teeth have been charted in Fig. 12-6. New decay was found on tooth 20. Recurrent decay was found around restorations in teeth 6, 7, 11, 15, 17, 18, 21, and 22. Part of a filling was lost on tooth 18. A clean, deep, erosive class 5 lesion was found at the buccal surface of tooth 13. A radiolucency with poorly defined borders was seen at the apex of tooth 11 in the roentgenograms; this tooth tested nonvital. The arch form, occlusion, and position of the remaining teeth all proved to be within normal limits.

Diagnostic summary

1. Patient in good health
2. Attitude presently very favorable
3. Extensive periodontal involvement
4. Much restorative work necessary replacing fillings
5. Edentulous spaces present; extraction of more teeth necessary

Prognosis

1. Hopeless for teeth 13, 15, 16, 23, 24, 25, and 26
2. Guarded for tooth 18
3. Moderately good to good for remainder of the dentition

Treatment plan
Summary

1. Extraction of teeth 13, 15, 16, 23, 24, 25, and 26
2. Extensive periodontal therapy on remainder coupled with home care instruction
3. Endodontic treatment of tooth 11
4. Much restorative work, including crowns on teeth 6, 12, and 29
5. Maxillary and mandibular partial dentures

Rationale

At first glance it might seem overly optimistic to plan for any extensive treatment procedures for Mr. T. in light of his rather poor track record. However, in light of Mr. T.'s recently improved attitude, apparent remotivation, and improved financial circumstances, it seems very appropriate to give Mr. T. the opportunity of restoring to health many of the remaining teeth. Of course, he will have to prove that his home care is quite satisfactory before the greater part of the work is commenced.

When a partial denture is being considered in an arch, it is always wise to condemn teeth for which the short-term prognosis is poor. In this regard we have chosen to condemn tooth 13 because of its rather poor bone support on the distal surface and its unfavorable root shape. It seems quite certain that this tooth would not last long as an abutment tooth. On the other hand, it was anticipated that tooth 18 would respond to periodontal surgery, and so it was not programmed for extraction.

Because of the anterior drifting of teeth 1 and 2, the edentulous span between these teeth and tooth 6 seems short enough for a bridge. However, in light of the fact that a partial denture would be required to replace teeth 13, 14, and 15, it was decided to make a bilateral partial instead of a bridge and a

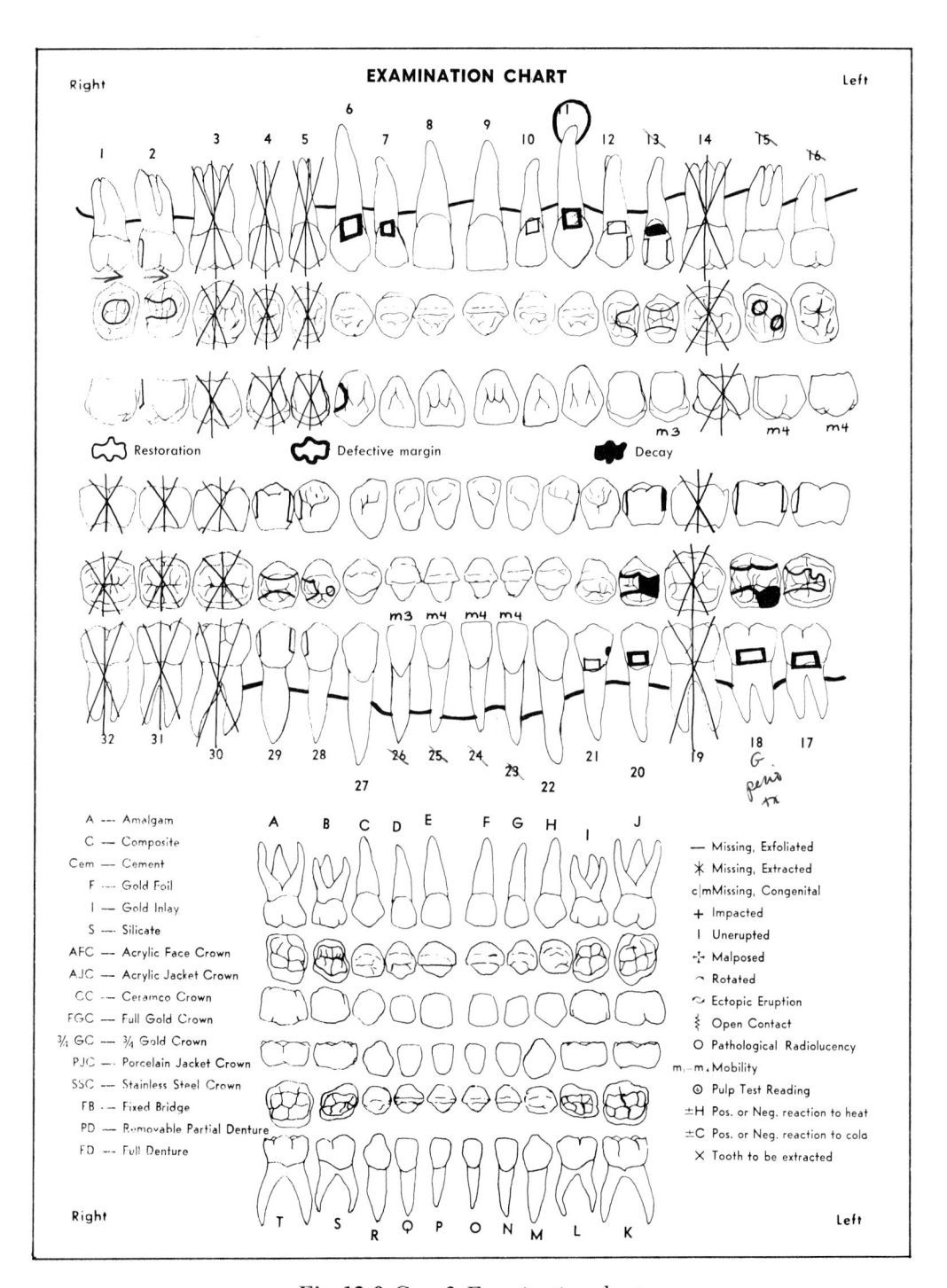

The interdisciplinary tooth replacement case 209

Fig. 12-6. Case 2. Examination chart.

unilateral partial. Also, it was thought that a fixed bridge would greatly complicate home care efforts and would quite likely discourage Mr. T.

Sequencing

It is crucial in a case like this to follow the sequencing order outlined in Chapter 10. It is essential to establish disease control in such a patient and to observe the patient's efforts in maintaining good oral hygiene before extensive restorative and replacement procedures are commended. In other words, the patient must prove that he is maintaining his mouth in a disease-free state during the monitoring period.

STABILIZATION (DISEASE CONTROL). As there are no life-threatening emergencies or real oral emergencies in this patient's case, the category of urgent care should be attended to first. This would include the following procedures in the suggested order.
1. Extraction of teeth 13, 15, and 16
2. Temporary MOD amalgams on teeth 18 and 20
3. Endodontic treatment of tooth 11

After the urgent care is given, the following procedures should be carried out to effect disease control.
1. Instruction and reinforcement of home care
2. Extensive therapeutic root planing on all remaining teeth
3. Periodontal surgery on tooth 18
4. The following teeth restored by quadrant: 7, 11, 17, 21, and 22

MAINTENANCE AND MONITORING. Mr. T. should be followed very carefully in order to evaluate his home care efforts and also to see if all the pockets have been reduced to acceptable depths.

REHABILITATION STAGE. If at the end of the maintenance and monitoring period Mr. T. has maintained satisfactory oral hygiene and stabilization, then the following procedures may be initiated:
1. Ceramco crowns on teeth 6 and 11
2. A full gold crown on teeth 18 and 29 (The crown on tooth 29 will correct the moderate supraeruption of this tooth as well as render the tooth more satisfactory as a partial denture abutment.)
3. Maxillary and mandibular partial dentures; extraction of teeth 23, 24, 25, and 26 when the immediate lower partial denture is ready for insertion

MAINTENANCE AND MONITORING. At this stage Mr. T. will be placed again on a monitoring program in order to provide reinstruction if necessary. In addition, the periodontal condition must be continually monitored, as must be the possible changes related to the partial dentures. The endodontic tooth (11) should be x-rayed 6 months after treatment and then at least every 2 years if it remains asymptomatic.

Case 3. FULL DENTURE UTILIZATION

Chief complaint

Mr. P., a 57-year-old man, presented saying, "I want this tooth pulled."

History of present illness

Mr. P. was seen in the emergency clinic seeking treatment for pain eminating from the mandibular left third molar. Paramont in the patient's thought was the relief of pain. A brief oral and written medical history, vital signs, and periapical x-rays were obtained to ascertain the patient's ability to undergo palliative treatment. Medical history revealed the patient has been treated for several years for coronary heart disease, hypertension, and chronic alcoholism. Blood pressure was recorded at 130/90. The patient's physician was contacted by telephone and certified that the patient was under treatment and could tolerate the proposed treatment. A written confirmation of this conversation followed several days later.

The severely carious, periodontially involved tooth was extracted; recovery was uneventful. At a following visit a routine examination of the patient was obtained.

Past medical history

As stated above, Mr. P. is under treatment for coronary heart disease, hypertension, and chronic alcoholism. He is taking methyldopa (Aldomet), 250 mg four times daily, as treatment for his hypertension.

Laboratory reports and vital signs were within normal limits with the exception of the serum glutamic-oxaloacetic transaminase, which was slightly elevated, possibly indicating compromised liver function. This finding would necessitate caution in using medicaments that would be detoxified in the liver. Bleeding studies did not reflect the suspected liver disease. Patient is 18 pounds underweight for his height, age, and build. However, he states that he is gaining "a little" weight because of his decreased consumption of alcohol. Patient denies any other medical conditions.

Social and family history

Mr. P. has been married for 33 years and has six children. At the present he is holding a laborer position at a local shipyard. Full-time employment has been difficult for him to obtain. The patient's wife has had permanent employment for 31 years. The patient states that he smokes two packs of cigarettes per day and that he is not presently using alcohol.

Past dental history

Mr. P. states that his past dental treatment consisted of "fillings," "cleaning," and "pulling." However, in the past 10 years he has limited his treatment to extractions as painful conditions occur. He has now reached the point where mastication is becoming more difficult.

Attitudinal considerations

Mr. P. has heavy family responsibilities and insufficient financial resources for anything but the bare necessities of life. Obviously saving his teeth receives a very low priority in his approach to life. The patient's main desire is to obtain full dentures so that he can chew his food properly.

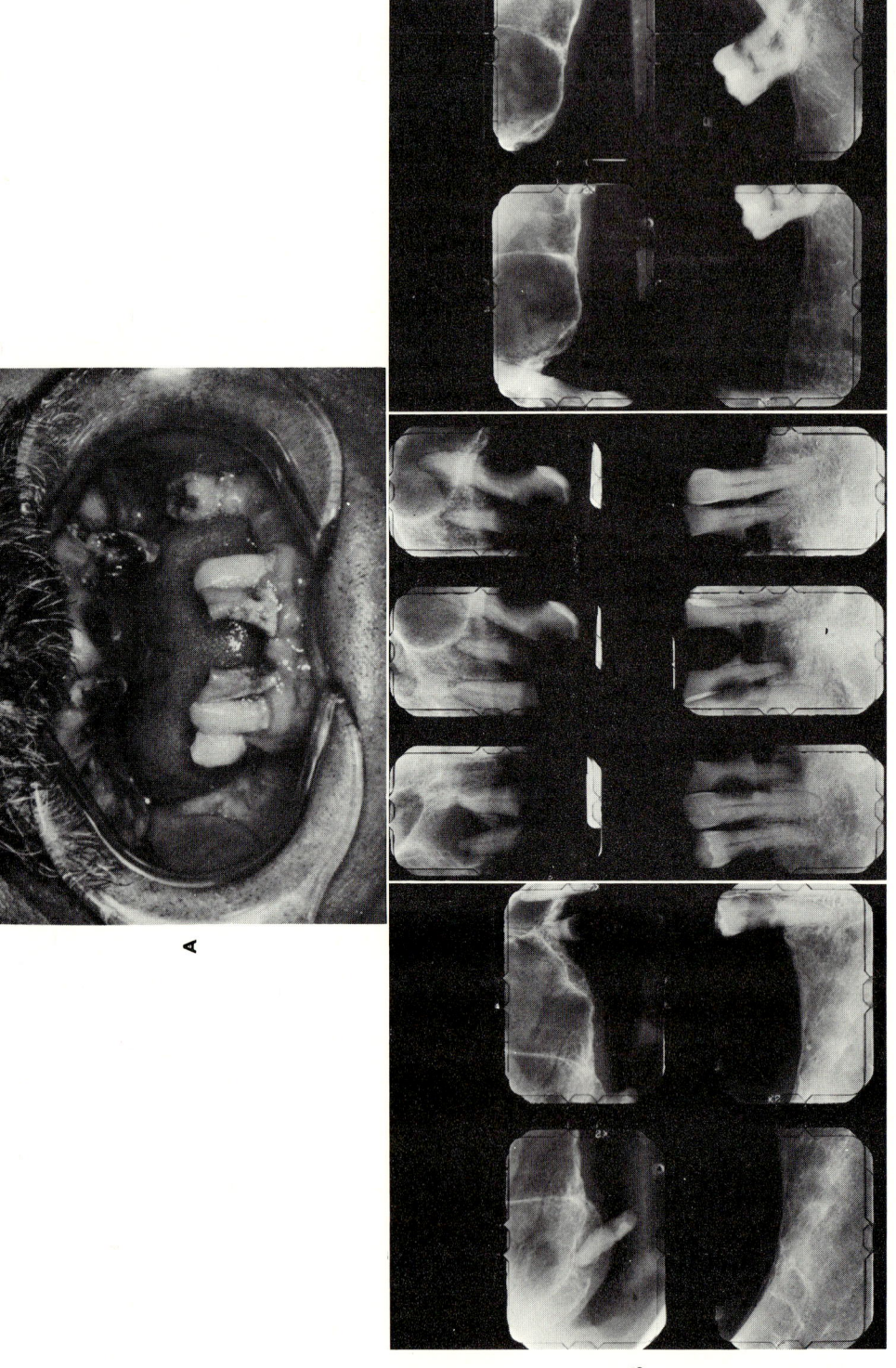

212 *Sequencing, classification, case analysis, and case treatment planning*

Fig. 12-7. Case 3. Complete denture case. **A,** Clinical photograph showing dentition. **B,** Full-mouth roentgenograms.

Clinical findings

Extraoral examination revealed no abnormal findings. Oral soft tissue examination revealed an exophytic lesion on the interdental papilla between teeth 22 and 23 and on the mandibular left labial mucosa opposite the canine area. (Both lesions were biopsied and diagnosed as squamous papillomas by the pathologist.)

Examination of all remaining teeth revealed extensive carious lesions (Fig. 12-7). Periodontal probing resulted in profuse bleeding and the calibration of pocket depths of 4 to 12 mm.

Roentgenographic examination revealed a large radiolucent area (later confirmed microscopically as a radicular cyst) at the apex of tooth 7 (Fig. 12-7). Heavy calculus was also apparent on the mandibular anterior teeth, as were carious lesions. The examination findings are illustrated in Fig. 12-8.

Diagnostic summary

1. Coronary heart disease, hypertension, chronic alcoholism
2. Pathologic lesions of soft tissue
3. Periapical radiolucency on tooth 7
4. Extensive carious lesions
5. Severe advanced periodontitis
6. Numerous missing teeth

Prognosis

Prognosis is poor for restorative procedures except for teeth 22, 27, and 28 (prognosis is guarded for these teeth) and fair to good for complete dentures.

Treatment plan
Summary

1. Maintain close consultation with physician
2. In hospital: (a) excise and biopsy soft tissue lesions and periapical radiolucency; (b) extract all remaining teeth

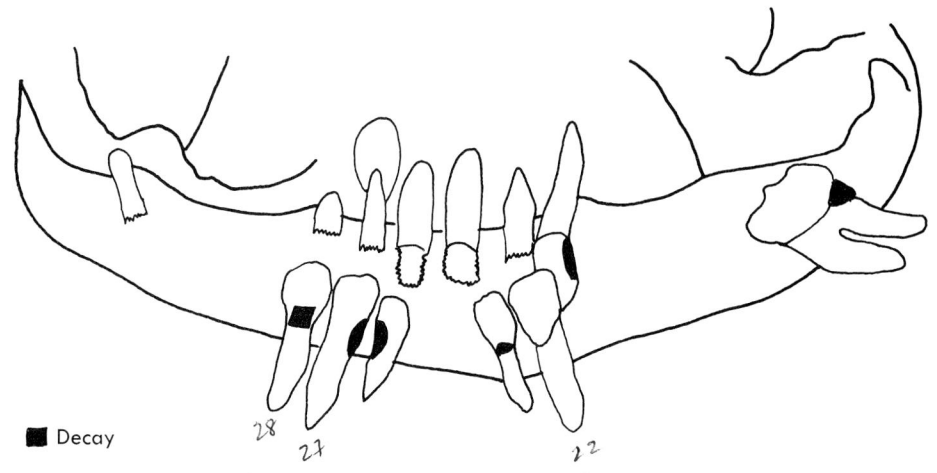

Fig. 12-8. Case 3. Examination chart.

214 *Sequencing, classification, case analysis, and case treatment planning*

    3. Complete maxillary and complete mandibular dentures
    4. Monitor

Rationale

As far as the maxillary arch is concerned, a full denture is the only feasible treatment. However, an alternative approach on the mandibular arch is to approach it as a transitional case. Thus teeth 22, 27, and 28 could be maintained and either an acrylic partial denture or an overdenture utilized. With such a plan the patient would enjoy the benefit of the added stability that these teeth would give the mandibular denture. Also, this approach would help to maintain alveolar bone height in the area of the retained teeth. Then too the experience gained by wearing a large partial denture or an overdenture for a while would aid Mr. P. in becoming accustomed to a complete lower denture. However, Mr. P.'s desire is to obtain a complete mandibular denture at this time so that he can get all the work over with at once and also because this route is the least expensive.

Sequencing

STABILIZATION. In order to maintain Mr. P.'s general health in a stable manner, it will be necessary to work very closely with his physician. Oral stabilization will be established by extracting the remainder of Mr. P.'s teeth in the hospital in addition to excision and biopsy of the two soft tissue lesions on the mucosa, as well as enucleation and biopsy of the periapical radiolucency on tooth 7.

MONITORING. After the extractions the patient will be reexamined to determine if the ridges are healing satisfactorily.

REHABILITATION. As soon as the alveolar ridges are sufficiently healed, appointments will be scheduled with the patient at mutually suitable times to begin the dentures.

MONITORING. After the dentures are inserted and adjusted to suit Mr. P., he should be reexamined at least every year in order to detect changes that require treatment.

13

The difficult case with alternative approaches

C. Daniel Overholser, Jr.

Perhaps nothing in dentistry is as challenging for the dentist as the design and execution of a complex treatment plan. Such a plan requires an intelligent and logical thought process, the development of good doctor-patient rapport, and the clinical skills so necessary for rendering proper dental treatment.

PARTNERS IN TREATMENT PLANNING

Naturally a patient for whom a complete workup is contemplated would be classified as "desiring complete oral care." It should be noted that even at this early point in the development of the dentist-patient relationship the patient has made a decision to seek "complete oral care." The dentist must continue to provide the information and data necessary for the patient to make informed decisions about his oral health. The dentist must afford the patient the opportunity to make these choices rather than persuade the patient to accept the wishes of the dentist. In this way a patient becomes a partner in the decision process. This is not to say that the dentist makes few or none of the decisions, for quite the opposite is true. The dentist should decide what is good and proper treatment for this patient by taking into consideration *all* the pertinent information he or she has gathered. If the dentist feels that there is only one proper form of treatment, then that is the treatment plan he or she should present to the patient. However, in these complex cases there may be several alternate treatments that are feasible, and these should be explained in detail to the patient along with their indications and contraindications. In this way the patient is able to make an intelligent choice.

Though it will not be expanded here, all treatment planning decisions are only as good as the accuracy of the data collected about the patient. Accurate findings that must be recorded include the patient's history, physical examination, results, roentgenograms, laboratory tests, personality profile, priorities, and financial status. Treatment recommendations based on most of the above findings are to be made by the dentist. Often in these complex cases the dentist will make such recommendations in concert with other dental specialists or the patient's physician. Some treatment areas particularly require that the patient participate in the decision-making process. For example, the patient should help make decisions that involve aesthetics, the ability to function with removable appliances, the acceptability of long appointments, or the psychological overtones associated with the loss of teeth via extraction.

Finally, some decision areas are solely the prerogative of the patient. These are mostly financial considerations, and the dentist's input should be in the form of fee amounts, acceptable payment schedules, and so on. While it certainly would be improper to "sell" a patient an expensive treatment plan, it is equally unjust to fail to inform the patient of proper treatment requirements just because the dentist feels they are too expensive for *this* patient. The decision as to whether a patient can afford dental care must be an educated one, but it must be made by the patient.

WHAT MAKES A CASE COMPLEX?

There are generally several problems present, such as caries, periodontal disease, missing teeth, and malocclusion, in a complex case. Each diagnosis requires a treatment decision, but more importantly each treatment decision must be coordinated not only with other treatment recommendations, but also with the many intangible aspects of treatment planning. For example, in addition to patient needs (as seen by the dentist), the dentist must be aware of the patient's desires. The chief complaint of the patient may concern aesthetics of a fractured maxillary central incisor, but the dental examination may reveal that periapical pathology associated with tooth 19 is the patient's most urgent need. If this were the only conflict, it would be relatively simple to explain to the patient why treating that "back tooth" is recommended before correcting the fractured incisor that is so disconcerting to the patient. Now let us add the facts that the patient is hypertensive (150/105 RASit), has poor oral hygiene, and was recently laid off from work. Suddenly a rather simple case becomes a complex one, for we have a patient who is seeking employment and who may require improved aesthetics as a consideration for hiring.

Following are several interrelated problems for this patient:
1. Chief complaint of a fractured maxillary central incisor (pulpal status considered normal)
2. Suspected hypertension
3. Necrotic pulp on tooth 19 with pulpoperiapical pathology
4. Poor oral hygiene; class 2 periodontitis
5. Unemployed (employment contingent upon correction of tooth 8)

ALTERNATIVE TREATMENT PLANS

A treatment plan based on the clinical findings alone for the case above could consist of the following:
1. Referral for evaluation of blood pressure
2. Endodontics on tooth 19
3. Periodontal therapy
4. Porcelain-fused-to-metal crown on tooth 8
5. Routine restorative work

However, considering the patient's financial and employment status, an alternative and a more realistic (pragmatic) approach for this patient could be:
1. Referral for evaluation of blood pressure
2. Extraction or initial endodontic debridement of tooth 19
3. Acid-etch resin restoring aesthetics to tooth 8
4. Prophylaxis; home care instructions
5. Patient to advise when financial condition allows him to receive the type of dental care that was presented in the first treatment plan

A patient who chooses the alternative treatment plan must be informed of the following:
1. Possible sequelae to the loss of tooth 19 (including loss of function, cost of replacement, and so on) or, if the initial endodontic debridement procedure is chosen, the potential problems associated with an incomplete endodontic procedure
2. Anticipated sequelae to the lack of complete periodontal therapy
3. Need for completion of therapy in the future

While certainly not the best treatment plan from a dental viewpoint, this alternate treatment plan is the best for this informed patient. A considerable degree of stabilization will have been attained, and hopefully the endodontic procedure required for the lower first molar could be completed within the next month or two. Often in such a case, if the work can be completed a little at a time over a longer period than usual, the patient can successfully reach the maintenance and monitoring stage and possibly even the rehabilitation stage where his care will be completed. With proper care and guidance, this can occur. However, if the patient had been originally presented with the choice between no treatment or "ideal" treatment, the patient would probably have chosen the former. In this manner we would be able to provide proper care for our hypothetical patient that is consistent with both the patient's and the dentist's objectives. It also allows the patient to obtain complete care in the future when he may be able to select that option.

FLEXIBILITY

Often complex cases hinge upon the success of some particular aspect of treatment. This may include successful endodontic or periodontal therapy for a strategic abutment tooth. The loss of this abutment could dramatically alter the plan of treatment from a fixed appliance to a tissue-supported removable partial denture. It is therefore imperative that the original treatment plan not only describe such contingencies, but also plan for them. This is often accomplished by dividing the treatment plan into treatment segments that allow for final decisions in the treatment plan to be made at appropriate times. These decisions usually occur after evaluating the success, and thus determining the prognosis, of the treatment rendered to date. Thus a treatment plan as illustrated in case 1 might consist of the following:
1. Periodontal therapy (case unit 3)
2. Provisional splint on teeth 2 to 14
3. Reevaluate after 6 to 12 months for the following:
   a. Present home care levels
   b. Fixed prosthesis for teeth 2 to 14
   c. Removable partial prosthesis on maxillary arch

Case 1

Chief complaint

Mrs. R., a 62-year-old woman, presents saying, "I would like to get my teeth fixed."

History of present illness

Mrs. R. has received much previous dental care and she has not been satisfied with it. It has included removable appliances that have been completely unsatisfactory. She felt that these interfered with her speech and that she could not function properly with them. Also included in her previous dental care were four endodontic procedures, which were performed at the patient's insistence because of her extreme fear at the loss of her teeth. She recalls having had a number of problems associated with these endodontic procedures, including retreatments and a surgical procedure on at least one of them. While she does not feel that her problem is an acute one, she is very upset because approximately 3 weeks ago her last dentist recommended extraction of all her remaining teeth and construction of complete removable dentures.

Past medical history

Mrs. R. states that her health is good. Her height and body weight appear within normal limits, and she denies any recent change in weight. The patient denies a history of scarlet fever, rheumatic fever, pneumonia, tuberculosis, or any infectious diseases. She does have a positive history of childhood diseases, including measles, mumps, and chickenpox. She denies any adverse sequelae or complications to these diseases or adverse reactions to the therapy for these diseases. The patient states that her only hospitalizations were for a tonsillectomy and adenoidectomy in 1920 and for the birth of children in 1936 and 1938. There were no adverse reactions to any of these admissions. She denies a history of operations and injuries requiring hospitalization. The patient also denies a history of serious illness, including diseases of the central nervous system, cardiovascular system, gastrointestinal system, genitourinary system, or musculoskeletal system. She does have a positive history of borderline diabetes, which is controlled by diet. She denies a history of other endocrine disorders or allergic or immunologic problems. She denies any diseases of psychologic or nervous origin.

Social and family history

Mrs. R. has been married for approximately 40 years and has two children, both of whom are grown and married. She is a citizen of the United States and appears to have no special social or financial problems. She considers herself a housewife and enjoys being a homemaker. She denies use of alcohol, tobacco, or drugs of any kind.

Mrs. R. denies any history of familial disorders including diabetes, other than herself, and has no history of infectious diseases such as tuberculosis or disorders of the cardiovascular system in her family.

Past dental history

The significant findings in Mrs. R.'s dental history have already been mentioned in the history of present illness.

Attitudinal considerations

Mrs. R.'s attitudinal considerations may be summarized by her fear of losing her teeth and that she will not be able to wear partial dentures. Mrs. R. states that she has sufficient funds to cover anticipated dental expenses.

Clinical findings

Extraoral examination, including the head, eyes, ears, and nose, revealed no abnormal findings with the exception of two small "lymph nodes" in the right submandibular area. These were firm, fairly movable, nontender, and appeared to be scarred in nature.

As far as the oral examination was concerned, the lips, buccal mucosa, major and minor salivary glands, hard and soft palate, tongue, and floor of the mouth all appeared normal. Muscles of mastication were not tender to palpa-

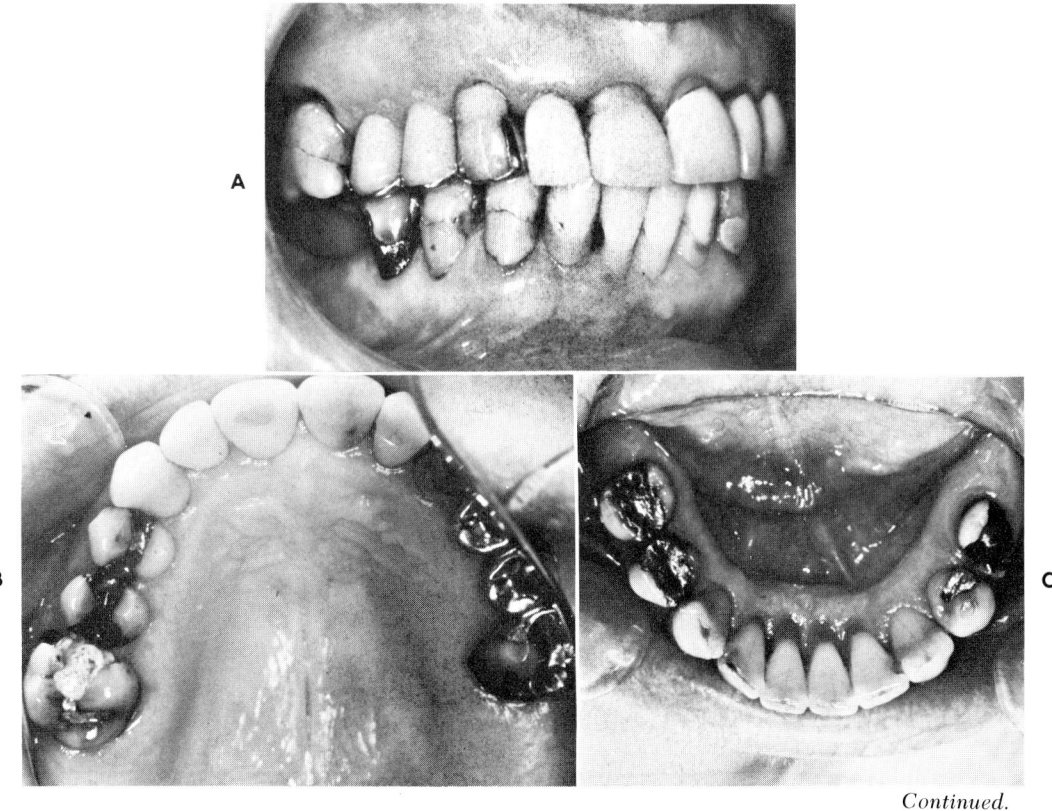

Continued.

Fig. 13-1. Case 1. Pretreatment views. **A**, Clinical view of teeth in occlusion. **B**, Occlusal view of maxillary arch. **C**, Occlusal view of mandibular arch. **D**, Full-mouth roentgenograms. (Courtesy Dr. Steve Somers, Baltimore, Md.)

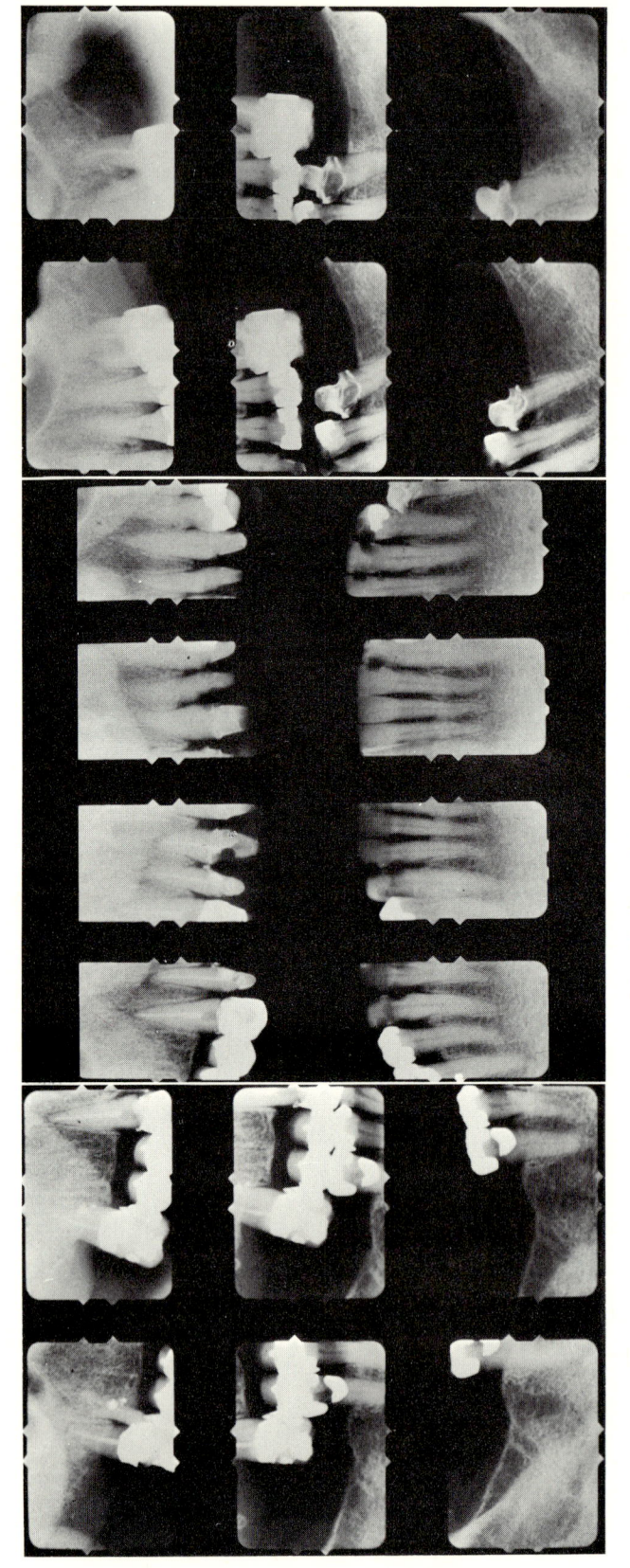

Fig. 13-1, cont'd. For legend see p. 219.

tion. Overall, the periodontium was classified as a case unit 3 with the exception of teeth 2 and 14, which exhibited 7 mm pocket depths and furcation involvement. Mobility was less than 2 mm in a buccolingual direction with the exception of tooth 2, which was a +2 mobility. However, tooth 2 was not depressable. Missing teeth included 1, 3, 4, 5, 15, 16, 17, 18, 19, 30, 31, and 32 (Fig. 13-1). Numerous defective restorations were observed and included a four-unit bridge from tooth 2 to tooth 6. The crowns on teeth 7 to 10 were also considered defective. No active clinical caries was noted. The dental findings are summarized in Fig. 13-2.

Medical consultation

A consultation was sought with Mrs. R.'s physician concerning the borderline diabetes, and her physician felt that she was adequately controlled. Her most recent glucose tolerance test taken approximately 1 month before was well within normal limits. Her physician stated that there were no medical contraindications to dental treatment at present.

Diagnostic summary

1. Borderline diabetes
2. Periodontal disease—moderate except for teeth 2 and 14, where it is severe
3. Numerous defective restorations, including a four-unit bridge and four single crowns

Prognosis

1. Guarded for teeth 2 and 14
2. Restorative work in maxillary right quadrant—fair to poor
3. Remainder of dentition—good with adequate home care

Treatment plan
Summary

The following treatment plans were presented to the patient in the descending order of preference:

Plan 1: complete upper denture; periodontal therapy for remaining mandibular teeth; splinted crowns on teeth 20 to 22 and 27 to 29; and a mandibular partial denture

Plan 2: extraction of teeth 2 and 14; periodontal therapy; and maxillary partial denture; treatment for mandibular arch same as in plan 1

Plan 3: complete maxillary denture; periodontal therapy; and minor restorative dentistry for the remaining mandibular teeth

Plan 4: initial periodontal therapy; provisional splint for remaining maxillary teeth, as well as teeth 20 to 22 and 27 to 29 in the mandibular to be reevaluated in approximately 6 months to determine the feasibility of splinting these with fixed prosthetic appliances at that time; bilateral splinting necessary because of buccolingual mobility patterns in maxillary arch

Plan 5: complete maxillary and mandibular denture

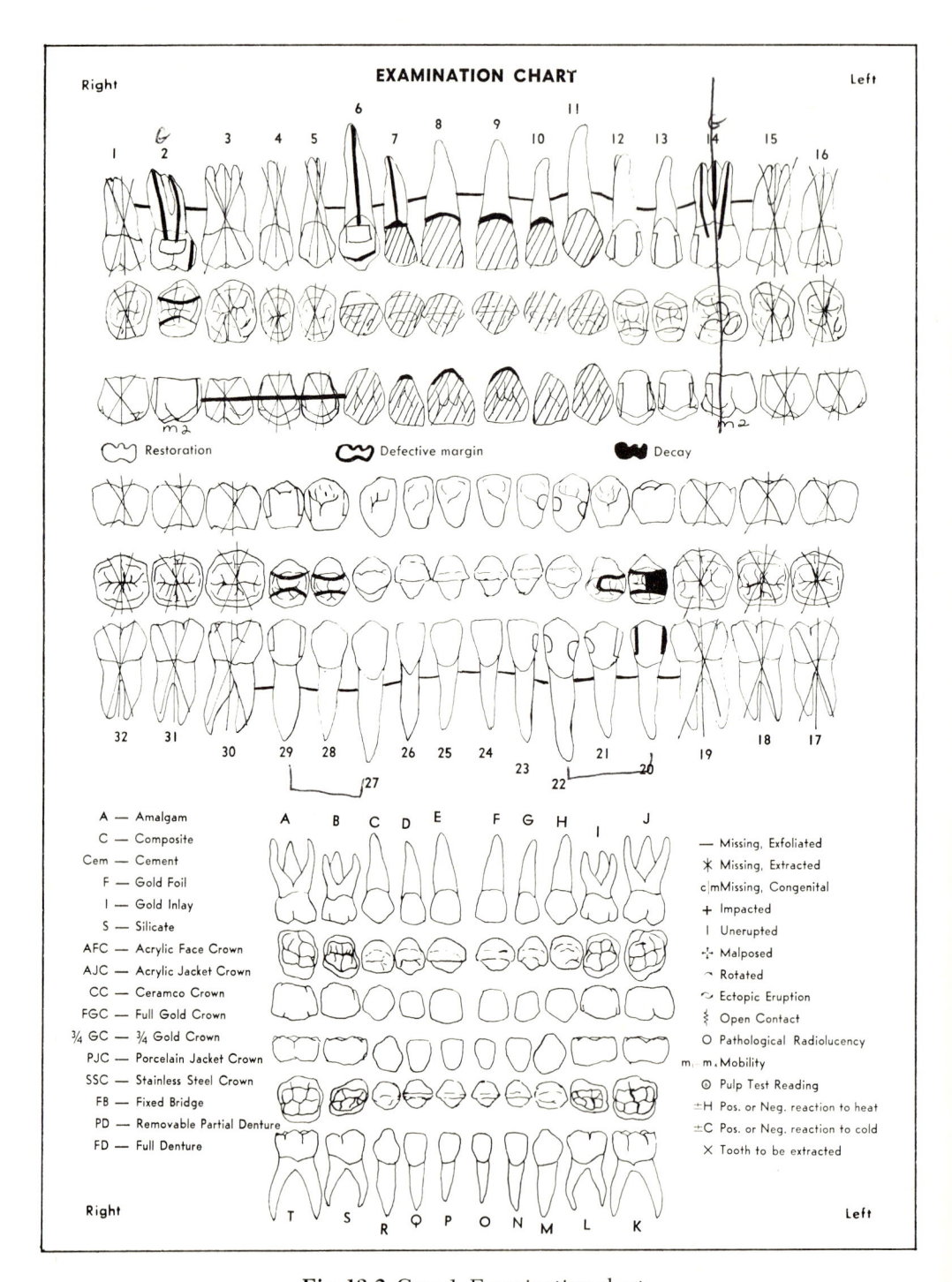

222 *Sequencing, classification, case analysis, and case treatment planning*

Fig. 13-2. Case 1. Examination chart.

Rationale

Treatment plan 5 appeared to be quite contraindicated and was never seriously considered in this case. Treatment plan 1 was the dentist's and consultant's early choice, but because of the patient's aversion to losing her teeth, fear of removable dentures, and her adequate finances, treatment plan 4 was offered with the understanding that everything was contingent upon improving oral hygiene and successful periodontal therapy of teeth 2 and 14.

Since the periodontal therapy was indicated in either treatment plan 2 or 4, little would be lost if the periodontal therapy failed to save teeth 2 and 14. Thus the only potential financial loss of any magnitude in the choice of treatment plan 4 was the construction of the provisional splint from teeth 2 to 14.

In the opinion of the treating dentist, periodontist, and endodontist, there was a reasonable chance (perhaps 50-50) that this would be successful. The patient felt the time and expense would be worth the potential gain. A joint decision was therefore made and treatment proceeded. While such treatment is not indicated for every patient, it was felt that it was indicated here. A change in any of the following variables would probably have resulted in a recommendation of treatment plans 1, 2, or 3:
 1. Uncontrolled diabetes (versus controlled)
 2. Average home care (versus good)
 3. Normal patient attitude toward loss of teeth (versus fear of loss)
 4. Less aversion to removable appliances (versus fear of removable appliances)

Sequencing

Attempts to obtain stabilization would include (1) home care instruction, evaluation, and reinforcement; (2) root planing of all teeth and periodontal surgery on teeth 2 and 14; and (3) a provisional splint for the maxillary teeth.

In 6 months, at the end of the maintenance and monitoring stage, if the prognosis for teeth 2 and 14 remained poor, then treatment plan 1 would be followed; that is, teeth 2 and 14 would be extracted and a maxillary partial denture made. On the other hand, if the prognosis for teeth 2 and 14 was sufficiently improved, then treatment plan 4 would be followed and a 12-unit fixed splint constructed for the maxillary arch. The design of the splint would incorporate the following features: decrease the occlusal table, platform the anterior crowns to provide positive vertical stops, and the mesiobuccal root of tooth 2 would be amputated to enable the patient to effectively clean this area. Also, the fixed appliance would be designed so that female attachments would be incorporated in the distal surface of tooth 6 and the distal surface of the pontic for tooth 14. Male attachments would be placed in the mesial pontic for tooth 5. Thus if tooth 2 was lost, a partial denture framework could be designed to incorporate this female attachment when it is constructed.

Results

In the stabilization phase of treatment, tooth 14 abscessed and had to be extracted. At the end of the monitoring period it was observed that home care had improved remarkably. Also, the periodontal condition on tooth 2 had improved considerably. With mobility decreasing to less than 1 mm, the 12-unit

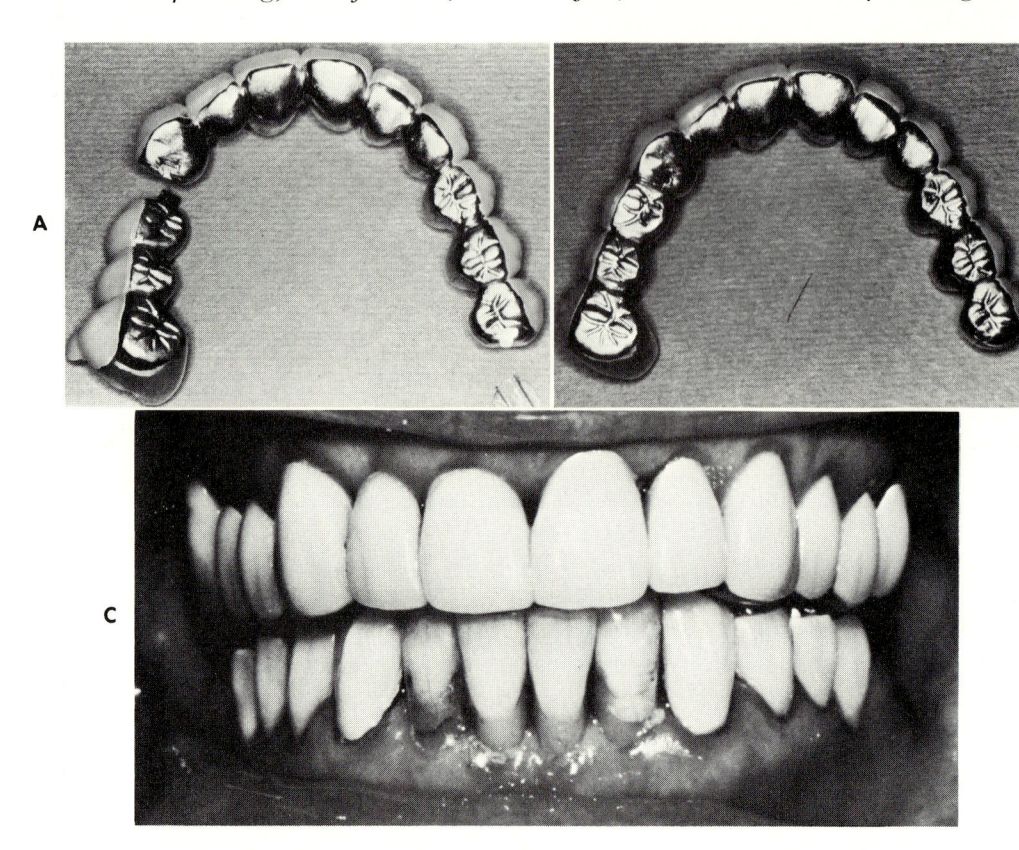

Fig. 13-3. Case 1. Fixed bridge constructed and ready to cement. **A,** Bridge is separated at precision attachment to show two segments. **B,** Precision attachment has been engaged. **C,** Teeth in occlusion after cementation of bridge.

fixed splint was designed, constructed, and inserted (Fig. 13-3). Also, cantilever bridges were constructed for the premolar–first molar regions bilaterally on the mandible by splinting the two premolars together.

One year after completion of the dental work the patient is still quite pleased with the function and aesthetics and is maintaining excellent oral hygiene. The treating dentist is also pleased with the treatment results up until the present time.

Case 2

Chief complaint

Mrs. S. is a 23-year-old woman who presents saying, "I have trouble chewing, and sometimes my gums bleed."

History of present illness

Mrs. S. has received regular dental care, including removable appliances, all of which she has found satisfactory. Recently she experienced difficulty with her lower partial denture, as her mouth has been dry as a result of her treatment for Hodgkin's disease. The gingiva began to bleed, and because she is unable to use her partial dentures, she has found it difficult to masticate her food. Her treating physician at the cancer center referred her for evaluation of her dental problems.

Past medical history

Mrs. S. states that her health had been quite good until recently. In December 1972 she was diagnosed as having Hodgkin's disease, and treatment was begun immediately. She received radiation therapy consisting of approximately 3,000 rads in the left neck area. Additionally, she received chemotherapy in the form of vincristine. Her dry mouth is chiefly a result of the radiation. A biopsy in the neck region approximately 6 months after therapy was negative for Hodgkin's disease, and the treating physician was somewhat hopeful concerning her prognosis. The remainder of her medical history was essentially within normal limits, as she denies a history of rheumatic fever, tuberculosis, pneumonia, and of any adverse sequelae from the normal childhood diseases, which she did have. She denies a history of other serious illnesses including diseases of the central nervous system, cardiovascular system, gastrointestinal system, genitourinary system, and musculoskeletal system. She denies a history of diabetes, other endocrine disorders, allergies, or diseases of psychological or nervous origin. She is taking no medications and has had no previous hospitalizations.

Past dental history

The patient gives a history of routine restorative dentistry, but no periodontal therapy to her knowledge. Extractions included teeth 2, 3, 15, 16, 17, 18, 19, 21, and 29 to 32. A partial denture had been constructed to replace the mandibular missing teeth and had functioned quite well until the therapy for Hodgkin's disease was commenced.

Attitudinal considerations

As is understandable, Mrs. S. is quite reluctant to undergo the expense and discomfort of having extensive dental procedures accomplished in view of the very guarded prognosis of her Hodgkin's disease. Her spirits have improved somewhat along with the regression of the Hodgkin's disease, and she feels that the dryness of her mouth has subsided somewhat since her initial therapy.

Clinical findings

The extraoral examination of the eyes, ears, and nose revealed no abnormal findings. Palpation of the neck revealed no palpable lymph nodes, and there was no evidence of erythema in the skin overlying the mandibular and neck regions that have received radiation therapy.

The intraoral examination revealed all soft tissues to appear normal though somewhat dry. Clear, viscous saliva was expressed from each salivary duct opening. The muscles of mastication were not tender to palpation. Overall, the periodontal disease was classified as a case unit 1-A. The gingiva around tooth 10 revealed 4 and 5 mm pockets associated with the poorly fitting porcelain-fused-to-gold crown on that tooth. Mobility was less than 1 mm on all teeth. Class 5 caries were noted on teeth 6, 11, and 22. Class 3 caries were noted on teeth 8, 23, 26, and 27 (Fig. 13-4). A summary of the dental examination is presented in Fig. 13-5.

Diagnostic summary
1. Hodgkin's disease
2. Class 1-A periodontal disease
3. Defective restorations and moderate amount of caries activity

Prognosis
1. Hodgkin's disease—guarded to fair
2. Periodontal disease—excellent with the establishment and maintenance of good home care

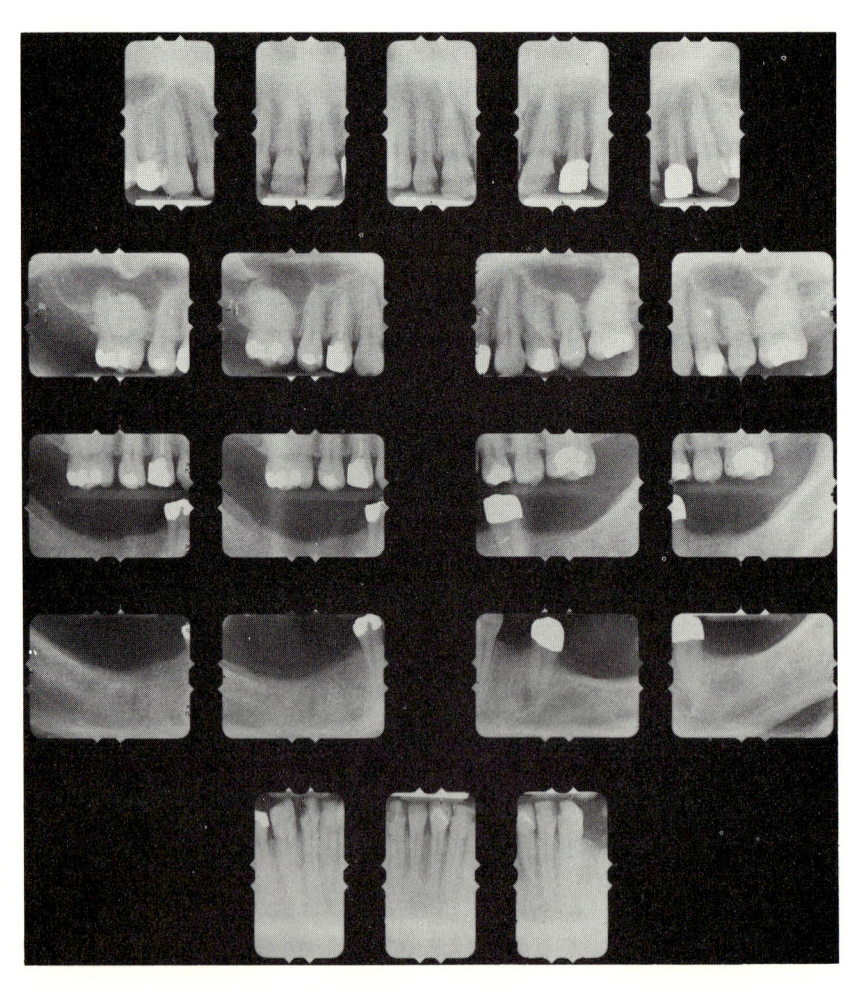

Fig. 13-4. Case 2. Pretreatment full-mouth roentgenograms.

3. Restorative problems—excellent with special fluoride treatments and the maintenance of good home care

The following two considerations render the prognosis of dental treatment quite unpredictable for this patient:
1. Long-term prognosis for the patient with regard to Hodgkin's disease
2. Ability of the salivary glands to function normally again to prevent numerous instances of recurrent caries and to allow the patient to provide adequate home care

Treatment plan
Summary

Consultation was sought with the referring physician, and the following recommendations for treatment were made at this time:

PHASE 1
1. Discontinue use of present partial denture altogether
2. Periodontal therapy: emphasis to be on improved home care and initial periodontal therapy
3. Minor restorative procedures for new caries and replacement of defective restorations
4. Weekly fluoride treatments to improve resistance to dental caries
5. Monitor recall approximately every 3 months

PHASE 2

In the future, if the prognosis for the Hodgkin's disease has changed to good, the salivary function has improved, and oral hygiene efforts have been maintained at a satisfactory level, then the following procedures are to be performed:
1. Porcelain-fused-to-gold crowns on teeth 10 and 28
2. Three-unit porcelain-fused-to-gold bridge on teeth 20 to 22
3. Crowns on mandibular arch designed to receive the lower partial denture, which was to be subsequently constructed

Rationale

The rationale for this treatment plan has been adequately discussed in the summary of phases 1 and 2 of the treatment plan.

Sequencing

The procedures were to be instituted according to the order listed in the summary of phases 1 and 2 of the treatment plan.

Results

Both the physician and the patient agreed to the treatment plan, and phase 1 therapy was accomplished. In October 1976 the patient's medical status progressed to the point where the physician recommended completion of all treatment. At that time the periodontal situation was reevaluated, and only minor therapy was needed, as the patient's home care had remained at a very high level. The patient's salivary function appeared normal. Phase 2 of the

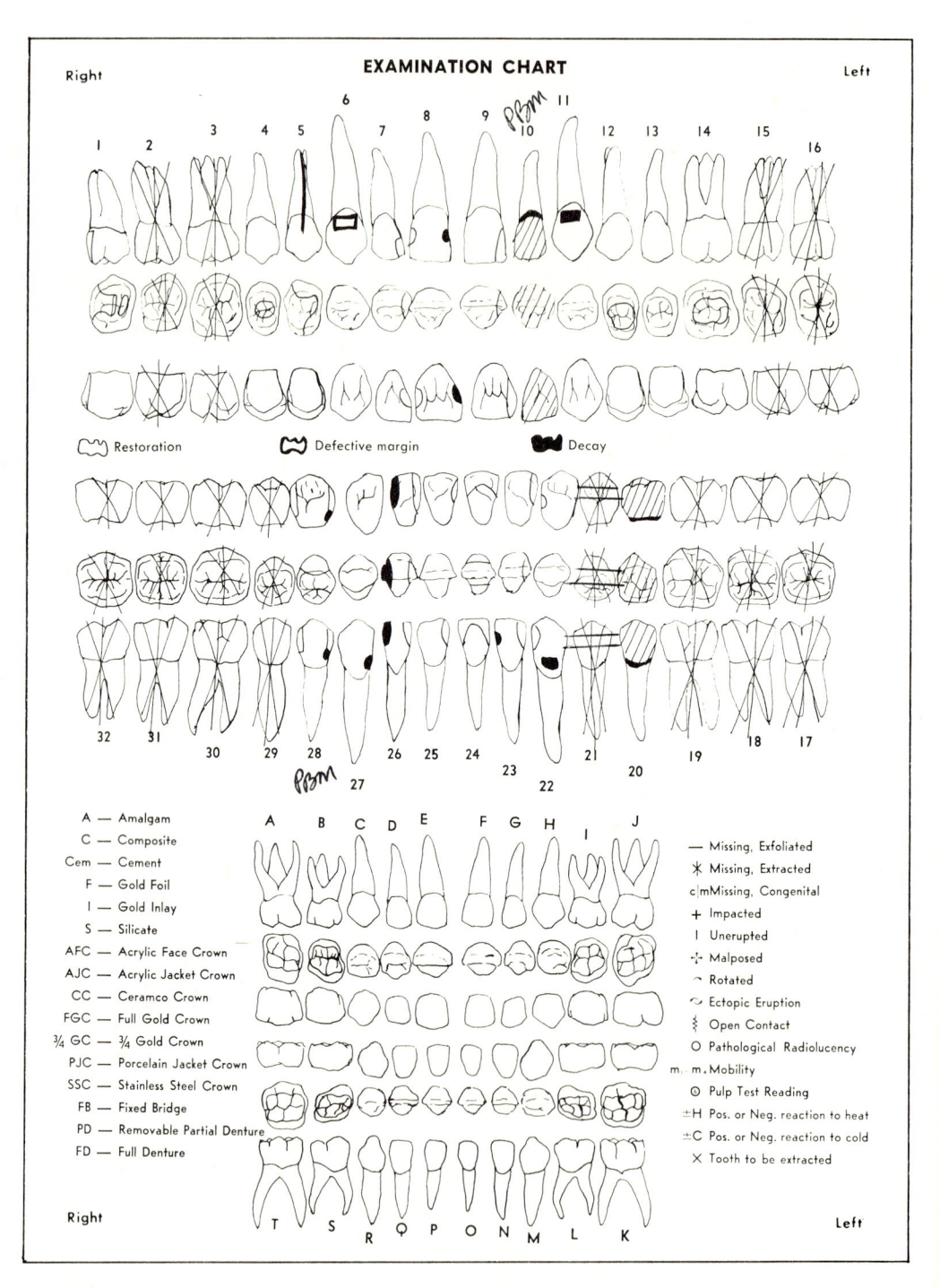

228 *Sequencing, classification, case analysis, and case treatment planning*

Fig. 13-5. Case 2. Examination chart.

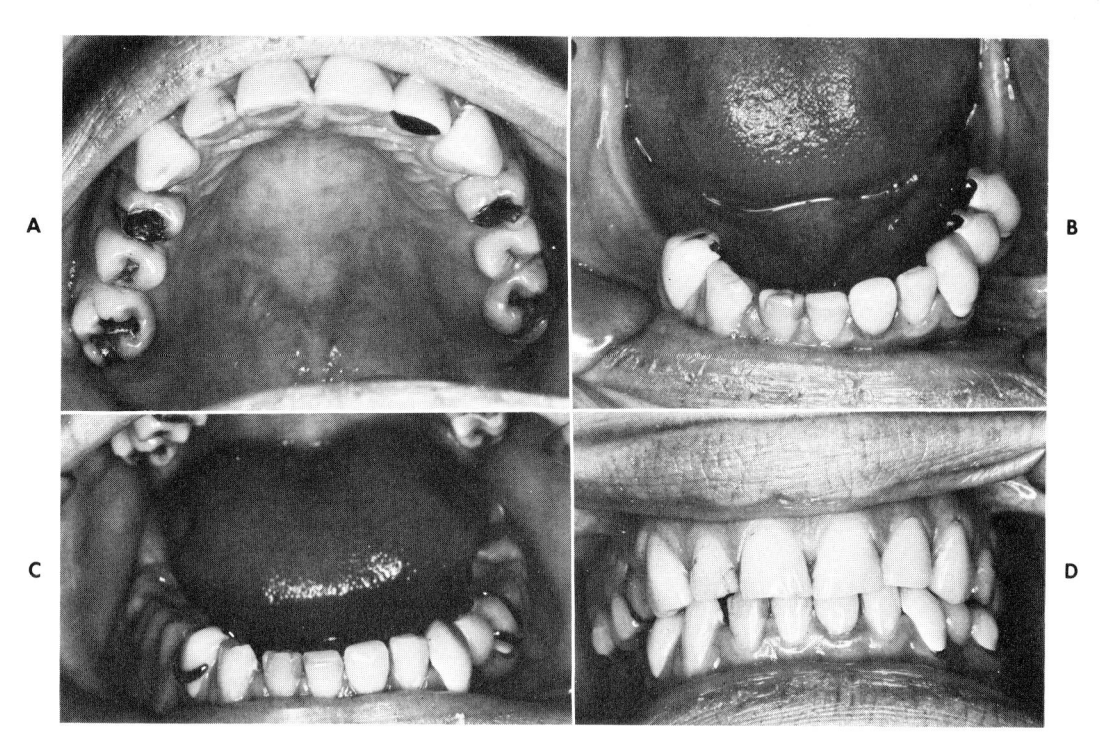

Fig. 13-6. Case 2. Posttreatment views. **A,** Clinical picture of maxillary arch. **B,** Mandibular arch. **C,** Mandibular arch with partial denture in place. **D,** Teeth in occlusion.

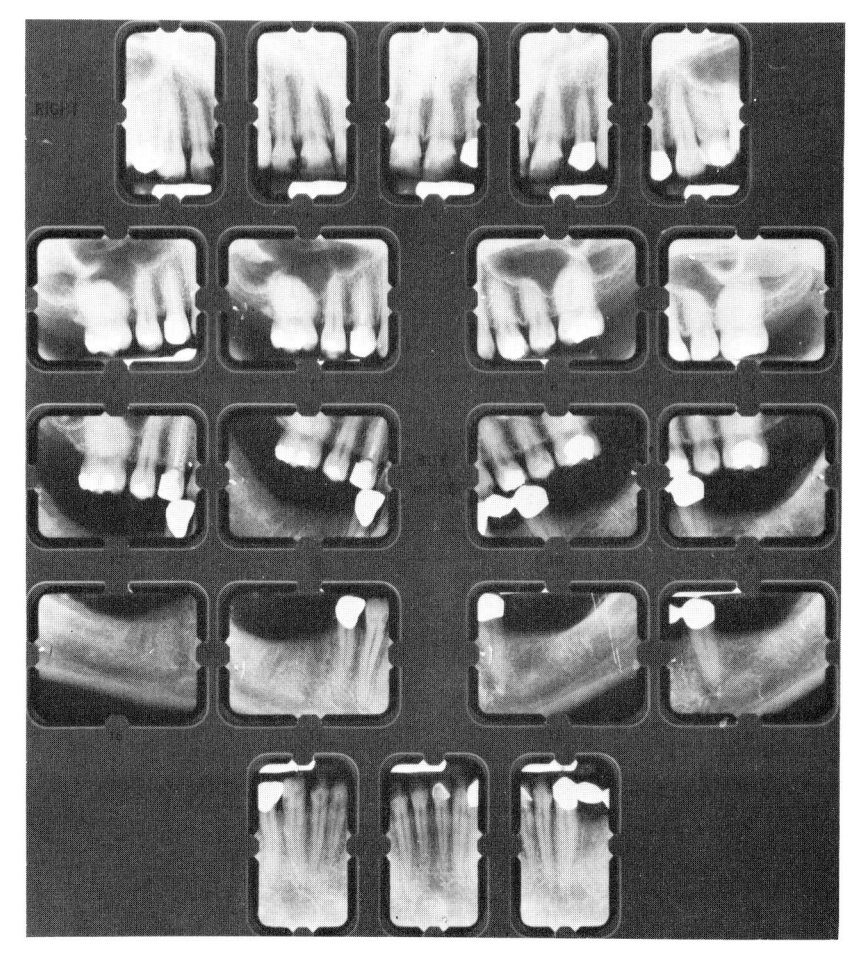

Fig. 13-7. Case 2. Posttreatment full-mouth roentgenograms.

treatment plan was instituted and completed as envisioned above (Figs. 13-6 and 13-7).

At this time, approximately 1 year after treatment, the dental and medical prognoses appear quite good. The patient is maintaining a high level of home care and is pleased with both the function and aesthetics of the prosthetic treatment.

Case 3

Chief complaint

Mr. M., a 71-year-old man, presents saying, "The recent extraction of an upper left tooth has made it very difficult for me to chew."

History of present illness

The upper left first premolar, which was the anterior abutment for a bridge from tooth 12 to tooth 15, was extracted approximately 1 month before by a local referring dentist because of lack of periodontal support. Since that time the patient has found it very difficult to masticate his food properly.

Past medical history

Diet- and medically controlled hypertension are the only significant findings in this well-developed, well-nourished man. He presently is taking hydrochlorothiazide, 100 mg per day, to control his hypertension. He reports that his blood pressure was 165/115 RASit at the time of initial therapy approximately 2 years ago. He denies a history of any other cardiovascular disease including myocardial infarction, angina, bleeding disorders, and so on. He also denies a history of gastrointestinal, genitourinary, musculoskeletal, endocrine, or dermatologic disorders. He also denies allergies to medications and is taking no medications other than the hydrochlorothiazide on a regular basis. He has never been hospitalized.

Past dental history

The patient states that he has received routine dental care on a fairly regular basis all of his life. Approximately 20 years ago a lower partial denture was constructed, which he was unable to tolerate. Approximately 10 years ago he had periodontal surgery prior to the construction of the bridge in the upper left quadrant. He has been satisfied with his previous dental care, with the exception of the removable partial denture. He states that he brushes two times a day, denies any oral habits, and does not smoke.

Attitudinal considerations

The patient demands that every attempt be made to preserve his remaining teeth. In addition, he states that he would not be happy with a partial denture.

Clinical findings

Mr. M.'s blood pressure was recorded as 140/90 RASit with a pulse rate of 76 beats per minute. Examination of the eyes, ears, nose, neck, and face revealed no abnormal findings. An intraoral exam revealed all soft tissues to be normal with normal salivary function. Muscles of mastication were not tender to palpation.

Examination of the periodontium revealed moderate bone loss with minimal pocket depth of less than 4 mm. Mobility was not significant except for tooth 11, which was mobile 1 mm in a buccolingual direction. Teeth 4, 12, 13, 14, 17, 30, 31, and 32 are missing. All teeth were found to be vital, and the anterior teeth exhibited severe incisal wear. Also noted was a severe anterior crossbite in the acquired centric relation (Figs. 13-8 and 13-9). No carious lesions were noted. A summary of the dental examination is presented in Fig. 13-10.

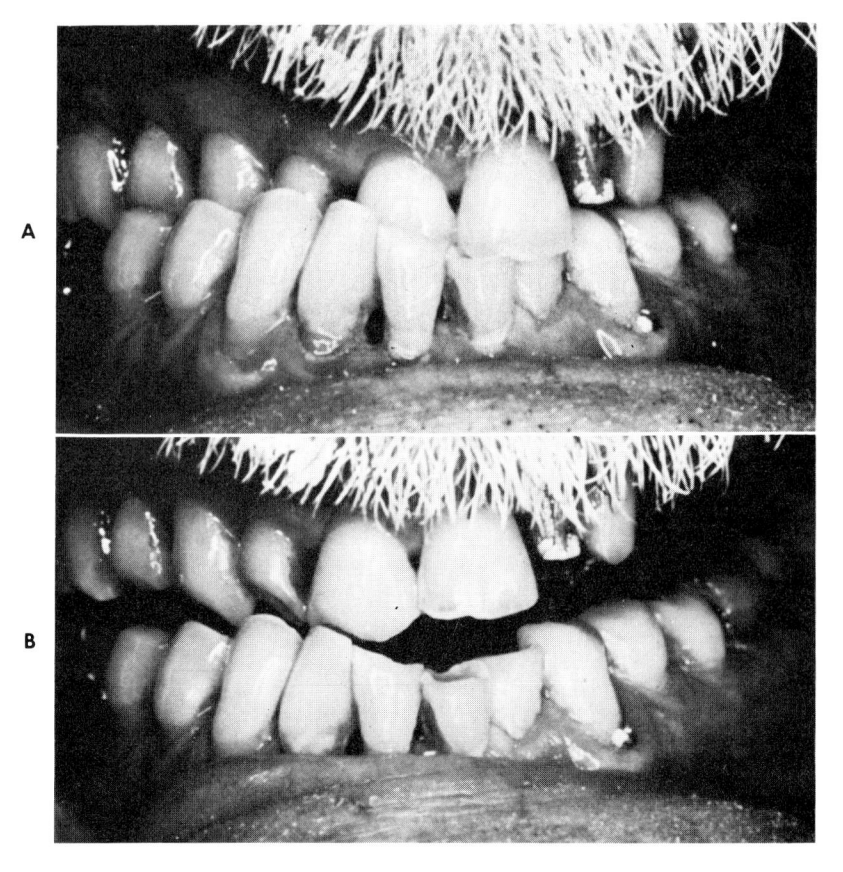

Fig. 13-8. Case 3. Pretreatment views. **A,** Anterior view of teeth in acquired centric occlusion. **B,** Teeth separated approximately 4 mm. (Courtesy Dr. Norton Brotman, Baltimore, Md.)

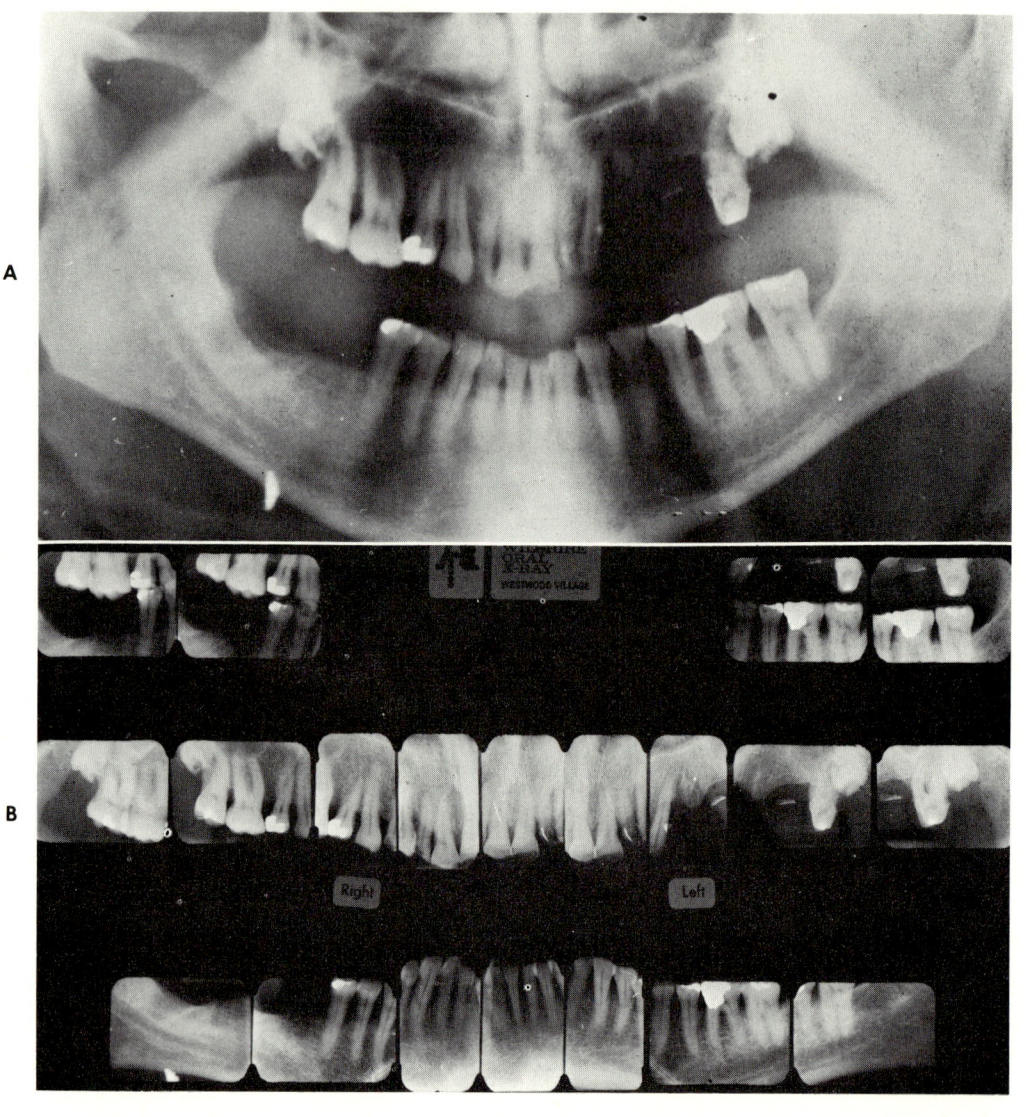

Fig. 13-9. Case 3. Pretreatment roentgenograms. **A,** Panoramic roentgenograms. **B,** Full-mouth roentgenograms. (Courtesy Dr. Norton Brotman, Baltimore, Md.)

Diagnostic summary

1. Hypertension controlled with medication
2. Mild chronic periodontal disease
3. Missing teeth in upper left quadrant
4. Severe incisal wear on anterior teeth with severe anterior crossbite in aquired centric relation

Prognosis

1. Patient in good health and hypertension well controlled
2. Excellent for periodontal disease

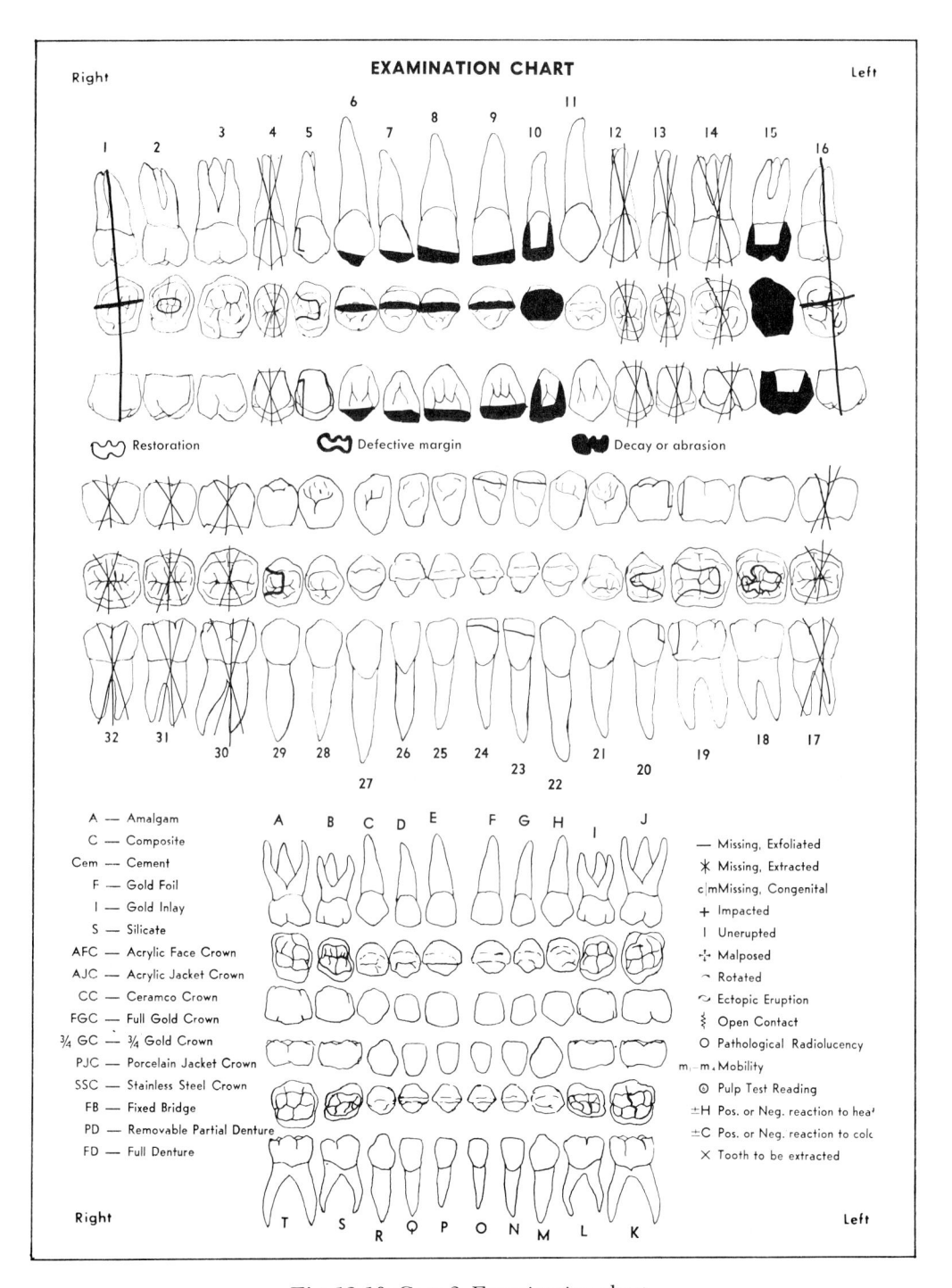

Fig. 13-10. Case 3. Examination chart.

3. Good for minor restorative procedures
4. Questionable to fair for bridge in upper left quadrant
5. Poor for major changes from present acquired centric relation

Treatment plan
Summary

A number of treatment plans could be outlined for this patient. They include the following:
1. Complete maxillary denture; complete mandibular denture
2. Complete maxillary denture; partial mandibular denture
3. Partial upper; partial lower
4. Fixed upper; partial lower
5. Fixed upper in the acquired centric relation
6. Complete reconstruction with fixed upper and fixed lower

Rationale

The patient ruled out any treatment plan that included removable appliances, which meant that treatment plans 5 and 6 were the remaining choices. Consultation was obtained with the periodontist who originally treated him, and it was felt that treatment plan 5 would have a reasonable prognosis if proper home care and maintenance and periodontial therapy was rendered. The magnitude of the work necessary, as well as its guarded prognosis, ruled out treatment plan 6 as a satisfactory choice.

Sequencing

In order to evaluate the results of a fixed bridge in the upper left quadrant, teeth 10 to 15 were prepared and a provisional acrylic splint was constructed. After a monitoring period of approximately 6 months, mobility in tooth 11 had decreased and there was no increased mobility in any of the abutment teeth. Treatment plan 5 was chosen, and a gold-acrylic bridge was constructed from teeth 10 to 15 in the acquired centric relation.

Results

At this time, approximately 7 years after treatment, the patient has been satisfied both functionally and aesthetically with this treatment.

14

The transitional case

Richard P. Cohan
Norman K. Wood

This chapter is devoted to the transitional case and concludes part three, which classifies and discusses approaches to the different types of cases. The term *transitional care dentistry* encompasses a wide variety of meanings and approaches. Temporary restorations could be considered transitional care, as could also temporary bridges. Some dentists consider all partial dentures to be transitional in nature. In complex cases one could consider the stages of stabilization and maintenance and monitoring to be transitional inasmuch as they represent stages passed through in hopes of reaching the rehabilitation stage. Other practitioners think of transitional care as "limited" care or less than "ideal" care. In this chapter the term *transitional case* is used to identify cases where dental treatment is designed to temporarily meet the functional or aesthetic needs of a patient whose short- to medium-term prognosis for retaining the remaining dentition is fair to poor.

As a general rule, the patient's dentition has been permitted to degenerate to the point that the chance of preserving some or all of the remaining teeth is small or completely nonexistent. In other cases the patient's health may be so precarious that much of the dental work needed to conserve the teeth cannot be rendered. Insufficient finances could be a third reason why a dentist and patient would have to opt for transitional-case care instead of the expensive procedures necessary to preserve the present dentition. The type of treatment intimated here is not a substandard form of care but is rather the best that circumstances permit.

Some practitioners, as well as some dental school clinics, do not offer this type of service. Their modus operandi is "First class dentistry for everyone or we don't do the case." We have no quarrel with this type of practitioner because every dentist has the privilege of deciding for himself or herself what type of practice he or she will maintain and what social level of patient he or she will serve. Nevertheless, there are a very large number of transitional-case type patients in this country who need dental care and who are delighted that there are dentists who will accept them as patients. At this juncture it is important to clarify that we are not contrasting *good* versus *poor* dentistry here. Nor are we considering the unscrupulous practitioner who routinely condemns readily salvageable teeth. Rather, we take it for granted that in the situations detailed above the procedures rendered by either practitioner are of the highest quality. What is really being discussed here is a contrast in the philosophy of patient care. As far as the general population is concerned, it is convenient and good that both types of practitioners exist because, given this choice, it is more likely that the individual's dental needs will be cared for with a treatment plan that has been tailored to meet the needs of the *total person.*

Unfortunately, whether a case is classified as a transitional case depends on the individual practitioner's judgment. Good judgment concerning prognosis of cases is only acquired through the experiences of several years of alert dental practice. Gross errors committed because of overanticipation of treatment success in complex cases are extremely damaging to a patient financially as well as psychologically. In addition, the doctor-patient relationship is severely jeopardized.

Following the principles of sequencing as presented in Chapter 10 helps to avoid greater disasters than would otherwise happen. This is so because in complex cases the <u>dentist does not initiate the rehabilitative phase</u> (usually the most expensive part) <u>until the stabilization and monitoring phases have been complete</u>d. Such an approach permits the dentist to evaluate whether disease control has been achieved. If the practitioner finds that disease control has not been achieved, then the expensive rehabilitative work is not commenced because of the poor prognosis.

Furthermore, it is imperative to mention at this juncture that conservative disease control cannot realistically be obtained and should not be attempted in some transitional-type cases. The dental practitioner who processes *every* patient through exactly the same treatment program, same disease-control program, same sequence, and same treatment for the same dental defects is a dismal person indeed. This type of practitioner rationalizes his or her streamlined operation by the cliché: "Every patient deserves a chance to save his teeth." This is a mindless motto used by some dentists as a substitute for the mental activity necessary to develop an approach tailored for *each* individual. Really, if treatment planning and its approach can be standardized in such a fashion, then the dental assistant is qualified to undertake it!

Every patient has unique needs and requires an approach unique for that individual. Nowhere is this more apparent than in the transitional case. For example, it would require an enormous outlay of time and money just to attempt to attain stabilization (disease control) in some of these cases. Perhaps there is gross caries in most of the teeth and severe generalized periodontitis. The extremely poor prognosis is evident. If a dentist were to process this patient through his or her standardized program, imagine the time and expense expended on the part of the patient for the full-mouth periodontal surgery and huge amalgam buildups of many of the teeth, not to mention the endodontic treatment required. What a disaster such an approach would prove to be in either the transitional or the completely hopeless case. Thus not every patient should be presented the option of saving all the teeth. <u>If the case is hopeless or the chance of success is small, the honest, mature dentist is able to recog-</u>

nize this and soon condemns the indicated teeth without causing unnecessary temporal or financial inconvenience to the patient. In summary, the point we are trying to make is that transitional-type cases present from time to time. These need to be recognized, and it should be understood that the approach to treatment planning for this type of case usually is quite different from that in the other categories.

In order to ensure that the foregoing discussion does not lend credence to the unscrupulous practitioner who routinely condemns *readily salvageable* teeth, it is important to stress that cases with moderate to good prognosis are *not* to be classified as transitional cases. There is *no* justification for approaching these individuals as transitional-case types when every effort has not been exhausted to educate and motivate such patients to appreciate the various treatment plans that may be available, their benefits and disadvantages, and the prognosis for each one.

GENERAL CONSIDERATIONS
Early identification

It is imperative to identify the transitional case as soon as possible. Such early recognition will pay big dividends in good patient rapport and will preclude the dentist from having the patient undergo and pay for extensive procedures that will likely fail in the near future. In addition, it will spare the dentist the embarrassment of having to change his or her approach in midtreatment after he or she has belatedly learned that he or she is working on a transitional case. Although midstream changes in treatment cannot always be avoided, the patient's confidence in the dentist may become eroded, and he may wonder if the dentist really understands his case after all.

General approach

The general overall approach of the treatment plan should be decided as soon as possible. For example, if the case is a severe generalized periodontitis and circumstances indicate that improved home care along with benign surveillance is the best plan for a year or two, this needs to be decided before conflicting treatment is introduced. If teeth are to be extracted and *temporary* acrylic partial dentures constructed, unusual heroic efforts should not be made to save a tooth or two. On the other hand, if overdentures are to be used, then endodontics and gold copings may be well advised for one, two, or more teeth.

Patient attitudes

Patients in this group possess various dental backgrounds. Some are from families who traditionally attach very little importance to retaining the natural dentition. Others have despaired of saving their teeth after having a great deal of dental work done over the years, much of which has not stood the test of time. In later years they have become so discouraged that they just let their teeth go altogether. Others have neglected their teeth out of fear. Another group is suffering from severe systemic disease, and the patients are just delighted to be able to chew comfortably and to be free of dental pain. Still others need an enormous amount of work, have a desire to save all their remaining teeth, but do not possess the necessary finances.

The members of this last group are usually the only patients of the transitional care group who present a real behavioral problem for the dentist. Frequently these are women approaching menopause who are concerned about their disappearing youth. Thus they are already concerned about losing their teeth. Now, let us consider, for example, that the woman in question needs full-mouth periodontal surgery, several teeth endodontically filled, and full-mouth splints and bridges constructed in order to conserve her natural dentition. However, her financial resources fall far short of the anticipated expense. Also, let us say that without the splints and bridges the periodontal treatment would almost certainly fail. The dentist needs to be *very* careful in his or her approach to such a patient. It is imperative that he or she obtain a good idea of the patient's finances before presenting his or her plan for treatment. The stage is set here for an emotional crisis of a large order. In our opinion, the dentist who tells *this* patient that if she does not have this work done she will become a "dental cripple" will almost certainly precipitate an unnecessary behavioral crisis. This situation calls for *downplaying* the importance of conserving all the remaining dentition rather than *increasing* the patient's dread of losing teeth. Rather than destroying this patient psychologically, the dentist should instruct the patient that it is not feasible to save *all* her teeth but that he or she is quite sure that she will be happy with the results of the financially feasible treatment that he or she envisions for her. As a result, the dentist will have a relatively happy patient who is able to function quite well with an aesthetically pleasing partial or full denture. This is in contrast to the unhappy *mental* cripple the dentist would have created with an ill-conceived push for total conservation.

Since patients of this type are frequently unresponsive, on the defensive, or easily upset, special effort is necessary to avoid a condescending attitude that would either "turn off," embarrass, or irritate them. Patients who fit into the transitional case mold often are among the more unreliable, fearful, unmotivated individuals that a dentist will treat. As a result, the dentist may find that such patients discontinue in the middle of treatment procedures. They may return at a later date or go elsewhere for another round of emergency or urgent care on the way to losing their entire natural dentition. One of my teachers once advised me never to provide a transitional care service that was too aesthetically pleasing, lest the patient never return for definitive care. He had in mind the kind of patient just described above. Germane to this discussion is the fact that among certain population groups with full dental insurance benefits, fewer than 40% of the insured individuals utilize any of the covered services!

Case presentation

As with all cases, the presentation is a critical step toward successful treatment. In these transitional cases the patient needs to be informed at as early a juncture as possible that his case lies within a "gray" zone: the prognosis is too poor to consider extensive procedures in attempts to maintain the complete dentition, but at the same time degeneration has not reached the stage where all the remaining teeth need to be extracted and full dentures constructed. The financially feasible options that would delay the day when full dentures would be needed should be clearly explained. It should be stressed that it is expected that these measures are of a temporary nature, that after a certain period of time further tooth loss will be experienced, that these teeth will be added to the existing partial dentures, and that eventually full dentures will be required. If the patient is uncertain about the dentist's recommended approach, he should be encouraged to seek a second opinion.

Case reevaluation and monitoring

As with other types of cases, reevaluation and monitoring is necessary on a periodic basis. The dentist should be alert for developments that would signal improvement in prognosis and a need to switch to a more permanent approach. Such developments would include improved health, finances, or perhaps drastically improved attitudes on the part of the patient concerning home care. Typically, an interim evaluation of these patients will call for "more of the same," and at times, for the condemnation of some or all of the remaining teeth because of the extremely poor home care demonstrated by the patient and a rapidly deteriorating oral condition.

Maintenance is not considered in the same light as it is with other types of cases. In transitional cases, disease control is usually not fully achieved and so cannot be maintained. However, remaining teeth are maintained as long as it is feasible. Of course, rehabilitation in the usual sense of the word is hardly a common denominator of the transitional case.

To reiterate, in this chapter we are discussing the case the practitioner judges as having such a poor prognosis that efforts to establish stabilization and maintenance are not warranted because failure is certain or very likely, but in which deterioration has not advanced quite to the stage where full dentures are indicated. This type of case represents an "in-between" or "transitional" situation. Following are case examples:

1. Complex case with severe medical problems
2. Complex case that has failed in the stabilization or monitoring stages
3. Gross caries with limited finances
4. Moderately severe periodontitis with limited finances
5. Severe periodontitis treated with a temporary partial denture (tx partial)
6. Transitional treatment to improve appearance only
7. Overdenture case

Case 1. COMPLEX CASE WITH SEVERE MEDICAL PROBLEMS

It is easily comprehended that severe medical problems such as recent coronary occlusions, congestive heart failure, or malignant hypertension will in most instances preclude the institution of elective dental procedures. Usually for such patients the physician will only permit dental treatment for infection and pain and then usually requires that such necessary work be undertaken in the hospital. Many such patients are not expected to live very long and so fall into the dental category of transitional-care cases. Usually the dentist's paramount concern is that the patient will not succumb during treatment or have his systemic problem worsened by the dental procedures. Thus all com-

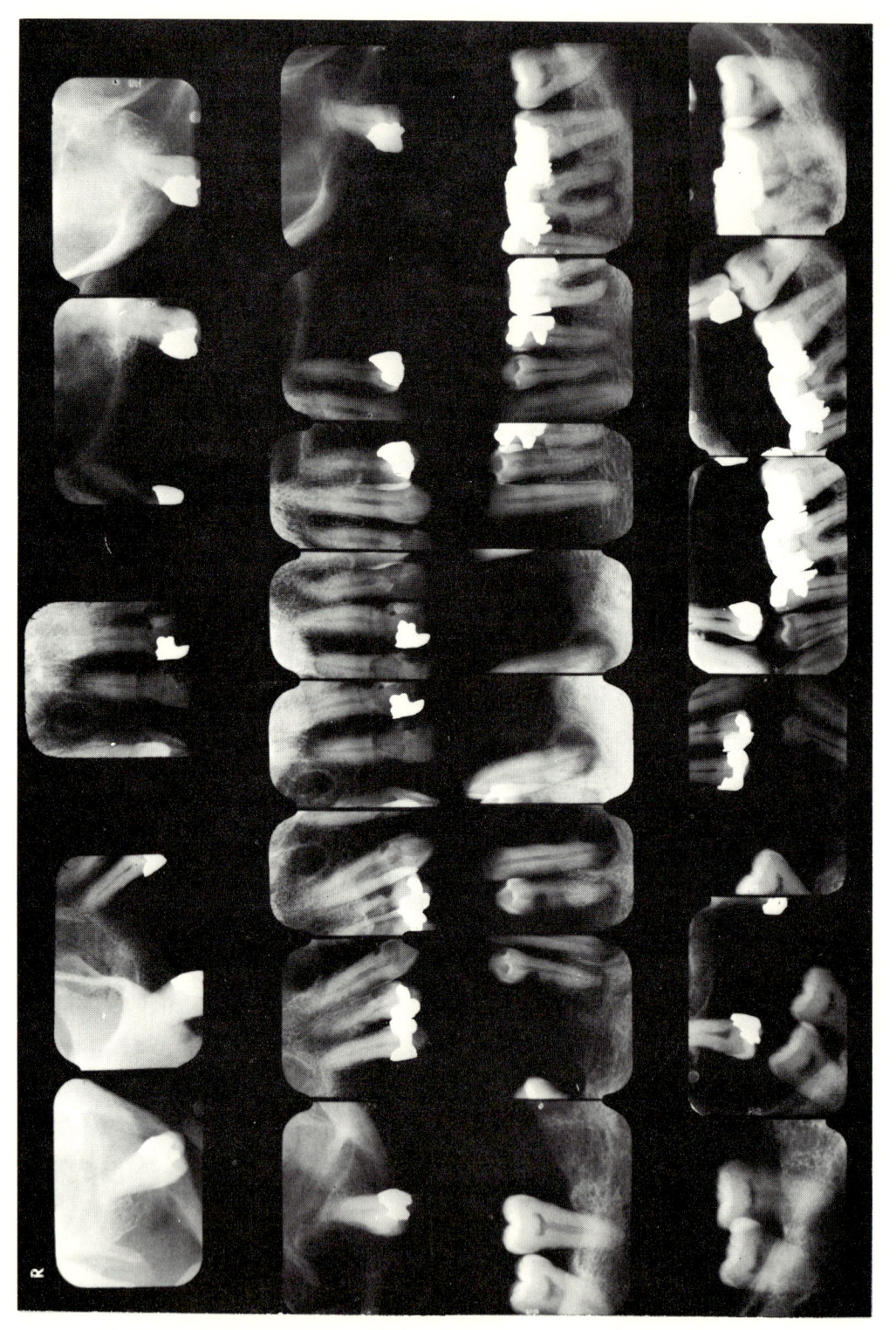

Fig. 14-1. Case 1. Full-mouth roentgenograms.

plex dental procedures such as unnecessary difficult extractions, surgical periodontics or endodontics, or crowns, bridges, and splinting procedures are not done.

In order to conserve space and also because a full case report is deemed unnecessary, we are showing only the full-mouth roentgenograms (Fig. 14-1) of a 60-year-old man who has suffered two myocardial infarctions within the last year. The physician advises that he will only permit dental treatment for pain and infection and that the patient would require hospitalization for this.

Chief complaint

The patient presents with a chief complaint of pain in the lower right canine.

Diagnostic summary

1. Critical cardiac condition
2. Abscess of tooth 27
3. Numerous dental problems of a complex nature

Treatment plan
Summary

Extraction of tooth 27 is required, with the patient hospitalized and the physician in attendance (in consultation with the physician, of course).

Rationale

If the whole mouth were being considered for treatment in a healthy individual who has adequate funds and appropriate desire, the case would be considered a complex tooth replacement case. Root canal therapy, crowns, extensive periodontal procedures, and partial dentures would be considered. However, none of these treatments should even be considered in this patient at this time. Attempts to instruct the patient in home care are indicated, and, if the patient's cardiac condition stabilizes in a year or two, in the absence of symptoms elective dental procedures could be considered at that time under the guidance of the physician.

Case 2. COMPLEX CASES THAT HAVE FAILED IN THE STABILIZATION OR MONITORING STAGES

Again, it seems unnecessary to illustrate this type of case with examples. What is being considered here is the patient who needs extensive periodontal therapy, deep restorations, and crowns and bridges. The dentist has mapped out his or her approach to the patient and the patient has accepted the treatment plan and also has sufficient funds. Let us consider that the dentist has completed the home care instruction and reinforcement, has excavated all the deep cavities, and has placed temporary fillings. However, the patient's home care efforts at this time prove to be grossly inadequate. The dentist should reinforce the need for and the techniques of adequate home care once again and check the patient in a month to see if the hygiene has improved. If significant improvement is not seen at that time, the case should be reclassified as a transitional case and the thought of extensive treatment abandoned. The patient should be told that since he has failed to take on his share of the responsibilities to help establish disease control, it is useless to pursue the planned treatment any further because he will gradually lose his teeth anyway.

Case 3. GROSS CARIES

Chief complaint

Mr. S. is a 21-year-old man seeking dental treatment because of several painful teeth. He states that he would like to have his teeth extracted and complete dentures made in order to obtain a more satisfactory appearance.

Medical history

The patient states that he is presently in very good physical condition. He is not taking any form of medication. There is a history of hospitalization for removal of tonsils and for fracture of a finger and a right elbow incurred during football games. He denies knowledge of the presence of any serious illnesses or symptoms of such.

Social and family history

The patient is single, is employed as a management trainee at a local savings and loan institution, and has a college education. He denies a family history of hereditary disease such as diabetes. No one in his family has ever had hepatitis B. He smokes about one and one-half packs of cigarettes per day and drinks alcohol only at parties.

Dental history

The patient has not been to see a dentist for 10 years. At that time orthodontic treatment was recommended to correct the buccal version of tooth 6, but treatment was never commenced. Mr. S. states that the only treatment he has received from a dentist has been a cleaning. He has experienced toothaches and drainage from sinuses in his alveolar mucosa and gingiva periodically over the last 4 or 5 years.

Attitudinal considerations

The patient was the last child in a family of 10 children. His father has worked steadily for years as a sanitary engineer at a local establishment. Financially it has been a struggle for the father just to provide the vital necessities of life. As stated previously, Mr. S. has not seen a dentist in 10 years. He attended the state university near his home and worked evenings during all 4 years of college to earn money to cover educational expenses. He has just begun his first postcollege job as a trainee in a savings and loan institution. Financially he figures that he can spend only $500 to $600 on his teeth over the next 2 years. He feels that his teeth are so bad that fixing them up satisfactorily would be a waste of money, although he says perhaps some of the better ones on the lower jaw could be maintained.

Clinical examination

Except for a firm, enlarged painless "node" in the right submaxillary space, the extraoral and neck examinations were unremarkable. All the teeth are present. Most show extreme amounts of decay (Fig. 14-2). Occlusion is basically class 1 with a cross-bite on the right side. The maxillary arch is narrow in comparison with the mandibular arch. There is much crowding in the

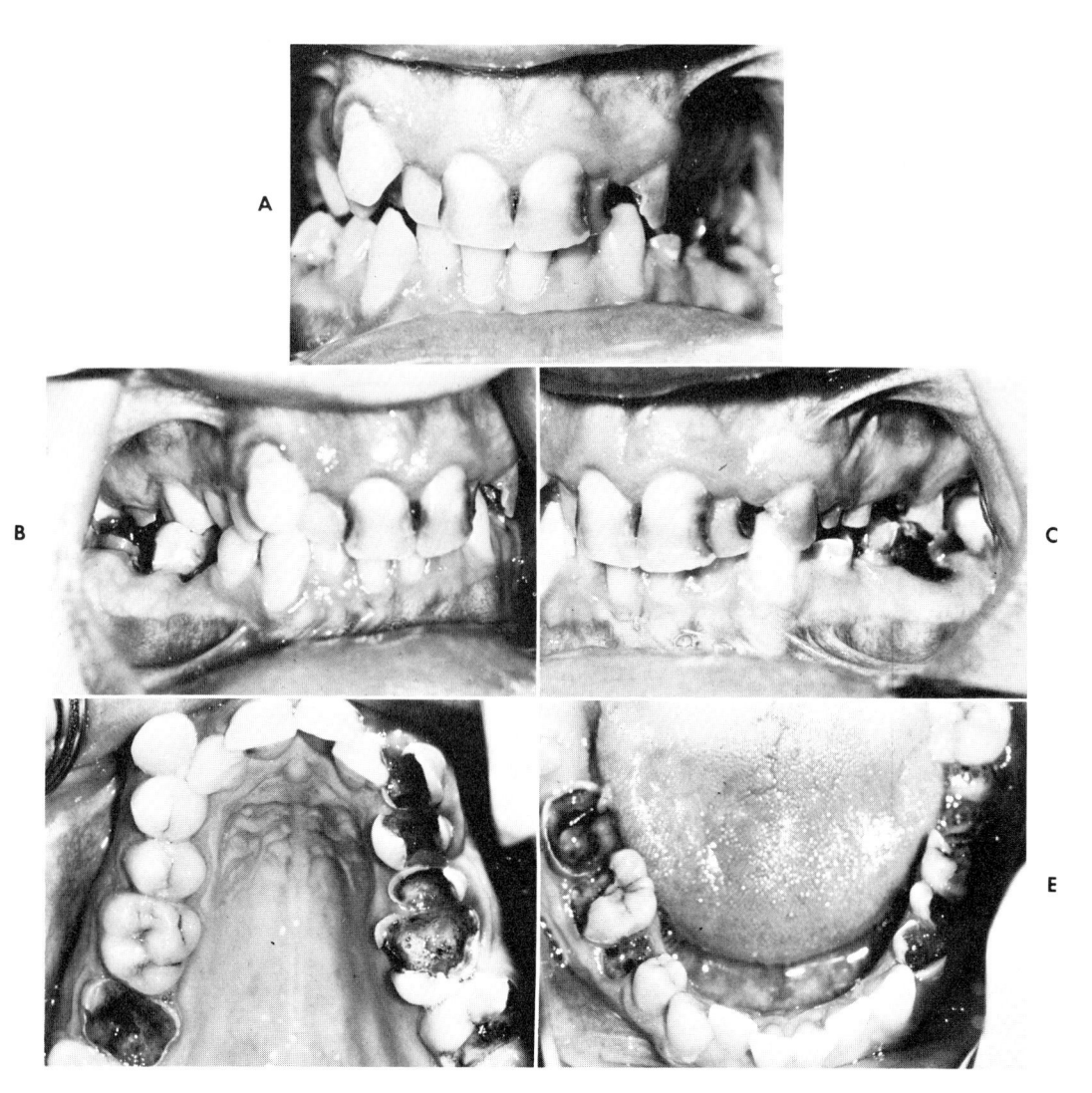

Fig. 14-2. Case 3. Clinical view of dentition. **A**, Anterior view of teeth in occlusion. **B**, View of right side. **C**, View of left side. **D**, Occlusal view of maxillary dentition. **E**, Occlusal view of mandibular dentition.

maxillary anterior region and a lesser amount in the mandibular anterior. Tooth 6 is severely malposed to the facial and is also somewhat superior to its normal position. The gingiva showed some imflammation in areas where the crowns are severely broken down. Roentgenographic examination showed periapical radiolucencies on teeth 2, 12, 13, 14, 20, 21, 29, 30, and 31 (Fig. 14-3). There is also a fourth maxillary molar impacted to the distal on the right side. Rampant decay is exhibited throughout the mouth—only tooth 6 and the six mandibular anterior teeth are spared. Fig. 14-4 shows the examination chart completed for this patient.

Diagnostic summary

1. Gross loss of much tooth tissue except for the upper right malposed canine and the six mandibular anterior teeth
2. Limited finances

Treatment plan
Summary

1. Complete maxillary immediate denture
2. Partial denture for the mandible, retaining the six anterior teeth

Rationale

Many of the strategic teeth are hopeless, having decayed to such extent that restoration is impossible. This fact, in combination with the patient's very stringent financial straits and also his desires, are indications for a complete upper denture. Because this patient must deal with the public every day, an immediate denture was selected. The condition of the lower arch prompted us to classify Mr. S. as a transitional case. His caries rate is currently so high that the prognosis of the lower teeth not yet severely involved with decay is in question. As a result, it was decided to preserve the lower anterior teeth and to place a partial denture as a transitional denture perhaps en route to a full denture in several years' time.

Sequencing

STABILIZATION. The lower left first and second molars were giving a great deal of pain, so the posterior teeth in this quadrant and the upper left quadrant would be extracted at the earliest opportunity. Then the posterior teeth to be extracted on the right side could be removed at the next appointment. After the extractions are done, home care instruction should come next. Then the necessary restorative work should be done on the mandibular anterior teeth prior to taking impressions for the immediate complete upper denture and the delayed mandibular partial denture.

MAINTENANCE AND MONITORING. Within 6 months the patient should be reexamined in order to determine if the patient is practicing adequate home care and to see if the upper immediate denture should be rebased at that time. Also, the remaining mandibular teeth will need to be monitored closely for decay activity. In addition, it is critical to ensure that the patient is wearing his lower partial denture because if he is failing to do so, the occlusal overload in the anterior region will produce an acceleration of loss of bone in the anterior region of the maxillary ridge.

The transitional case 245

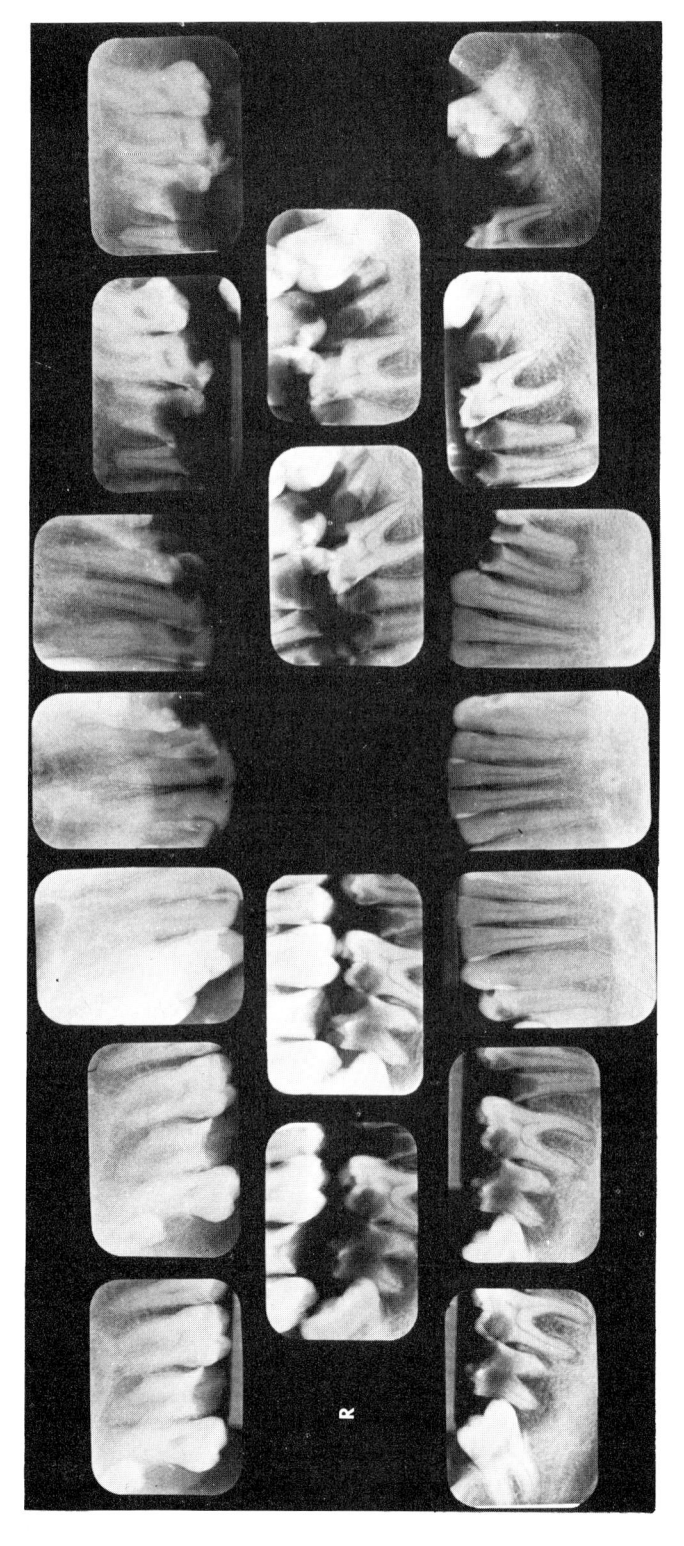

Fig. 14-3. Case 3. Full-mouth roentgenograms.

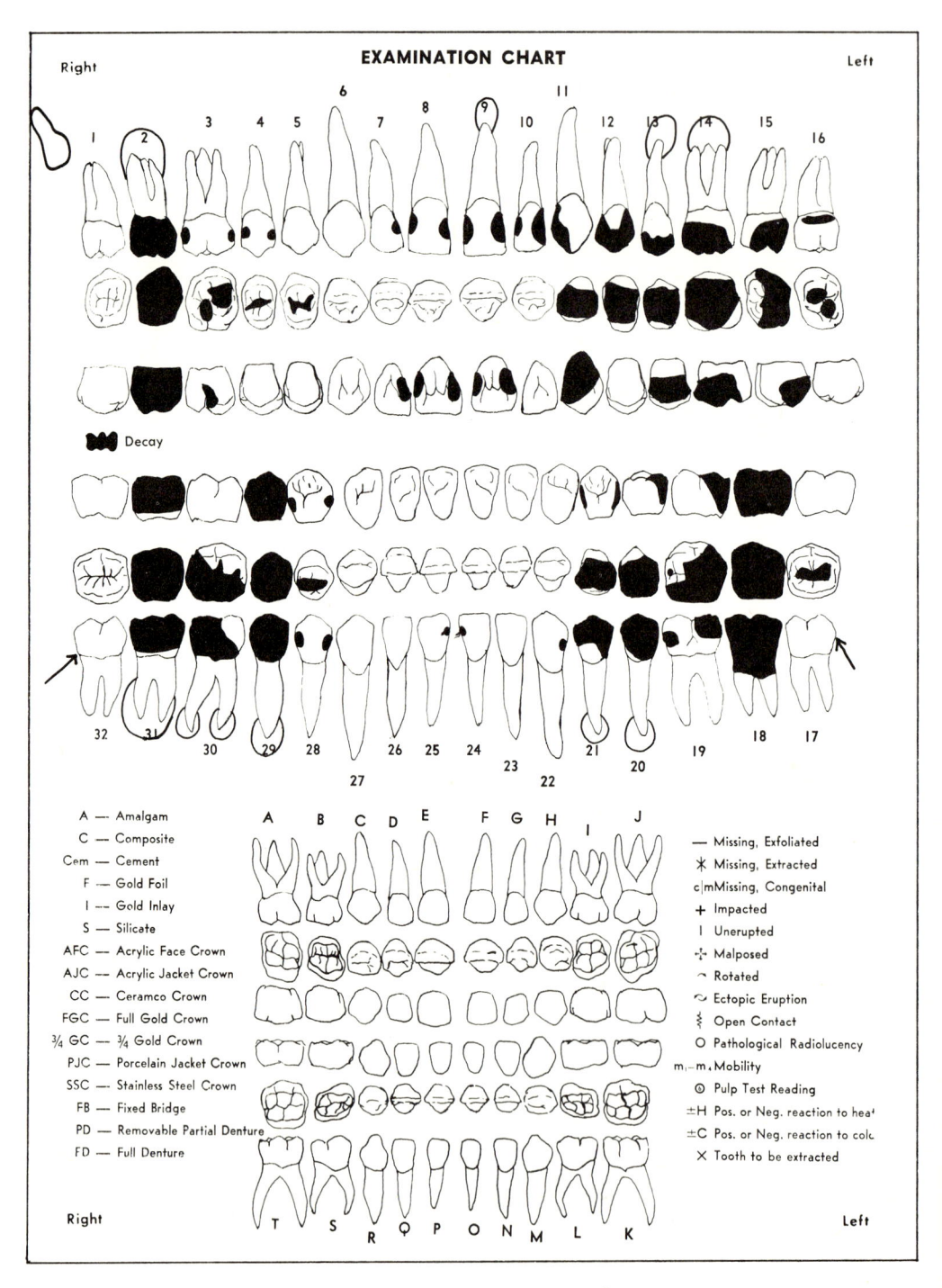

246 *Sequencing, classification, case analysis, and case treatment planning*

Fig. 14-4. Case 3. Examination chart.

Case 4. MODERATE TO SEVERE PERIODONTITIS IN PATIENT WITH LIMITED FINANCES

In this instance the patient is an elderly widow whose finances are so limited that she has only $100 or $200 to spend for dental treatment over the next year or two. The patient has all of her dentition except for the third molars. Unfortunately, extensive full-mouth periodontal surgery in conjunction with some splinting will be necessary to achieve stabilization. The patient obviously cannot afford this approach, nor does she anticipate that her financial position will ever improve. About the only option available is to treat the case as a transitional-care case. Home care instruction is mandatory, but only emergency procedures would be done as she presents with problems.

Case 5. HOPELESS PERIODONTITIS WITH TOOTH REPLACEMENT

The type of case that is envisioned here is the patient who presents with hopeless generalized periodontitis yet has so far retained all his teeth. This is obviously a transitional case no matter what the financial situation of the patient is. One approach would be to have the patient maintain all his remaining teeth until the presence of pain or infection dictates the need for immediate extraction of a tooth or two. In my opinion, a better approach is to extract most of the teeth immediately and go to temporary partial dentures before any more of the alveolar bone is lost. This approach is illustrated below.

Chief complaint

Mr. J. is a 72-year-old man who presents for full-mouth extractions and complete dentures.

Medical history

Mr. J. reports that he experienced the usual childhood diseases. He was hospitalized four times: in 1917 for influenza, in 1921 for the reduction of a fractured femur, in 1929 for an appendectomy, and in 1972 for a hemorrhoidectomy. He does not experience residual symptoms from any of these experiences. He states that he currently is enjoying good health and has not taken any medication for years except aspirin, which he takes for an occasional headache.

Social and family history

Mr. J. denies a family history of diabetes, cancer, or other hereditary diseases. He admits to smoking one pack of cigarettes per day and says he has done so for the last 50 years. He states that he does not drink alcohol except on certain occasions such as Christmas and the Fourth of July.

Dental history

Throughout his lifetime the patient has sought dental care only for relief of pain, and then he has requested that the offending tooth be extracted. His most recent extraction was tooth 31. It was removed 6 months ago because it became so loose that he was afraid he would aspirate it.

Attitudinal considerations

Mr. J. comes from an immigrant European family that has never placed much emphasis on maintaining teeth. He used to brush his teeth once a week, but reports that he gave that up some 30 years ago. He states that most of his forefathers have had all their teeth extracted by 50 years of age and have had good experiences with full dentures. He expresses some concern about the lower denture because his wife had experienced a very difficult time getting used to one. Mr. J. is a retired mail clerk.

Clinical findings

A firm, freely movable, enlarged "node" was found in the right submaxillary area. The examination of the face was unremarkable except for a rough-surfaced dark-brown mass just lateral to his left eye in the temple region. The exophytic mass was about 2 cm in diameter and was raised about 0.5 cm above the surface of the skin. It felt greasy on palpation (impression was seborrheic keratosis).

Intraoral examination showed varicosities on the undersurface of the tongue that were within normal limits for a patient of Mr. J.'s age. All of the remaining maxillary and mandibular teeth demonstrated marked mobility caused by the severe generalized periodontitis. Gross calculus deposits were present on all the teeth. Caries were present on teeth 2, 3, 4, 5, 6, 7, 11, 12, 15, and 31. The roentgenographic examination verified the clinical impression of generalized advanced bone loss (Fig. 14-5).

Diagnostic summary

1. No apparent medical problems
2. Seborrheic keratotic lesion on left temple

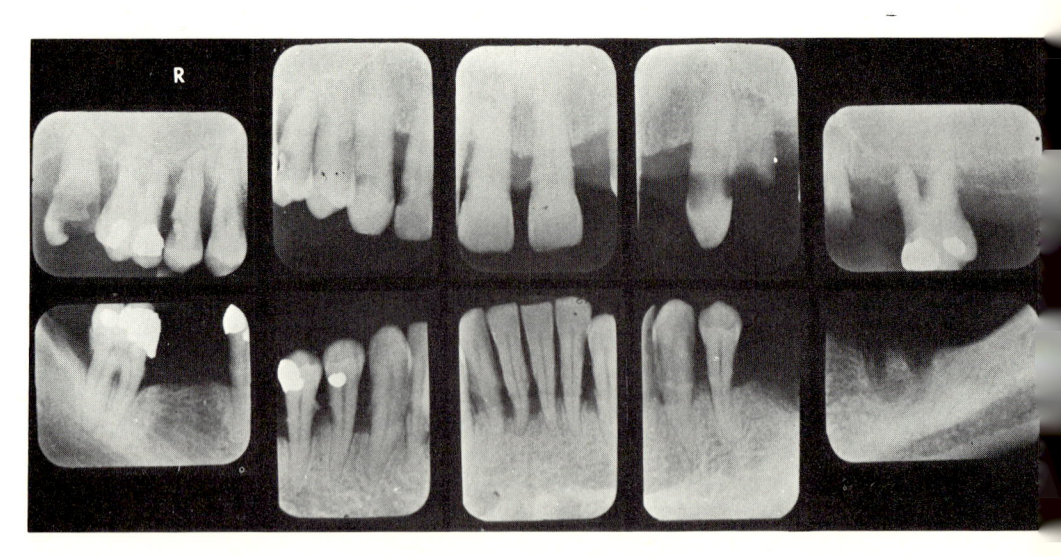

Fig. 14-5. Case 5. Full-mouth roentgenograms.

3. Severe advanced generalized periodontal disease in all remaining teeth; gross caries present on several teeth; smaller cavities present in others

Treatment Plan
Summary

1. Extraction of all remaining maxillary and mandibular teeth except the mandibular canines
2. Full upper denture and temporary mandibular acrylic partial denture with wrought-gold clasps on lower canines

Rationale

It was decided to provide a complete upper denture for at least two reasons: (1) this is what the patient desired; and (2) all the posterior teeth were hopelessly involved periodontally and, in addition, some were involved with gross caries. The maxillary anterior teeth, although not as involved periodontally as the posterior teeth, still demonstrated marked mobility. One option would have been to extract the left maxillary canine, save the four maxillary anterior teeth, and place a temporary acrylic partial denture. However, these teeth would probably not last longer than a year, and also the aesthetics would be inferior to that provided by a full denture. Furthermore, inasmuch as patients usually adjust quite well to a complete maxillary denture, it was decided to go this route. Another option is to go to an overdenture, with endodontics on the maxillary canines and placement of gold copings. This approach was decided against because in this practitioner's opinion maxillary overdentures at this age provide very few advantages, if any, over the complete denture.

It was decided to provide an acrylic partial denture on the mandibular arch with wrought-gold clasps on the retained canines. Although the practitioner and patient understood that the canines might not last the year, they were retained in order to train the patient in the use of an "almost" complete denture. It was anticipated that within 6 months to 1 year these teeth would become so mobile that they would have to be extracted, and at that time they could be added to the temporary partial denture, and the temporary partial denture could be converted into a complete denture. An overdenture was considered but rejected because it was felt that the bone support on the premolars and canines was inadequate. A complete lower denture could have been made immediately; however, both the practitioner and the patient believed the training period with the transitional partial denture would be quite helpful.

Sequencing

Since Mr. J. volunteers 1 day per week in the community hospital, he did not wish to go without anterior teeth. Thus it was decided to provide immediate maxillary and mandibular dentures. Thus the posterior teeth 2, 3, 4, 5, 12, 15, 21, 28, 29, and 31 were to be extracted first. Then in 4 weeks, if the ridges were healed adequately, the construction of the dentures would be begun. When the dentures were ready, the anterior teeth 6, 7, 8, 9, 10, 11, 23, 24, 25, and 26 would be extracted and the dentures placed.

DISEASE CONTROL. In this case, stabilization (disease control) was achieved through extraction of the periodontally involved teeth. In addition, therapeutic root planing was carried out on the retained mandibular canines, attempting to reduce the periodontal condition as much as possible.

MAINTENANCE AND MONITORING. After necessary postinsertion adjustments are made, the patient should be seen again in 6 months for a reexamination for the purpose of determining if all is maintained in order. Particularly, it will be necessary to evaluate the dentures for possible rebasing at that time. In addition, the mandibular canines need to be evaluated to determine if they should be retained for a longer period or if they should be extracted at that time and added to the partial denture, thus converting it into a full denture.

Case 6. COMPLEX CASE: TRANSITIONAL TREATMENT TO IMPROVE APPEARANCE ONLY

This case is typical of a large cross section of the population who seek dental care when aesthetics become a matter of concern to them, their family, or, occasionally, their friends or employers. Quite frequently such patients present when it is already too late to save those very teeth that have become unsightly. The physical condition of the patient, the status of the remaining dentition, motivation, and financial capability for care influence any course of treatment proposed.

Chief complaint

Mr. S. is a 60-year-old man who presents for treatment of a loose central incisor and also to improve the appearance of his front teeth.

History of present illness

Mr. S. first became aware of his gum problems about 8 years ago, but he doubted the sincerity of the dentist who informed him about his condition, so he delayed treatment. Approximately 1 year later he noticed that tooth 9 was loose. This same tooth had been traumatized some 2 years before, and he assumed that there might be some relationship between that accident and its current mobile state. About a year ago, Mr. S. went to a new dentist who examined him, also noted his periodontal condition, and presented a treatment plan at a subsequent appointment. Mr. S. was shocked to learn that virtually no treatment of the gum problems was included in the plan—only crowns and bridges. This appeared unwise to him in view of the fact that tooth 9 and now tooth 8 as well were considerably more mobile than they had ever been and were getting worse, not to mention the fact that they had drifted from their original positions. He decided not to go through with treatment. The condition was annoying, but it never caused him any pain.

Past medical history

Mr. S. is a member of the Kaiser-Permanente medical health plan and has had physical examinations on an annual basis for many years. He had all of the usual childhood diseases, but he denies a history of rheumatic fever, tuberculosis, diabetes, or heart disease. All systems are within normal limits at present; however, in 1949 Mr. S. had pneumonia and pleurisy, and in 1973 he was hospitalized for surgical correction of a hernia and varicose veins. At age 16 he fractured his right collarbone, but there had been no adverse long-term effects. For the past 4 years Mr. S. has enjoyed exceptionally good health.

Social and family history

Mr. S. has been married for more than 30 years and has three grown children. He does not smoke tobacco or drink alcohol and denies taking any drugs. He brushes once or twice a day with a fluoride toothpaste, but he never has received formal instruction in these techniques. He does not use dental floss, but he has heard about it from his family. Mr. S. cannot recall any diseases that have run in his family.

Dental history

The patient has had no dental care over the past 9 years. Previously Mr. S. had several silver alloy restorations placed (three of which are still present) and a number of extractions done because of extensive caries or periodontal disease.

Attitudinal considerations

Mr. S. is a retired building contractor who indicates he could budget approximately $200 for dental care over the next 6 months to 1 year. He states that he is aware of problems with his gums, and he would like to save his teeth but cannot financially afford to. He is very anxious to improve the appearance of his upper front teeth.

Clinical findings

Examination of extraoral structures and cranial nerve functions confirmed that these systems are all within normal limits.

All tissues appear normal except for the gingiva, which is only slightly stippled and receded 2 to 4 mm generally. The free gingival margins are rounded and ischemic, especially around tooth 9 (Fig. 14-6). Pocket depths range from 1 to 9 mm. Plaque is heavy in many gingival sulci, and gingival atrophy is particularly notable at teeth 5, 6, 7, 8, 9, 13, 21, and 22; less than 1 mm of attached gingiva is present at the latter two sites.

Teeth 5, 15, and 18 exhibit occlusal caries. Teeth 21 and 29 have slight distal pit caries, and recurrent caries is notable on the facial surfaces of teeth 18 and 31, and on the occlusal surface of tooth 31 as well. Incipient caries is evident on the mesial surface of tooth 7, and recurrent caries and partial breakdown of the composite restoration in tooth 9 are also apparent. Teeth 1, 2, 3, 14, 16, 17, 19, 20, 30, and 32 are missing. Plaque is heavy in some areas, especially interproximally. Mandibular teeth exhibit no mobility, but eight of the ten maxillary teeth are mobile.

Fig. 14-7 demonstrates the hand-articulated diagnostic casts of Mr. S. The canines are in a class 1 relationship on the right side and a class 2 relationship on the left side. Note the space present distal to each canine. The left side is slightly collapsed posteriorly where teeth 19 and 20 have been lost. Also note

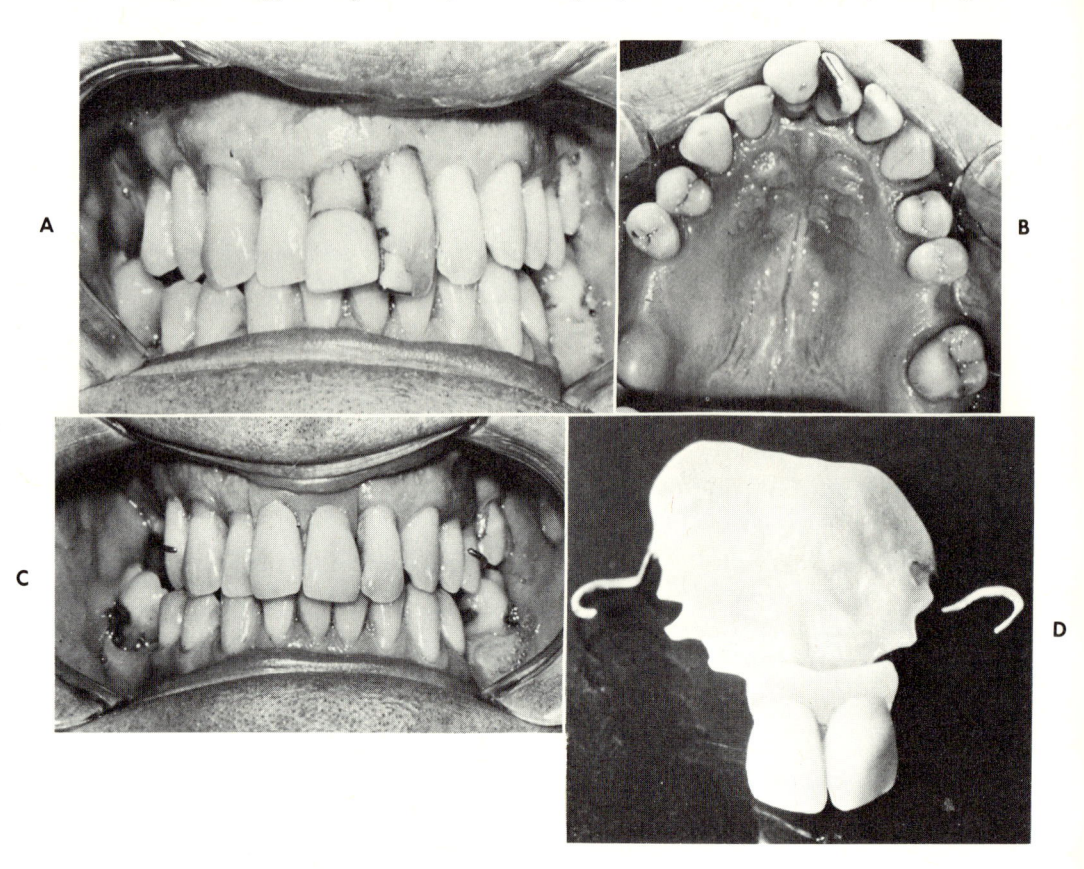

Fig. 14-6. Case 6. Clinical view of dentition. **A** and **B**, Pretreatment views. **C**, Partial denture in position. Note improved appearance. **D**, Transitional partial denture.

the supraeruption of tooth 31 and its relationship to the enlarged maxillary tuberosity above, which can be seen in Fig. 14-7, *B*. The overbite of tooth 9 is approximately 12 mm, and that of tooth 8 is about 9 mm. On closing, a 5 mm horizontal and 2 mm vertical shunt is observable. Wear is greatest on the canines (incisal edges) and least on the premolars and molars. The patient has no occlusal complaints, but tooth 9 is undergoing obvious secondary occlusal trauma.

Roentgenographically, furcation involvement was suggestive on teeth 18 and 31 (Fig. 14-8). This was confirmed during the clinical examination. Fig. 14-9 depicts the examination chart for this patient.

Diagnostic summary

1. Severe generalized periodontitis, localized periodontal atrophy, and occlusal trauma
2. Poor aesthetics in upper central incisors

Prognosis

The prognosis is generally fair, but hopeless for teeth 4, 8, and 9 and guarded for the remaining maxillary teeth and for teeth 18, 24, and 31.

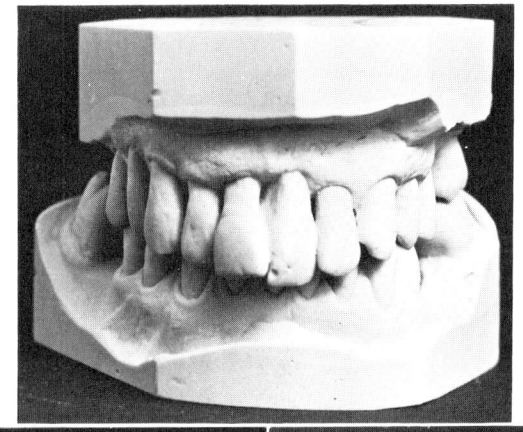

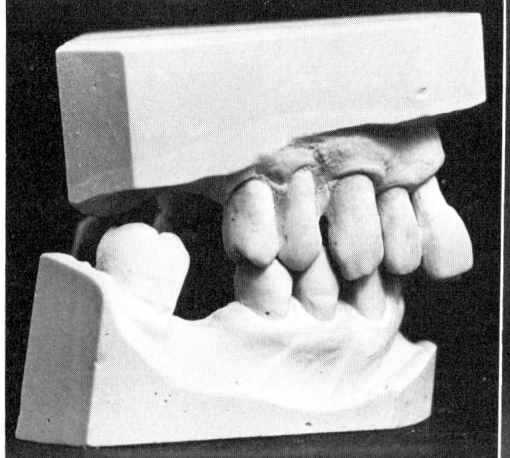

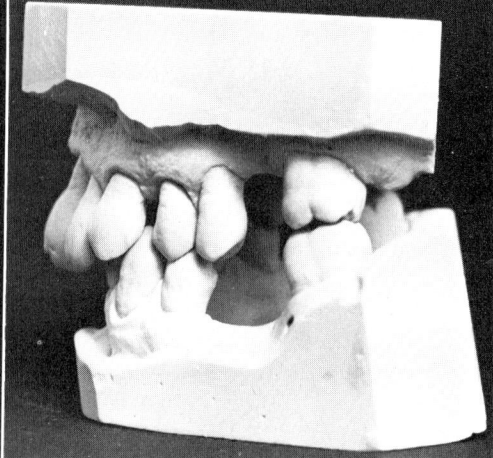

Fig. 14-7. Case 6. Hand-articulated models. **A,** Anterior view. **B,** Right side. **C,** Left side.

Treatment plan
Summary

1. Oral home care instruction
2. Therapeutic root planing on all teeth
3. Extraction of teeth 4, 8, and 9
4. Temporary maxillary partial denture to replace teeth 8 and 9

Rationale

It was proposed that Mr. S. be given oral hygiene instruction and that four quadrants of root planing be carried out. A diagnostic mounting was done to evaluate the occlusion and locate the centric relation position prior to constructing any prosthesis that would occlude with the remaining dentition. It also was determined that surgical correction of areas exhibiting periodontal atrophy be considered only if Mr. S.'s financial situation improved, if oral hygiene was substantially improved, and if the gingival tissues appeared otherwise healthy.

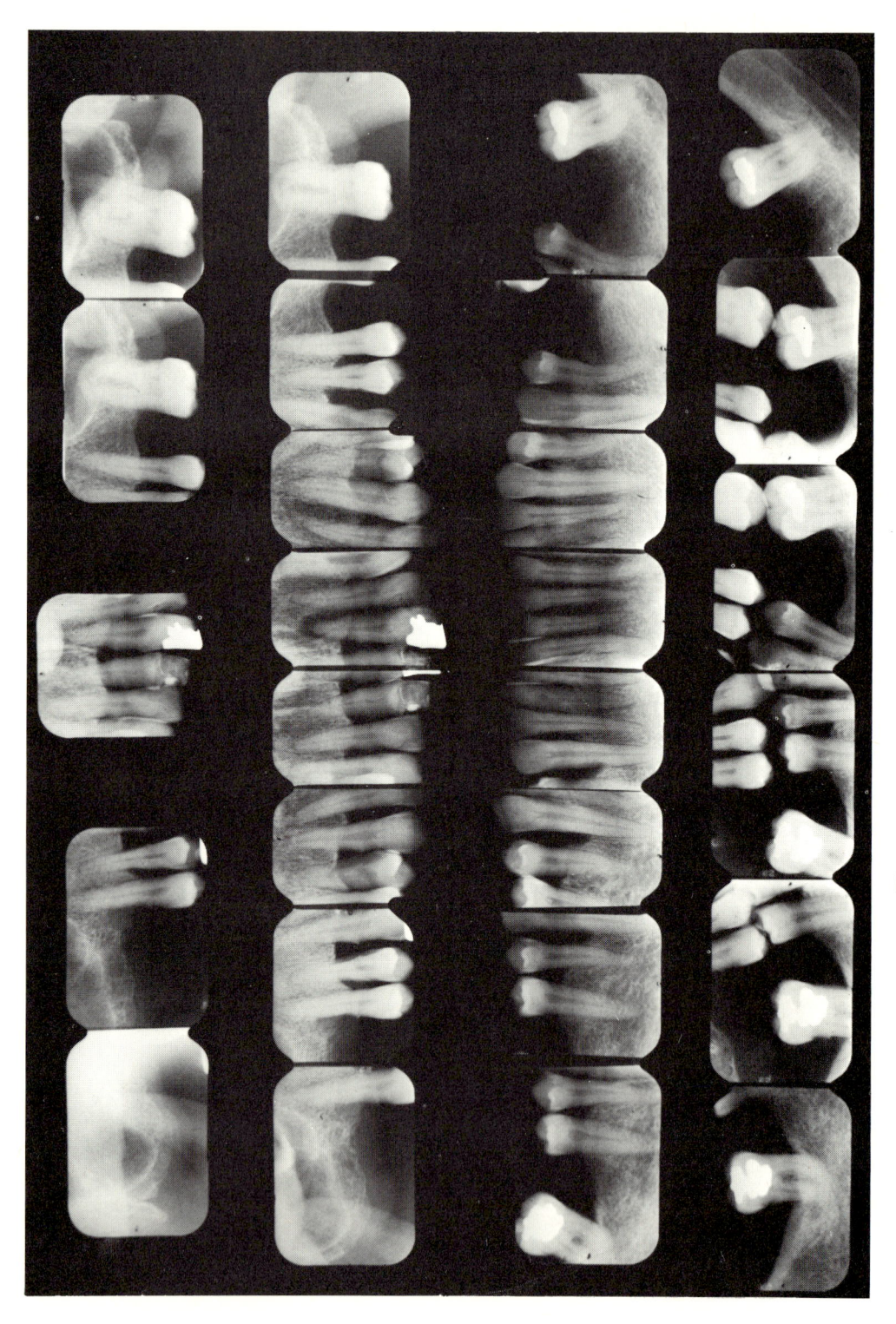

254 *Sequencing, classification, case analysis, and case treatment planning*

Fig. 14-8. Case 6. Full-mouth roentgenograms.

The transitional case 255

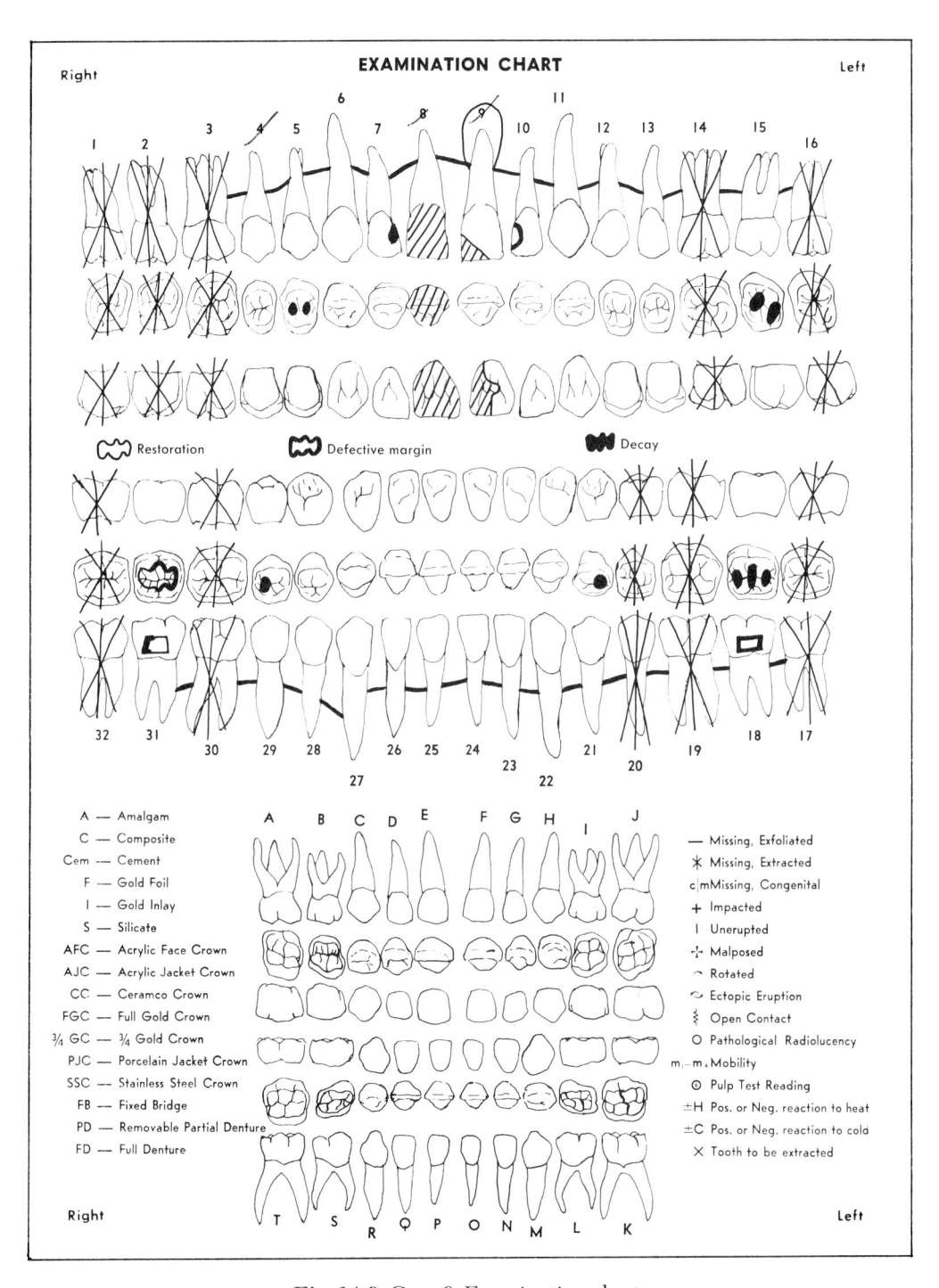

Fig. 14-9. Case 6. Examination chart.

An immediate provisional maxillary partial denture was planned to replace teeth 8 and 9 following their extraction, but not to replace tooth 4, which was extracted at the same time. The appliance was designed so as not to interfere with the existing occlusion. Semicircumferential wrought-wire clasps were fabricated to retain it. Since occlusal stresses borne by the partial denture would be minimal, no rest seats were fabricated in this case (Fig. 14-6, *D*). Note the substantial improvement in aesthetics (which was the key reason that this patient sought dental care) by contrasting the appearance of the patient in the postextraction photograph (Fig. 14-6, *C*) with his pretreatment appearance (Fig. 14-6, *A* and *B*). Following delivery of the temporary appliance, replacement of the defective restorations and an occlusal amalgam to repair the carious lesion on the occlusal surface of tooth 15 were completed. Simultaneously, healing of the extraction sites was monitored and explicit instructions for care and removal of the appliance, especially while sleeping, were reviewed on more than one occasion. It was felt that should the patient demonstrate outstanding home care, the prognosis for the maxillary teeth would be improved enough to consider a permanent maxillary partial denture. If, however, improvement did not occur, a suitable alternative treatment would be an immediate complete maxillary denture, following reduction of the enlarged tuberosity, and a distal-extension mandibular-cast partial denture, assuming the loss of teeth 18 and 31. Mr. S. was apprised of these alternatives. This case currently is undergoing the evaluative phase described above.

Sequencing

Stabilization or complete disease control was not attempted in Mr. S.'s case because he did not have the necessary funds to pay for the extensive periodontal therapy required even if he was able to demonstrate the required home care improvement. Mr. S. was first to be instructed in home care techniques, and then therapeutic root planing was to be initiated on all the teeth. Later, teeth 4, 8, and 9, the most severely periodontally involved teeth, were to be extracted when the temporary partial denture was ready for insertion.

As far as maintenance and monitoring is concerned, Mr. S. should be reexamined in 6 months to evaluate his home care. If he has shown remarkable improvement in this aspect and has sufficient funds, then consideration should be given to the possibility of instituting the necessary periodontal surgery in an attempt to achieve stabilization. With the improved prognosis for retaining the remaining maxillary teeth, thought should be given to providing a more permanent type of partial dentures that, in addition to carrying teeth 8 and 9, would also replace teeth 2, 3, 4, and 14.

On the other hand, if the monitoring process revealed continuing deterioration of the remaining maxillary teeth, then it would be anticipated that a full denture would be required in the not-too-distant future.

Case 7. OVERDENTURES

There is another type of case that deserves special mention—the transitional-care patient who might receive an overdenture. At least one entire text has been devoted to this subject,[1] so this discussion is meant only to be an introduction. Although there are some who may argue that overdentures constitute a permanent rather than a provisional form of care, we consider them a temporary diversion on the road to a complete denture. Furthermore, because of wearing of the appliances and changes that occur in oral tissues, overdentures require far more supervision and maintenance than truly permanent dentures.

Advantages of overdentures

In choosing between definitive, permanent dentures and overdentures, or between overdentures and conventional partial or complete dentures, the following factors and considerations are noteworthy:
1. Dramatic results with overdentures are often achieved at relatively low cost.
2. The overdenture treatment time is favorable when compared to more elaborate treatment modalities.
3. Overdentures generally are easily fabricated and modified.
4. Malalignment problems that cannot be resolved with fixed prostheses or conventional partial dentures are more readily concealed and overcome with ovendenture appliances.
5. Preservation of some condemned teeth and of the adjacent alveolar bone can be accomplished with overdentures.
6. With overdentures the patient is prepared for the possible eventual loss of all abutments should their condition continue to deteriorate.
7. The prognosis is often improved with overdentures, as compared to a more costly treatment plan, since the risks in the former case usually are less and modifications are more easily and rapidly accomplished when necessary.
8. The overdenture technique is equally applicable to the maxillary and mandibular arches, and virtually every tooth is a potential overdenture abutment.

While overdentures, like any other denture, should ideally be prepared only when a patient has a healthy mouth, in reality, patients who often need such appliances cannot be counted on to maintain a healthy oral environment. As outlined above, a distinct advantage of the overdenture is that loss of an abutment tooth requires only the addition of a small amount of plastic resin. In comparison, if a partial denture abutment tooth is lost, it may be necessary to construct a new crown as well as a new partial denture.

Indications

There is a considerable range of situations in which overdentures are utilized. The usual overdenture patient may have only two abutment teeth, preferably canines or premolars (Fig. 14-10). It is more favorable but not essential that the supporting teeth be present bilaterally. Such teeth are usually not suitable to serve as abutments for bridges or partial dentures because of their poor bone support. Yet the crowns of such teeth can be reduced considerably and used successfully to support an overdenture.

On the other extreme, a potential overdenture patient may have a *full complement of teeth* that have undergone severe attrition or abrasion. If pres-

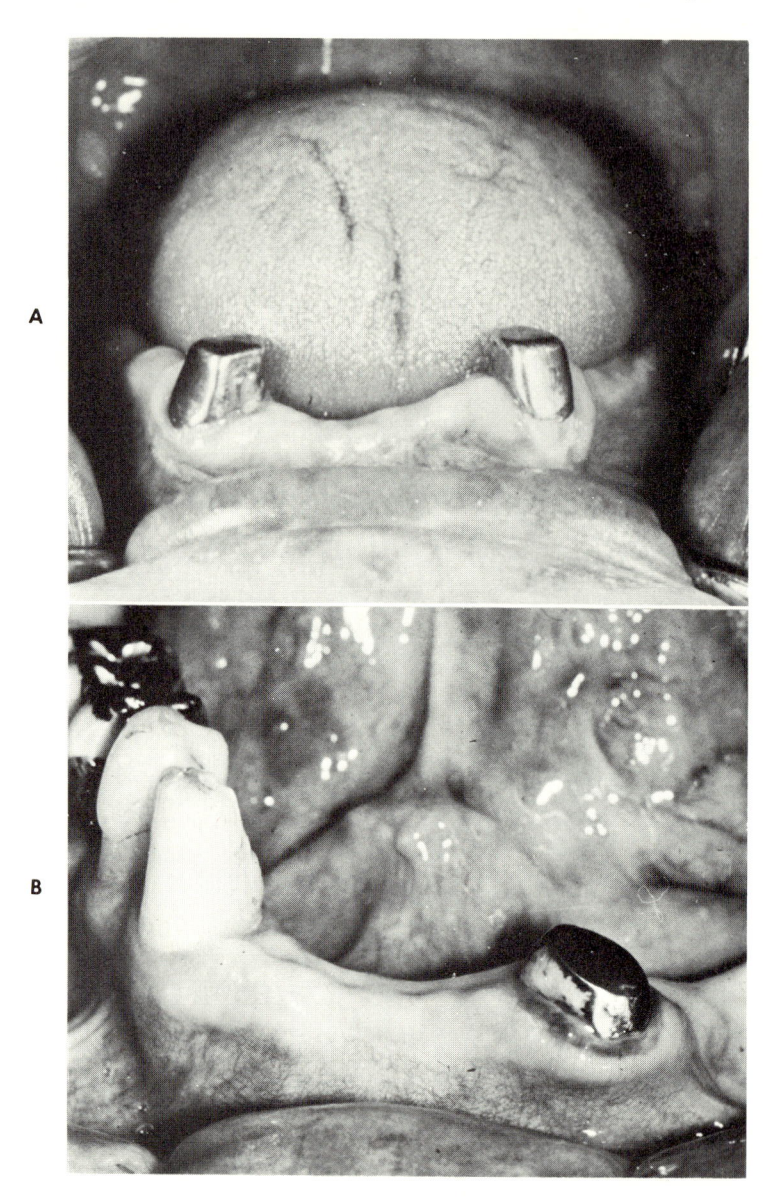

Fig. 14-10. Overdenture cases. **A,** Mandibular canines have been preserved bilaterally, and gold copings have been placed in order to prevent caries and erosion. **B,** This case represents a combination of an overdenture and a removable partial denture.

ent, caries and periodontal disease are eliminated first. Then severe undercuts in the dentition are blocked out and an overlay denture is fabricated that restores aesthetics, the approximated original intermaxillary occlusal dimensions, and much improved function—all without altering the dentition itself. Typically such an overdenture is fabricated with a short flange, since retention of the overdenture in this case is not dependent on a seal at the depth of the vestibule, as is the case with a conventional denture. Rather, retention is

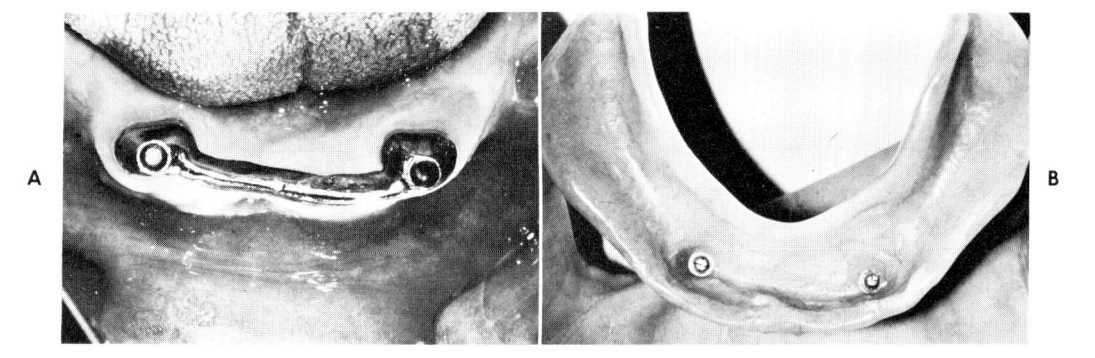

Fig. 14-11. Overdenture case with Baker bar and precision attachments. **A,** Bar with female attachments. **B,** Overdenture with two bilateral male attachments.

accomplished by means of the interdigitation of the teeth with the undersurface of the denture.

Abutment design

The methods of treating these remaining teeth vary from more or less elaborate telescoping gold-thimble crowns and intracoronal precision attachments, to interconnecting case (Dolder or Baker) bars that splint crowns that are one-half or less the height of the original teeth in order to reduce stress on the periodontium, to gold or silver restorations that seal the root canal(s) of therapeutically or intentionally endodontically treated teeth that have been reduced, often to a height only slightly above the residual ridge (Figs. 14-10 and 14-11). Frequently the telescoping crowns are cast or residual teeth altered so that distinct shoulders provide a definite seat for the denture; however, controversy exists regarding whether the overdenture should be relieved partially or completely in these abutment areas. The overdenture is fabricated sometimes with reciprocal telescoping crowns or a "clip" to further enhance retention and stability.

Contraindications and maintenance

Indiscriminate treatment planning for overdentures, such as placing them over abutments that have caries or periodontal disease, will end in failure. In addition, maintenance of both the prosthesis and the remaining abutments is crucial to successful management of these cases. Daily application of fluoride to all residual abutments is necessary in addition to thorough cleansing of the denture itself. Also, immaculate home care of the abutments and periodic scaling are mandatory. In the absence of such care, it can be predicted with certainty that destruction of the teeth or the periodontium or both will be accelerated. In all cases the overdenture should be considered as a transitional prosthesis that will require modifications from time to time, depending on changes in the individual patient and on the condition of the overdenture itself.

REFERENCE

1. Brewer, A. A., and Morrow, R. M.: Overdentures, St. Louis, 1975, The C. V. Mosby Co.

PART IV

Miscellaneous

15

Innovative approaches

Ronald E. Gier

A basic requirement that will generally ensure success in dental treatment is that the treatment rendered is desired by the patient and requires a minimal amount of patient involvement. This means that successful dental treatment is frequently the simplest that can be prescribed. As a general rule, the more complex the treatment the greater the chances for failure. Notwithstanding, there are times when drastic measures or innovative approaches are indicated in order to maintain teeth, to preclude the need for removable prosthetic appliances, to ensure aesthetics, and to correct anatomic defects. Innovative approaches may be defined as methods of dental treatment that are more dramatic, complicated, difficult, or heroic than are the usual conventional procedures.

Examples of innovative approaches currently being used in dentistry include surgery and surgical orthodontics, ridge extensions, implants, hemisection and root amputations, precision- or semiprecision-attachment partial dentures, bar bridges (Andrews bridges), and overlay dentures. These innovative approaches to treatment planning require much thought by the dentist performing the procedures and are never prescribed in a hasty manner. A thorough evaluation of the patient is imperative in each case before it can be determined if the procedures are warranted. This chapter will deal with the patient evaluation for such procedures and the indications for prescribing such types of restoration as well as the contraindications.

SPECIAL CONSIDERATIONS

An important factor to consider when contemplating the use of these innovative approaches to treatment planning is the dentist's training and ability. The dentist must have the ability and facilities to provide the recommended treatment or be willing to refer the patient to a specialist he or she knows is competent in providing the recommended treatment. Attempts by unqualified clinicians to provide these services usually end with unsatisfactory if not disastrous results. Anyone wishing to learn the techniques for these varied treatments can do so by attending continuing education courses that provide the information in lecture, laboratory, and clinical settings.

264 *Miscellaneous*

An equally important factor to consider when contemplating the use of innovative methods is the patient evaluation. In other chapters the general evaluation of patients has been discussed. This chapter will discuss additional evaluations that need to be made when considering these particular procedures.

The patients must be evaluated psychologically to determine if they are willing to accept the complicated procedure and to face the fact that the procedure is not always successful and may indeed fail. This evaluation must determine what effect the loss of the teeth or not doing the procedure will have on a particular patient. Complicated procedures may be indicated when the patient is unable to accept the loss of teeth. The strategic importance of the teeth in the reconstruction of the mouth is another factor to consider. The procedures to save one tooth whose loss would cause the patient to require a removable prosthesis or possibly lose the rest of his teeth may indicate the need for greater efforts on the dentist's part to maintain a particular tooth. The next factor to consider must be the economics. For all extensive and high-risk procedures that are attempted, there is a fee attached that is compatible to the difficulty of the procedure. The patient must be able and willing to assume this fee in order for the dentist to successfully provide the treatment. The placement of removable prosthetic appliances, including complete dentures, is still an indicated and acceptable dental treatment. If the patient is unwilling or unable to pay for the extensive procedures, then less complicated, more conventional treatments are indicated.

SURGERY AND SURGICAL ORTHODONTICS

Major oral surgery procedures are available to correct many of the growth, developmental, and anatomic jaw-relation discrepancies. These same procedures can also be used to correct acquired anatomic defects and deficiencies. These procedures include the well-recognized surgical procedures for correction of mandibular prognathisms that involve surgical sectioning of the mandible in different areas (depending on the problem) and repositioning of the mandible to produce a more satisfactory occlusion. Newer procedures are available for increasing mandibular jaw length by augmentation of the chin area, such as sliding the segments of the mandible forward to move anterior teeth into a more favorable position, or by depressing segments of the mandible, especially in the anterior region in order to reduce overbit relations (Fig. 15-1). Procedures are also available for correction of cross-bites: (1) splitting

Fig. 15-1. Surgical orthodontics case in which bilateral sagittal osteotomies were performed in combination with sliding geneoplasty to correct severe overjet and overbite and also to improve facial aesthetics. **A** and **B**, Presurgical full-face and lateral profile views showing severe class II deformity. **C**, Orthodontic appliances in place and pretreatment open bite. **D**, Postsurgical occlusion. **E** and **F**, Postsurgical full-face and lateral profile views showing marked aesthetic improvement. (Courtesy Dr. W. R. Hiatt, Kansas City, Mo.)

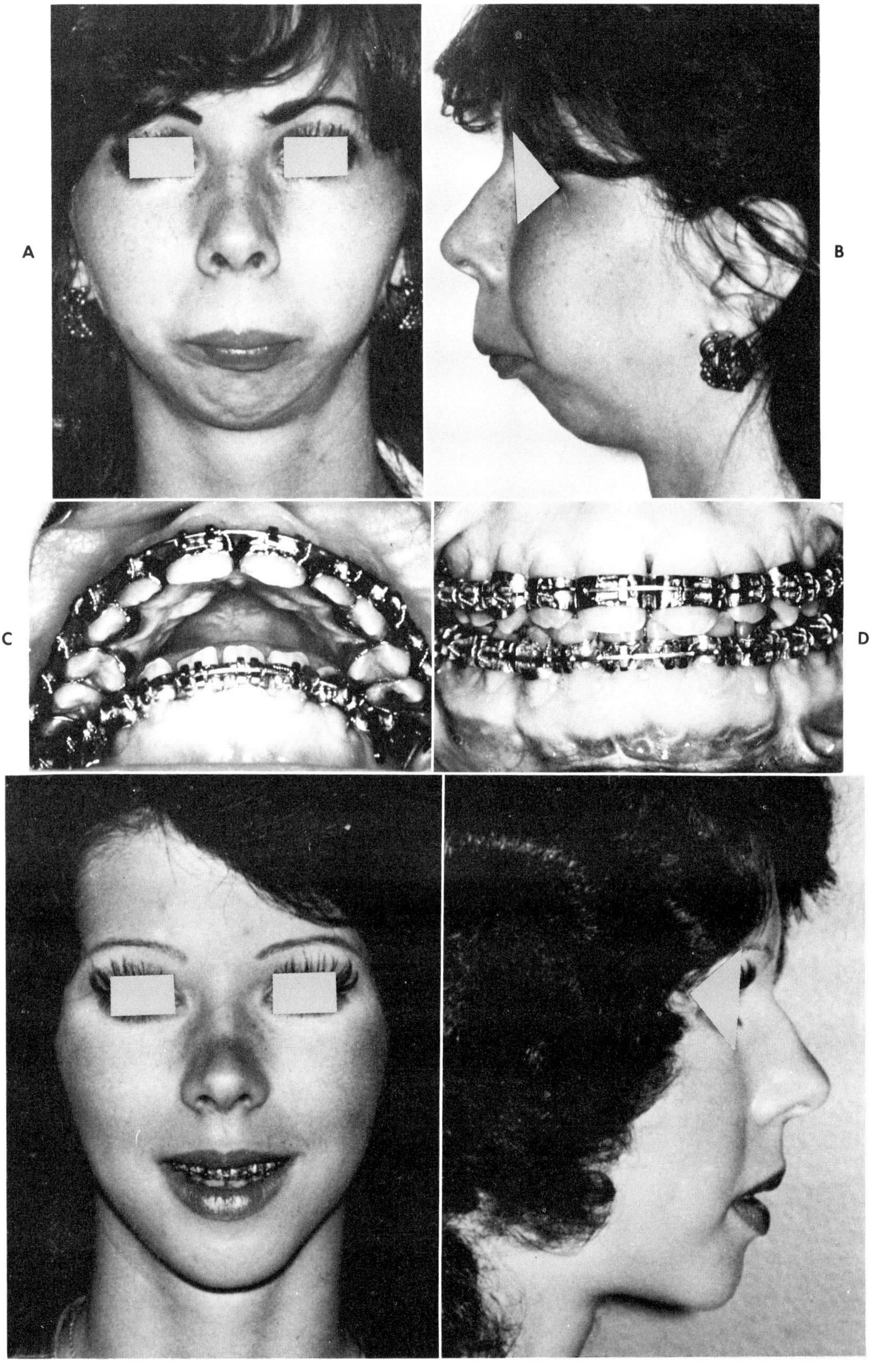

A B C D F

and spreading of the mandible or (2) moving complete sections of the mandible buccally or lingually. The same types of procedures are available for the maxillary arch in which segments or even half of the maxilla can be moved. The palate may be split along suture lines either to expand the arch or to move the anterior segment forward. Posterior segments may be moved buccally, lingually, superiorly, or occlusally. The anterior segment may also be surgically repositioned to correct extensive open bites, gross overjets, overbites, and maxillary deficiencies. Bone grafts or metallic implants can be used to correct bone loss due to injury, birth defects, or surgical procedures.

Surgical procedures alone can correct the problem in some cases, but frequently it is necessary for the surgeon to work in cooperation with an orthodontist in order to obtain ideal placement of teeth.

Major surgical procedures are best handled by a team approach. The dentist recommending such a procedure will need to serve as coordinator of the team, since he or she will be responsible for the final restorative phase of treatment. In the initial phases the dentist should contact the surgeon or orthodontist and evaluate the conditions together and decide if additional specialists will be needed on the team. The treatment should be completely designed prior to initiation of any procedures if possible. Most of the time the procedures discussed will take several years to complete, especially if orthodontics is involved. Surgical phases usually take only a matter of a few weeks to months to accomplish, and the restorative phases then take only the length of time necessary for the dentist to fabricate whatever appliances are necessary.

It is important for the general dentist to ensure that the mouth is disease free prior to initiation of these procedures. This is essential because both the surgical procedures and orthodontics will involve placing appliances in the mouth that will make home care more difficult. Also, it is much more convenient to place restorations before the appliances are placed in position. The degree of restorative dentistry done prior to surgery and orthodontics needs to be coordinated with the team. The treatment plan must take into consideration what teeth will be sacrificed for either orthodontic or surgical reasons. The possibility of devitalization of teeth as a result of the surgical procedures and repositioning of teeth must be considered. The dentist will also need to follow the patient for regular dental checkups throughout the surgical and orthodontic phases.

Indications

Severe prognathism, major cross-bite, severe anterior open bites or posterior open bites, major overbite and overjets, narrow palates, narrow mandibles, deficient base-bone support, and skeletal deficiencies are all indications for major surgical repositioning. As a general rule, if orthodontics or other prosthetic procedures can correct the malocclusions or deformities, then surgery is not done.

The psychologic aspect of the patient must be taken into consideration. Many of the patients with severe facial deformities caused by discrepancies in arch relationships have developed emotional problems. Most of the time the improvement that can be obtained is highly gratifying to both the surgeon and the patient. However, patients who expect too much improvement through the surgical or orthodontic procedures are not good candidates. A clear understanding should be worked out between the patient and the team providing the treatment as to what degree of improvement the patient can expect from the treatment.

Contraindications

The patient must be in satisfactory health to undergo the extensive anesthesia and surgical procedures for these corrections. Patients with severe cardiovascular disease, diabetes, other significant systemic diseases, or those taking medication (e.g., steroids) that would make them a surgical risk, delay healing, or increase the susceptibility to infection generally are not good candidates.

Psychologic considerations may rule against the procedure being undertaken. For instance, the patient that expects too much and cannot be convinced that the procedure will give improvement but not perfection should be eliminated as a candidate for this type of procedure.

RIDGE EXTENSIONS

The ridge extension procedure is one in which the denture-bearing surface of an edentulous patient can be increased through surgical techniques. This procedure involves surgical repositioning of the mucosa and muscle attachments in order to deepen the labial and buccal sulcus of the maxilla and mandible and the lingual sulcus of the mandible (Fig. 15-2).

Indications

Patients who have extensive bone loss of the maxillary or mandibular edentulous ridge are potential candidates for this procedure. Since many such patients function very adequately with their dentures, it is necessary to state that only those for which a satisfactory conventional denture cannot be made are considered as serious candidates for the procedure. There must be an adequate amount of mandibular or maxillary bone remaining to give support for both muscle attachment and mucosal attachment. Patients must be willing to undergo this procedure and be willing to accept the fact that this procedure will only improve their ability to wear dentures but will not provide them with a large denture-bearing surface and, therefore, any greatly added retention or stability to the denture. At best, surgical ridge extension procedures will only make difficult a once impossible denture situation.

Contraindications

The major contraindications for the alveolar ridge extension procedure is a lack of bone structure. Patients who have "pencil-thin" mandibles are not satisfactory candidates because there is inadequate bone support for muscle and soft tissue reattachment. Also, patients who have compromised mental foramina because of excessive ridge resorption will be unsatisfactory candidates because the denture and procedure will impinge on the mental nerve. Excessive loss of the bone on the maxillary arch in the zygoma region will cause failure. The patient must be in satisfactory health to undergo the extensive anesthesia and surgical procedures for these corrections. Patients with severe cardiovascular disease, diabetes, some other systemic diseases, or

268 *Miscellaneous*

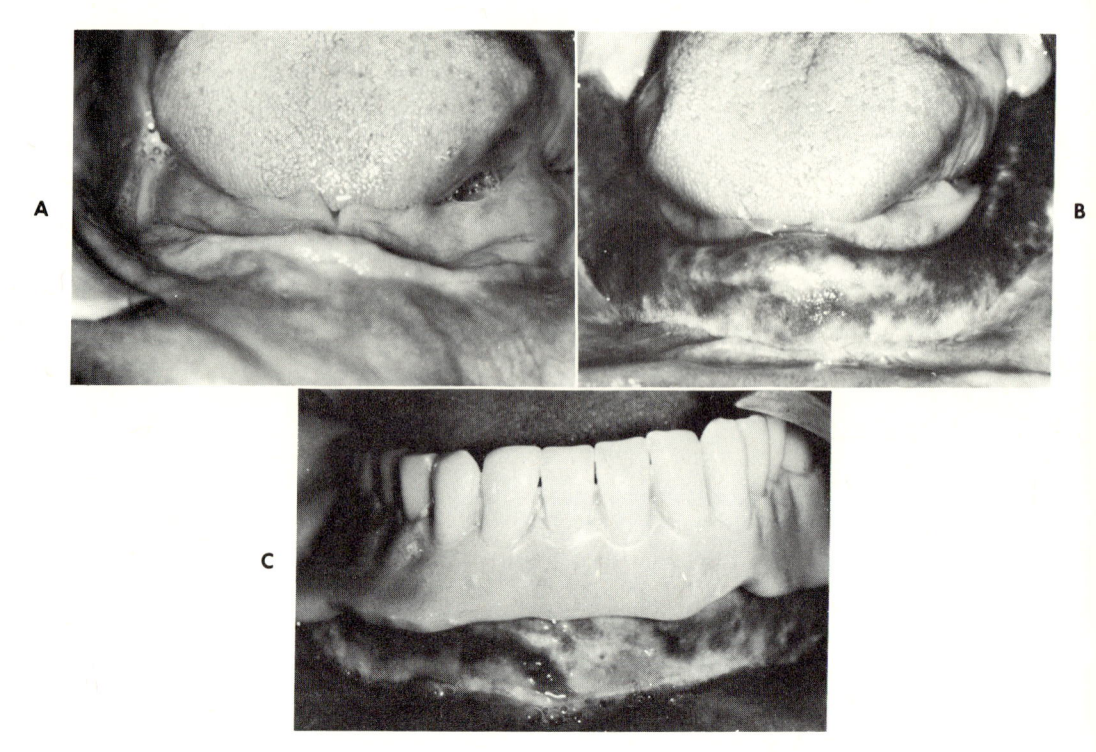

Fig. 15-2. Surgical ridge extension case. **A,** Minimal mandibular ridge and sulcus prior to surgery. **B,** Marked increase in ridge and sulcus 2 weeks after ridge extension and skin graft procedure. **C,** Old denture in place on postsurgical ridge showing increase in sulcus depth. Unfortunately, in most cases only some of the depth gained will be retained in a year's time. (Courtesy Dr. W. R. Hiatt, Kansas City, Mo.)

those taking medication (i.e., steroids) that would make them a surgical risk, delay healing, or increase the susceptibility to infection generally are not good candidates. The patient who expects dramatic results from this procedure should be eliminated from consideration.

IMPLANTS

There are two basic types of implants: subperiosteal and endosseous. The subperiosteal implant is used for support of complete dentures. The endosseous implant is primarily used for the support of fixed prostheses.

Subperiosteal implants

The subperiosteal implant involves insertion of a metal framework between the bone and the periosteum with extensions or posts through the mucosa to support and retain dentures (Fig. 15-3). The subperiosteal implant is primarily used in patients where the mandible has undergone severe and rapid ridge resorption. Following placement of the implant, a denture is made with female attachments to fit on the protruding portions of the implant.

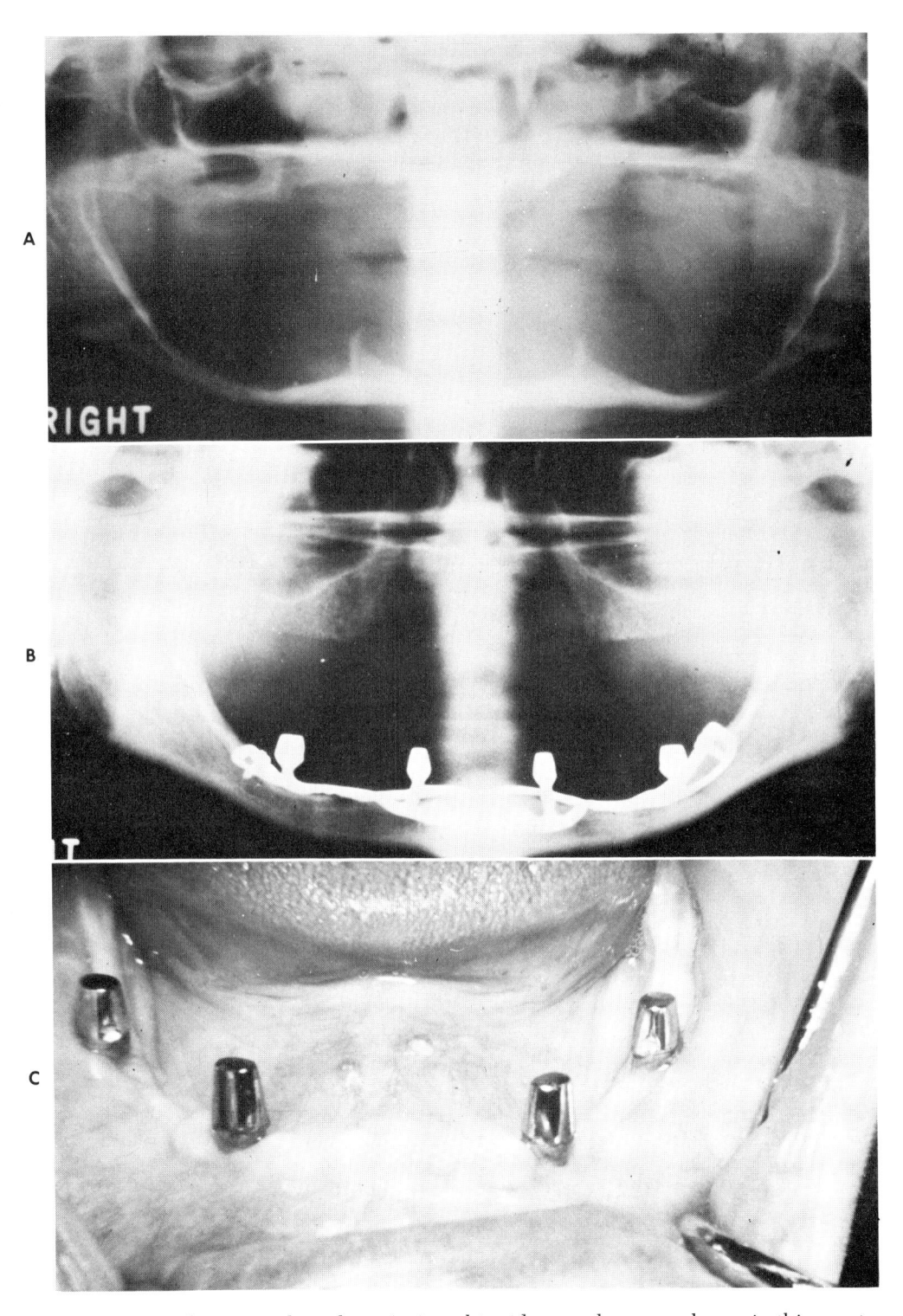

Fig. 15-3. Subperiosteal implant. **A,** Atrophic ridges such as one shown in this roentgenogram may be candidates for subperiosteal implants. **B,** Panograph showing subperiosteal implant in position. **C,** Intraoral photograph showing four supporting posts of subperiosteal implant protruding through mucosa. (Courtesy Dr. Phillip Jones, Kansas City, Mo.)

INDICATIONS

The subperiosteal implant is indicated for use in patients who have severe atrophy of the mandible. The implant procedure is done only after patients have been unable to wear a conventional lower denture. The patient must be willing to accept the fact that he is a dental cripple and that the implant procedure is done only when all else fails. Implants do fail even when very judicially placed. The patient must be willing to accept this possibility.

CONTRAINDICATIONS

Unrealistic patients should not be considered for this procedure. Patients with severe medical problems that render them a poor surgical risk should not be considered. Diabetics, unless well controlled, are not good risks for this type of procedure. Patients with heart-valve defects will need to be evaluated carefully because conceivably these patients could experience frequent transient bacteremias produced by contamination through the open pathway around the protruding posts of the implant.

Endosseous implants

Endosseous implants have been attempted for several years. Many materials have been developed for use, but at the present time the blade implant appears to be the most successful. Research work is being done on a glass implant that does have some promise. Vitreous carbon has been used, but results generally have been disappointing. Stainless-steel pins inserted through endodontically treated teeth for the purpose of stabilizing individual teeth are another form of implant.

The endosseous implant involves the surgical placement of a retentive framework into the bone with the post protruding through the mucosa to provide an abutment for the placement of a prosthetic device (Figs. 15-4 and 15-5). As stated previously, the blade implant is the most successful of these types. It consists of a chrome-cobalt steel blade that is placed in the bone with a post protruding through the mucosa (Figs. 15-4 and 15-5). Most of the blade implants are inserted to provide posterior abutments for fixed bridges or intermediate abutments for long-span bridges (Figs. 15-4 and 15-5). Variations on this have been proposed, for example, the pterygoid extension implant and the ramus implant.

INDICATIONS

Endosseous implants may be indicated whenever there is a missing tooth. The most common indication is when there is a free end situation with no posterior abutment available for fixed prosthesis. The placement of such an implant permits the patient to wear a fixed prosthesis instead of a removable prosthetic appliance (Fig. 15-5).

Prior to insertion of an endosseous implant the patient must be carefully evaluated roentgenographically and clinically to determine if there is adequate bone support between the alveolar crest and the sinuses or mandibular canal to permit insertion of the implant.

Radiopaque grids have been manufactured to place over x-ray films prior to exposing the film so that a grid is superimposed. This grid then gives a pattern by which the amount of bone available for the implant can be deter-

Innovative approaches 271

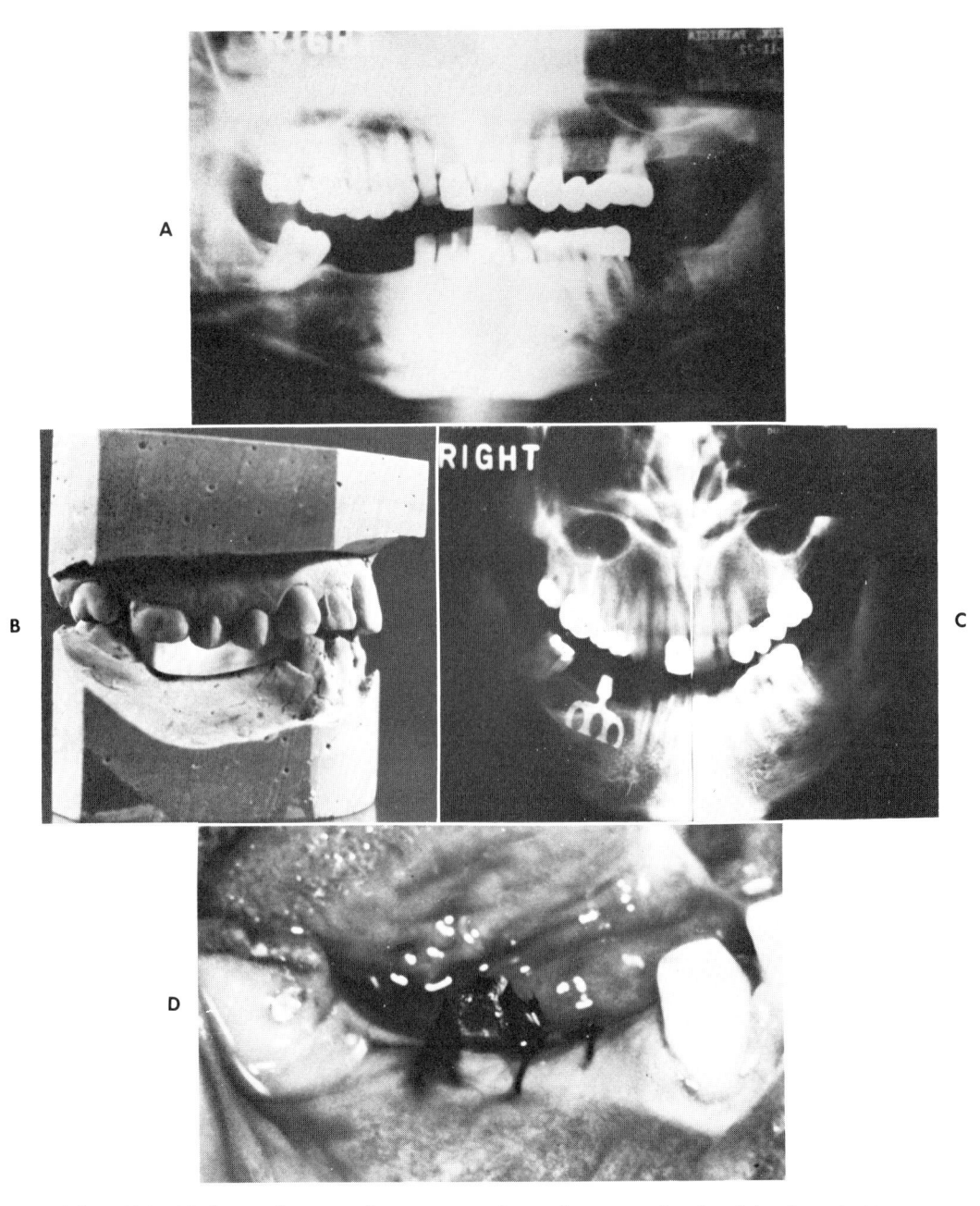

Fig. 15-4. Blade implant used as intermediate abutment for fixed bridge. **A,** Panograph showing edentulous span in mandibular right quadrant between canine and second molar. **B,** Diagnostic casts illustrating case. **C,** Panograph showing blade implant in intermediate position after surgical insertion. **D,** Intraoral appearance of blade implant immediately after insertion. (Courtesy Dr. Robert Chappell, Kansas City, Mo.)

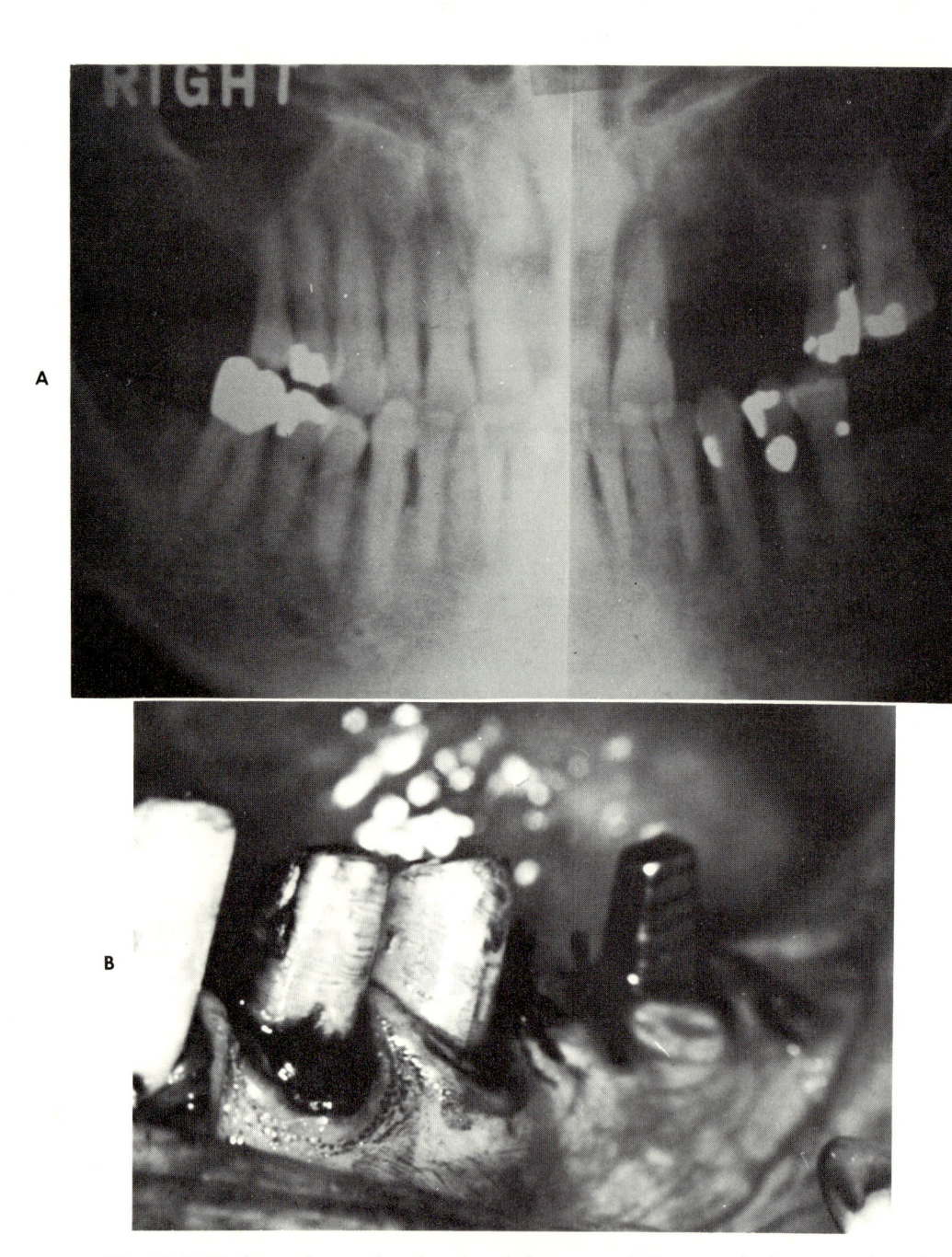

Fig. 15-5. Blade implant utilized as distal abutment. **A,** Panograph showing edentulous mandibular left molar region. **B,** Intraoral picture showing implant in place immediately following surgery. **C,** Panograph showing bridge and blade implant in place. **D,** Intraoral photograph of bridge after cementation. (Courtesy Dr. Robert Chappell, Kansas City, Mo.)

Innovative approaches 273

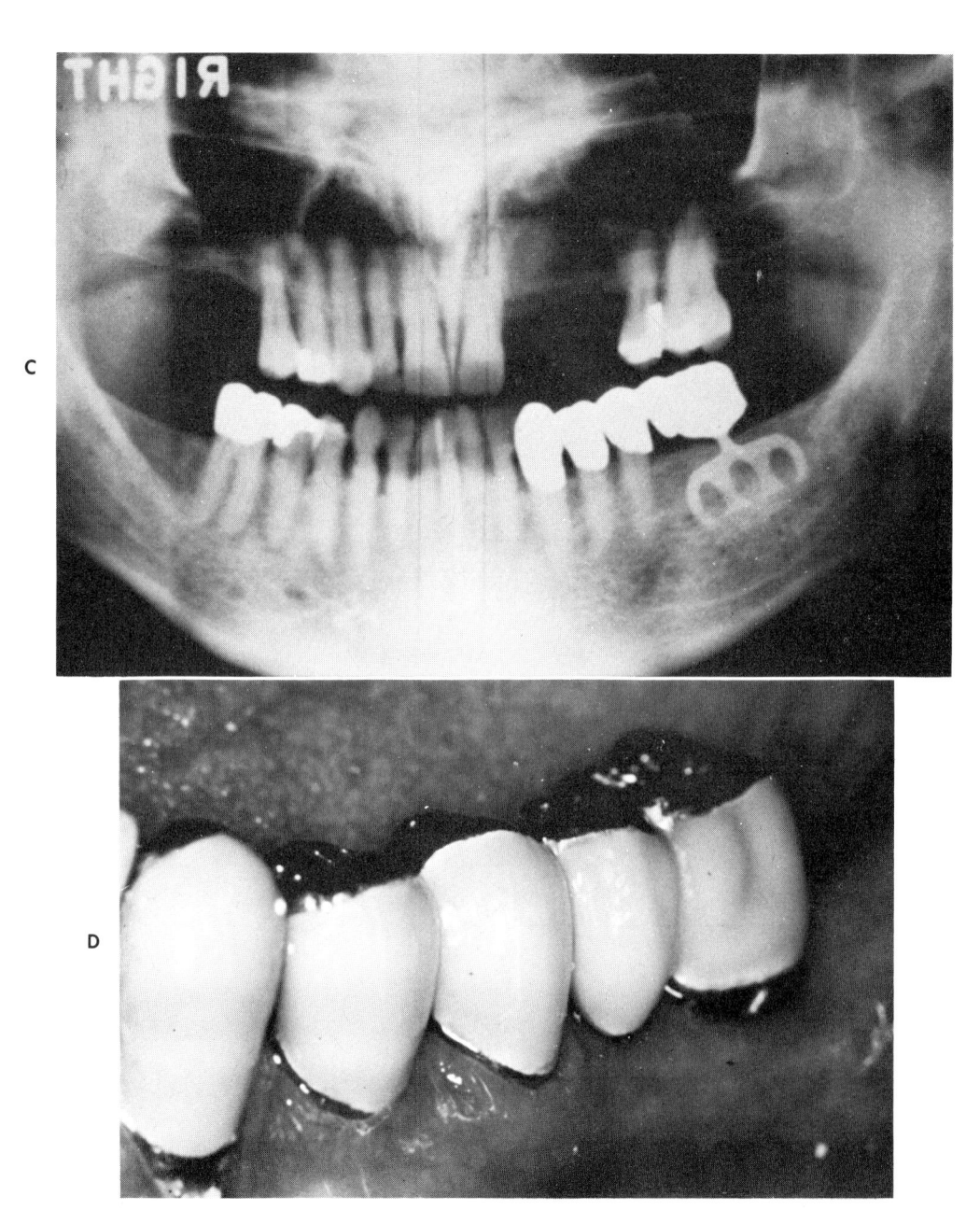

Fig. 15-5, cont'd. For legend see opposite page.

mined. The patient must be evaluated psychologically and must be willing to accept the trauma of the surgical procedure as well as the possibility of failure.

CONTRAINDICATIONS

Patients suffering from systemic diseases that render them poor surgical risks should be excluded from further consideration for endosseous implants. Patients with diabetes or patients on steroids or with decreased healing abilities also are not good candidates. Psychologically patients must be willing to accept the surgical procedure and the possibility of failure of the implant. They must not expect to obtain the same function from the implant that they enjoyed with their natural teeth. However, they can expect adequate function. Patients who have oral habits such as clenching and grinding should be ruled out as candidates for implants. It is our experience that such patients will dislodge an implant even if their dentition is protected with a night guard.

HEMISECTIONS AND ROOT AMPUTATIONS

Hemisections and root amputations will be considered together. They represent different procedures, but the indications and contraindications are similar.

A hemisection generally involves the removal of one root and one-half of the crown of a mandibular molar (Fig. 15-6), and the remaining root is treated periodontally and endodontically. Occasionally both roots of a mandibular molar can be endodontically treated and the crown split. Such a tooth has been converted into two single-rooted teeth. Root amputation involves the removal of one or more roots of a maxillary molar with periodontal-endodontic treatment rendered on the remaining roots (Fig. 15-7).

Indications

Hemisections and root amputations are performed on teeth that have periodontal involvement of the furcation which is so severe or otherwise of such a character that periodontal treatment would not be expected to be successful.

These procedures are indicated when retention of the tooth or a portion of the teeth will retain arch integrity or else permit the patient to wear a fixed bridge instead of a removable prosthesis. The patient must demonstrate a desire to maintain the gingival health around the remaining tooth and root structure.

Contraindications

Root amputations and hemisections are contraindicated in patients with uncontrolled periodontitis. They are also contraindicated when less than half of the root remains supported by bone. Teeth with poor crown-to-root ratios also should not have these procedures done unless the ratio can be improved through appropriate restorative measures.

Patients who are unwilling to maintain adequate oral hygiene should be eliminated as candidates for root amputations or hemisections. Patients who are unwilling to accept the possibility that they will eventually lose the tooth that is treated also make poor candidates. Patients with uncontrolled diabetes or on antimetabolite or steroid therapy are not good candidates for these pro-

Innovative approaches 275

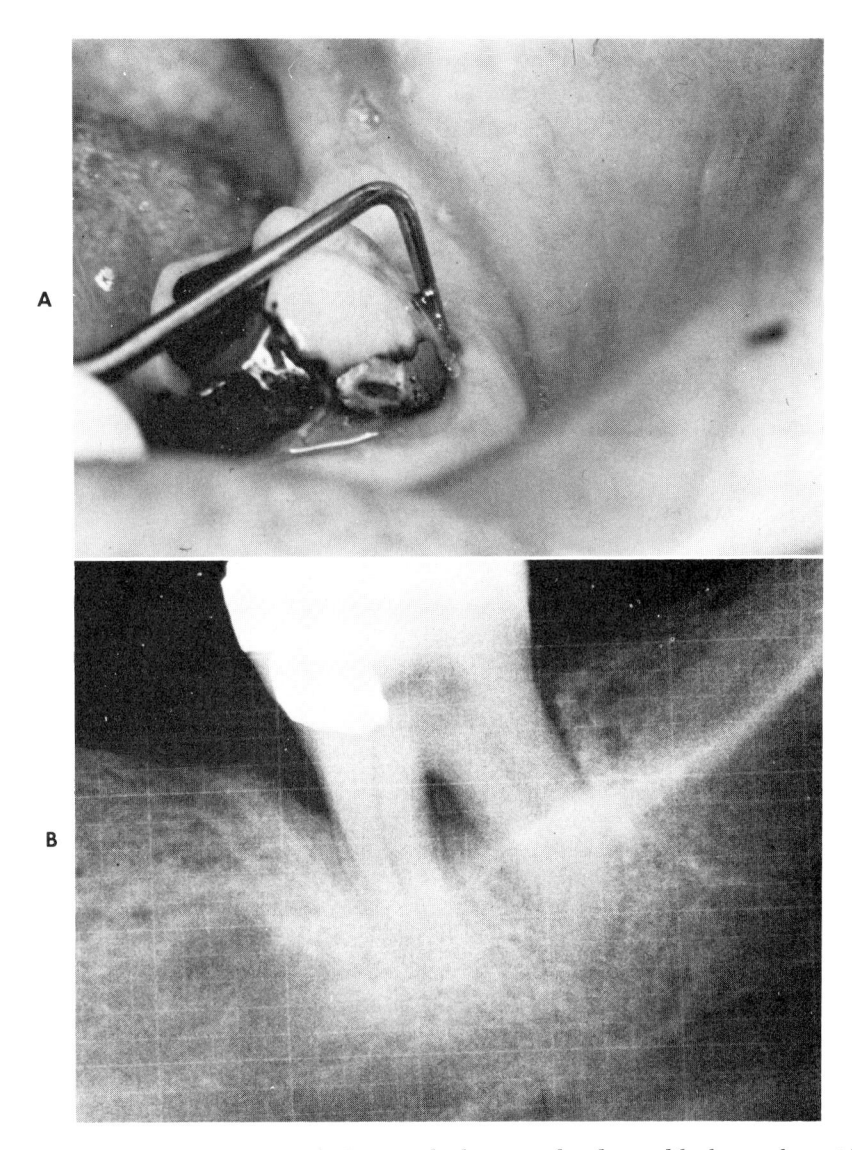

Fig. 15-6. Hemisection case. **A,** Intraoral photograph of mandibular molar with furcation involvement as well as deep mesial periodontal pocket. **B,** Roentgenogram of tooth illustrated in **A,** showing bone loss around mesial root and furcation involvement. **C,** Surgical view showing bony defect. **D,** Intraoral view of molar following hemisection and endodontic and periodontal treatment. (Courtesy Dr. Robert Lockhart, Kansas City, Mo.)

Continued.

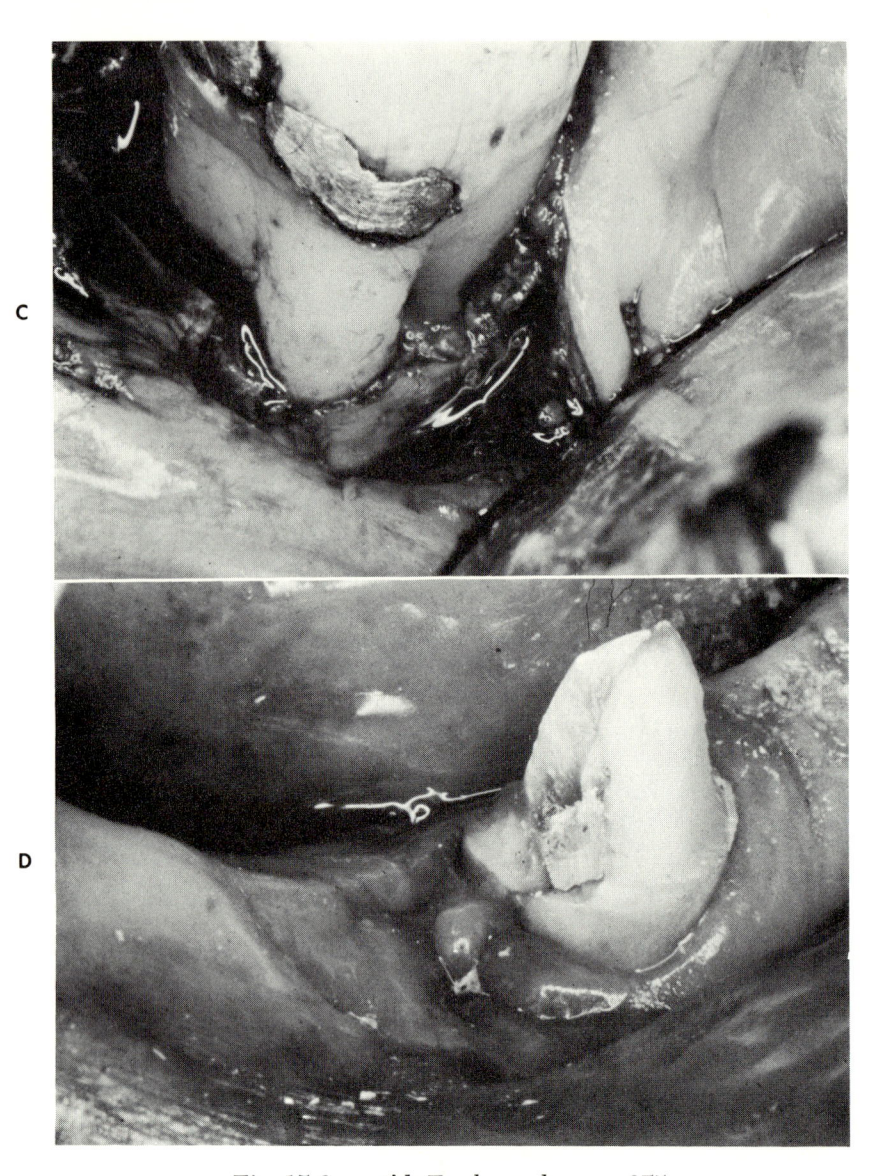

Fig. 15-6, cont'd. For legend see p. 275

cedures. Hemisected or root-amputated teeth will not serve as adequate abutments for long-span bridges. Usually they do not make good partial denture abutments, and so such teeth should be considered for extraction and included in the partial denture rather than doing hemisections or amputations and permitting them to stand alone.

PRECISION- OR SEMIPRECISION-ATTACHMENT PARTIAL DENTURES

An alternative method for making removable partial dentures is to use precision or semiprecision attachments instead of the conventional rests and clasps. The precision attachment is a finely machined, preformed device. The

Innovative approaches 277

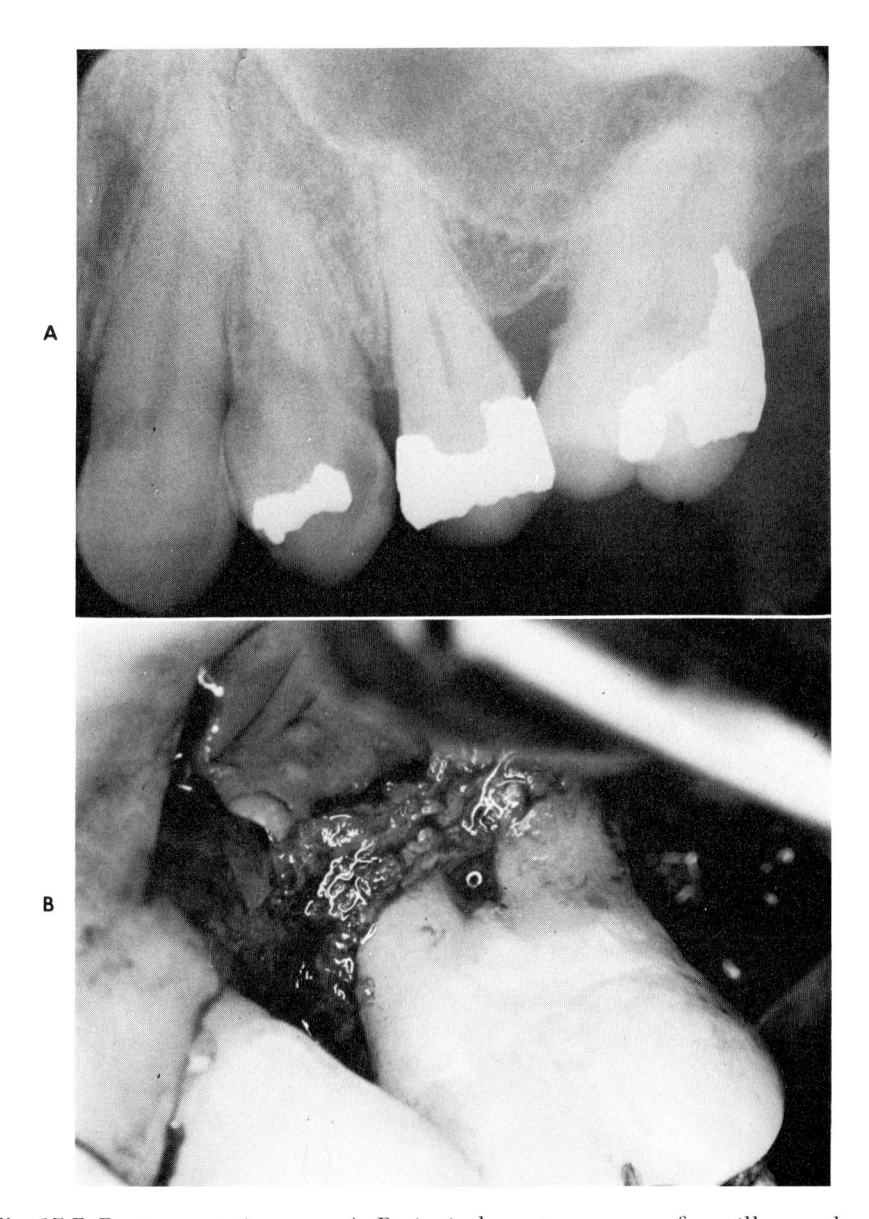

Fig. 15-7. Root amputation case. **A**, Periapical roentgenogram of maxillary molar with severe bone loss at distal aspect of distobuccal root. Although not evident in this roentgenogram, trifurcation is also involved. **B**, Surgical view. **C**, Clinical view (through mirror) of tooth 2 weeks after amputation of distobuccal root. **D**, Periapical roentgenogram showing root-amputated molar serving as splint abutment. (Courtesy Dr. Robert Lockhart, Kansas City, Mo.)

Continued.

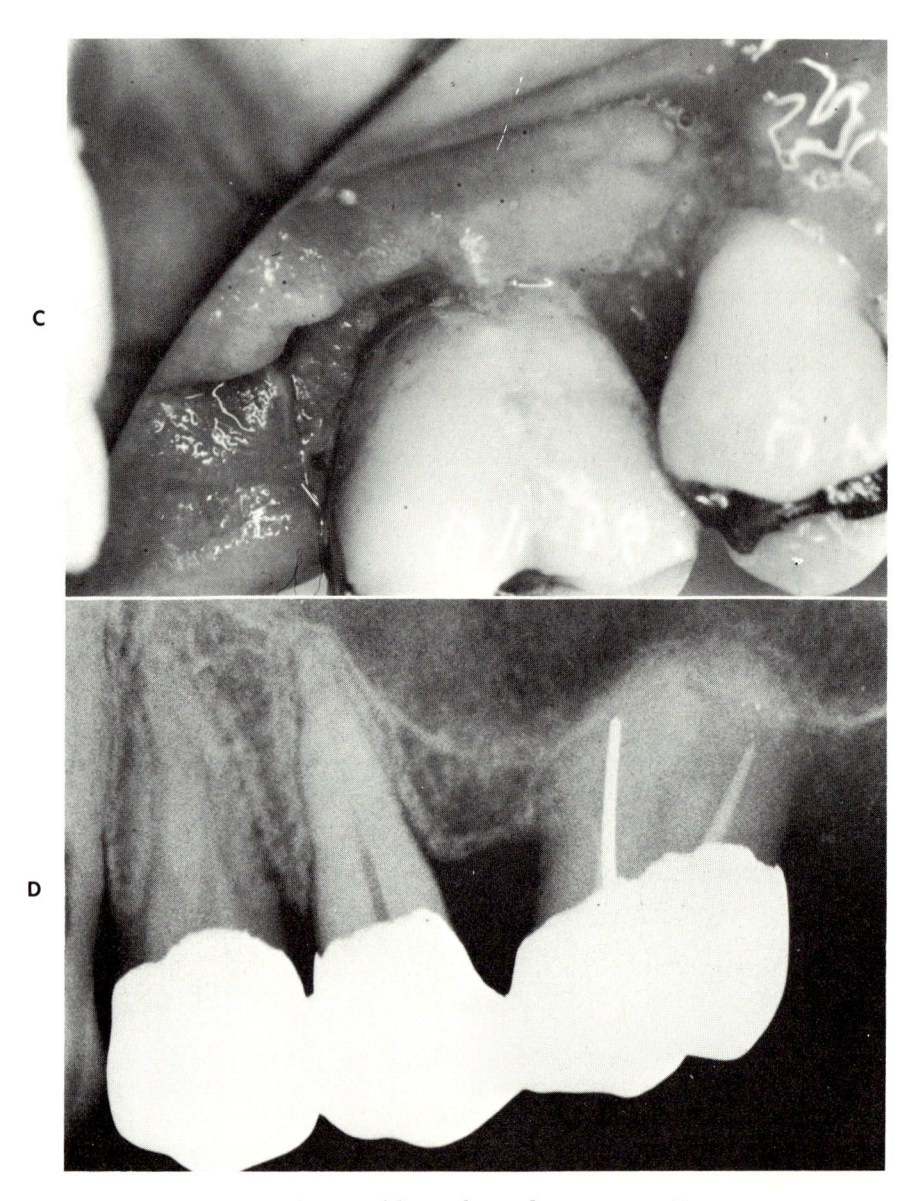

Fig. 15-7, cont'd. For legend see page 277.

female portion is soldered onto an abutment crown while the male attachment is soldered into a precast slot on the removable partial denture.

Semiprecision partial dentures are made by placing a female attachment dovetail in an abutment crown before the partial denture impression is taken. The resulting partial denture framework has a male dovetail attachment as part of the casting. Usually a lingual bracing clasp is utilized for supplementary support. The partial denture casting may be either chrome-cobalt or gold.

Indications

Precision- and semiprecision-attachment removable partial dentures can be considered when aesthetics is a prime factor in patients requiring removable partial dentures. It is essential that the abutment teeth be crowned, and frequently the abutment teeth must be splinted to provide adequate support. The periodontium must be in good health and the crown-to-root ratio of the proposed abutment teeth must be satisfactory. Patients must be willing to include immaculate oral hygiene as part of their lives. Patients must be willing to accept the additional expense and additional chair time necessary to crown all abutment teeth and have additional try-ins and other procedures that are necessary.

There also are additional expenses involved in the precision-attachment partial dentures because the attachments are finely machined, have an additional charge placed on them, and must be of cast gold. The tooth support and periodontal support for precision- and semiprecision-attachment partial dentures must be at least as good as that required for conventional partial dentures.

Contraindications

Precision- and semiprecision-attachment partial dentures are contraindicated in patients who are not devoted to keeping their mouths immaculately clean. They are contraindicated in patients who are unwilling to pay the additional fees necessary to allow the dentist to insert these appliances. Otherwise there are no contraindications for these appliances that would not also apply to the conventional removable partial denture.

BAR BRIDGES (ANDREWS BRIDGES)

Bar bridges are a modification of a removable prosthesis and actually combine features of both fixed and removable appliances. The basic principle behind the bar bridge is that the abutment teeth on either side of the edentulous space are crowned and a gold bar that follows the ridge contour is soldered to each abutment. This whole unit is cemented into place. A removable partial denture with a clip that fits over the bar is then fabricated to replace the missing teeth (Fig. 15-8).

Indications

Bar bridges are indicated when abutment teeth are available on either side of an edentulous space, particularly when the space is in the anterior region. The edentulous space is generally deficient in bone and soft tissue so that a fixed prostheses would not provide an adequate aesthetic result. The abutment teeth must have adequate bone in order to support a fixed prosthetic appliance, and the patient must be successfully motivated to maintain satisfactory oral hygiene, remembering that the cementation of the fixed appliance will render this chore much more difficult.

Contraindications

Bar bridges are contraindicated in the patient who is not willing to maintain adequate oral hygiene. They are also contraindicated when the abutment teeth have inadequate bone support.

280 *Miscellaneous*

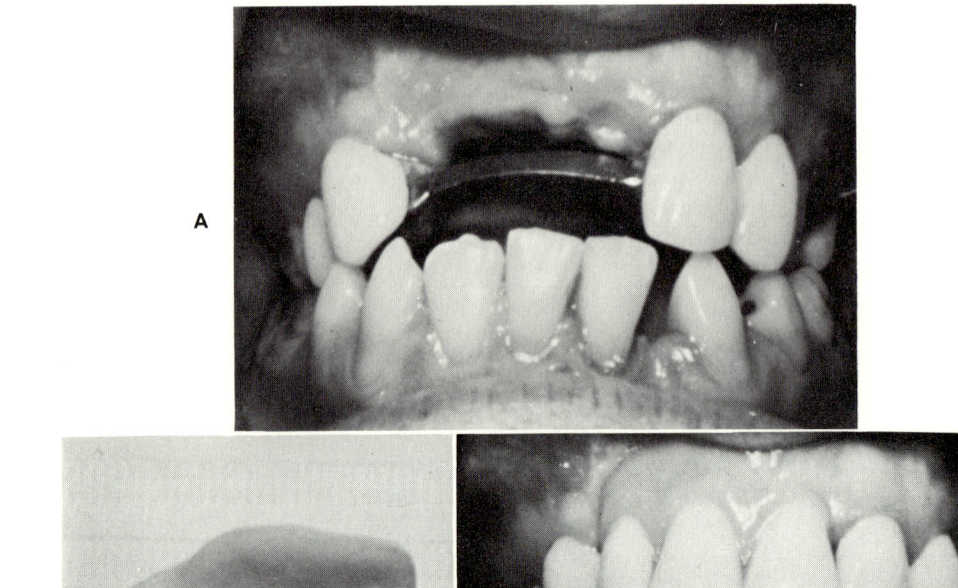

Fig. 15-8. Bar bridge (Andrews bridge) case. **A,** Clinical photograph showing cast section of bar bridge cemented in place. Note deficient alveolar crest, which would make satisfactory aesthetics with conventional bridge very difficult if not impossible to obtain. **B,** Ridge side of Andrews denture showing clip-type retainer that will engage bar illustrated in **A**. **C,** Andrews appliance in place. Note that acrylic flange hides bony defect. (Courtesy Dr. Norman Schwartz, Kansas City, Mo.)

OVERLAY DENTURES

Overlay dentures are completely removable dentures that are fabricated over the retained tooth roots. The tooth roots partially support the denture, and hopefully this situation will impede alveolar bone resorption. Following are two basic ways in which the remaining root structure may be treated:

1. The simplest method is that of amputating the crowns of the remaining teeth and treating the roots endodontically. The access preparation is then filled with amalgam or direct gold, and the root surface is polished. A conventional denture is then constructed.
2. The second method is that of reducing the crowns of the remaining teeth and cementing the copings (conical gold crowns) in place. The tooth may or may not require endodontic treatment. A conventional denture with a clip to fit over this conical crown is then constructed.

Indications

Overlay dentures may be indicated on the mandible when there are one or more retained teeth. These teeth must have at least one-half of the root supported by bone, and periodontal health must be good. The teeth frequently must be amenable to endodontic treatment, and the patient must be willing to maintain adequate oral hygiene. It is best if the remaining teeth are bilateral. Mandibular canines are most frequently used, but premolars, incisors, and even molars may be utilized. Some clinicians have proposed the use of hemisectioned molars as residual roots for overlay dentures. Generally overlay dentures are not indicated on the maxilla, but some practitioners like to maintain canines or premolars in the maxillary area for overlay denture support.

Contraindications

Overlay dentures are contraindicated in the patient who is not willing to maintain some degree of oral hygiene of the remaining roots. They are also contraindicated when the remaining root cannot be adequately endodontically treated and when it has major periodontal pockets that cannot be eliminated.

The patient's health is a factor to consider when determining whether to utilize overdentures. Generally speaking, if the patient is able to withstand the physical and emotional trauma of the extraction of these teeth, he is also able to withstand endodontic treatment or crowning of two teeth. Medical aspects are considered in detail in Chapters 5 and 6.

16

Case presentation

John C. Ebinger
Earl E. Sommers

After a dentist has examined a new patient and developed the treatment plan, an appointment time should be arranged so that the dentist can explain the findings of the examination and suggest a feasible solution to the patient. This meeting is called the case presentation. The purpose of the case presentation is threefold: to inform the patient of his current oral health status, to discuss reasonable therapeutic solutions, and to finalize a mutually acceptable treatment plan.

Case presentations that are managed correctly can be extremely valuable to the dentist and the patient. So often patients are unaware of the nature and magnitude of their oral problems. By utilizing simple visual aids, the dentist can easily *educate* the patient with regard to the various disease processes that are taking place. In addition, procedures such as root canal therapy and periodontal root planing will no longer remain a mystery after giving a simple explanation with good visual aids.

By allowing the patient to participate in planning his own care, a great deal of the mystery in dentistry can be eliminated. With proper education concerning his oral needs and the possible technical methods of solving his problems, the patient can aid the dentist in selecting the best plan that will also fit his particular life situation. Patient involvement is an essential key to case success. When the patient is allowed to participate in planning care, there is added incentive for cooperating with the instructions given by the dental team. The patient will want the plan that he helped construct to work.

Quite often the source of a number of patient-dentist misunderstandings is a breakdown in communication. The dentist performs a service the patient does not desire or the service rendered is not the service anticipated by the patient. By spending time and carefully explaining and agreeing upon each phase of treatment, the dentist and patient can avoid many midtreatment and posttreatment misunderstandings.

In the recent past the dentist-patient relationship has often resembled the parent-child relationship. The dentist was the unquestionable authority who knew enough to be able to make all the dental-related decisions for the patient. Today, however, the patient expects to be made aware and be given the opportunity to participate in the decision-making process. Consequently the dentist needs to seriously work on developing open lines of communication. An excellent time for the dentist to establish the policy of open communication is at the case presentation.

Many patients have a great fear of the dental profession. Extreme anxiety and apprehension resulting from past painful experiences and distrust cause many individuals to avoid necessary treatment. The new patient deserves an opportunity to meet with the dentist and relate his anxiety or distrust over dental care before being subjected to the environment that causes his apprehension. The patient will be less likely to have problems during treatment if a good rapport has been established. New patients need to understand that many new technical changes in dentistry have occurred that can make the total dental experience more enjoyable. In addition, the apprehensive patient must have a feeling that he is in capable, concerned hands.

The case presentation should be a time when the specifics of future treatment are discussed and agreed upon. There should be no question in the mind of the patient or the dentist with regard to future treatment, how it will be managed financially, and so on. The plan to solve the patient's problems must be one that is agreeable to both parties and that can be considered as an informal contract.

Case presentation affords the dentist time to get to know the patient on a personal basis, determine the patient's personal priorities, and understand the patient's life situations. Information about the patient's life is essential before a realistic plan can be finalized. For instance, students who are living on financial shoestrings will most likely want urgent care and less likely desire expensive rehabilitative care.

CASE PRESENTATION FORMAT

A formal case presentation can be subdivided into a number of categories. This discussion will involve each of the following categories in some detail:
1. Introduction
2. Areas of concern
3. Consequence of neglecting treatment
4. Treatment plan proposal
5. Establishing mutual goals of therapy
6. Policies
7. Conclusion

Introduction
GREETING

The dentist sets the tone of the meeting by the way in which the patient is greeted. It is the objective of a case presentation to encourage the patient to actively participate in his own treatment. Therefore creating a friendly, relaxed, nonthreatening atmosphere is essential.

Patients are often influenced more by what they observe than by what they hear. The dentist must be very aware of his or her nonverbal gestures such as a good handshake, taking the patient's coat, offering a comfortable chair, and a pleasant smile. Gestures such as these will let the patients *see* that the dentist is pleased to spend this time with them.

Determining level of receptivity

The dentist must next determine whether the patient is ready to listen and talk about the treatment plan. He or she must determine if the patient is relaxed, uptight, or if there is something the patient needs to mention before beginning. There are many situations in life that will cause a patient to have a difficult time concentrating on the topic of discussion; for example, patients with successive appointments will be concerned about their time limitations, patients with family problems may not be able to listen, and patients who need to go to the bathroom will be restless. It is important to read the patient's nonverbal messages and be sensitive to his level of receptivity before beginning a conversation. Two people must be concentrating on the same subject before they can productively communicate with each other.

Agenda

The dentist should very briefly tell the patient that he or she would like to review the case with the patient, establish mutual treatment goals, and answer any questions; for example, "Mrs. Hillary, I would like to review your case with you briefly today so that we can establish a plan suitable to your needs." Be sure that all attempts are made to encourage the patient to participate.

Areas of concern

The dentist should summarize the existing areas of concern in laymen's language and attempt to discern patient understanding of each area. Those conditions that are obvious to the patient will not require extensive explanation. For example, large carious lesions on labial surfaces of the maxillary anterior teeth are usually self-evident, whereas horizontal alveolar bone loss might not be as apparent. Spend additional time clarifying the areas of concern that the patient does not understand.

Patients usually want to know the extent or severity of their condition. By using descriptive terms such as "beginning", "moderate," and "advanced" to describe areas of concern, the dentist helps the patient develop a dental frame of reference. Occasionally patients will not be able to grasp the significance of their level of disease. Then it is extremely important for the dentist to explain, with the use of visual tools such as periodontal models and roentgenograms, the actual destructive process so the patient develops a clear mental picture.

Consequence of neglecting treatment

The patient needs to be aware of the probable long-term consequences of neglecting therapy. The dentist should objectively explain the final result of continued disease progress. Once the patient understands the relative significance of each area of concern and the consequences of procrastination, then he is ready to consider the dentist's treatment plan proposal.

Treatment plan proposal

After the dentist has described the various problems and explained the possible consequence if therapeutic intervention is neglected, then it is appropriate to present the proposed treatment plan. There are a number of concepts that should be included in this phase of the case presentation that will be beneficial to the patient's understanding.

It is often helpful for the patient to realize that dental therapy should be delivered in a logical order and that there are progressive phases of treatment. The dentist should explain stabilization, maintenance and monitoring, and rehabilitation (see Chapter 10) as three discrete entities. Often patients are delighted to discover that they can receive the highest quality of care and not be required to have it all completed at one time.

Each phase of treatment should be described in the same order as it will occur. In other words, the dentist should describe the urgent treatment before directing attention to the rehabilitation phase. Patients should be reassured that the most urgent needs will be the first to be resolved.

When describing the management of restorations, it is best to avoid a tooth-by-tooth explanation. It is usually adequate to mention that a certain number of teeth will receive "silver fillings," select front teeth will require "tooth-colored" fillings for cosmetic reasons, and specific structurally weak teeth are candidates for cast-gold restoration. So often the dentist's elaborate description of the restoration required by each tooth is soon forgotten by the patient. The dentist should be certain the patient understands the basic form and advantages of the various restorations if there is any question in the patient's mind. For instance, if an aesthetic area is to be restored with cast restorations, the dentist should be certain that the patient has a good mental picture of the treatment options.

When the patient is not familiar with a specific therapeutic technique, the dentist should give a *simple* verbal and visual explanation. Often treatments such as endodontics, occlusal equilibration, and nonsurgical periodontics will require a word of clarification. A *clear, concise* explanation seldom includes many details.

Patients like to know the length of appointments and the number of times they will need to be seen. A single sentence with the appropriate information can satisfy this need.

Because dentistry is a very technical service, the tendency in many case presentations is to emphasize the details of each dental technique rather than the improvements the patient will experience after therapy is completed. For instance, patients should be reminded that once urgent care has been rendered, the threat of pain and swelling will be removed.

Establishing mutual goals of therapy

One of the objectives in a case presentation is to help the patient develop a better understanding of his present oral health status and the possible therapeutic solutions to his oral needs that require treatment. By spending the time to educate the patient, the dentist helps the patient develop an appreciation for the relative worth of dental care. The patient will now be able to more realistically evaluate the need for dental care in light of his personal priorities. By utilizing patient education effectively, the dentist shares the responsibility of decision making with the patient and assumes the role of an advisor rather than a dictator.

Now that the patient has a basic understanding of his needs and the possible services available, he can actively participate with the dentist in making necessary alterations in the plan that will satisfy his personal life situation and also fulfill the dentist's concept of oral health. Mutual goals of therapy might be elimination of urgent needs or complete stabilization, maintenance, and fabrication of one aesthetic porcelain crown. It is imperative that both the dentist and the patient anticipate the same end product; otherwise problems will inevitably develop.

Occasionally patients will have ideas that are contrary to sound dental science. An example would be the patient with severe periodontal disease who wants crowns and bridges but refuses to accept periodontal treatment. If the dentist is unable to incorporate the principles of oral health with the patient's desires, then it will be impossible to formulate mutually agreeable goals, and the patient and dentist should not continue their professional relationship.

Finances usually become a point of consideration when mutual goals are being established. The dentist can help the patient by explaining the cost of each phase of treatment and allowing the patient to decide how much care he can afford. Options should be based on the various phases of treatment. For instance, the patient should know how much it will cost for stabilization, maintenance, and total rehabilitation. By not placing the patient in the "all-or-none" situation, the dentist has removed finances as an obstacle to beginning dental care. For some patients, treatment can be rendered over a longer period of time to help decrease the monthly financial burden. Personal finance is a very sensitive issue that must be managed with care. The dentist must avoid causing the patient any embarrassment.

Some patients will require additional time to consider the mutual goals of therapy and to discuss them with others, for example, parents, spouse, and employer. The dentist should encourage a future meeting time to continue the discussion. Patients who are placed under pressure to make a decision will often be unable to objectively evaluate the points of consideration adequately and will make poor decisions.

Policies

Each dental office will have a number of policies that have been developed to ensure smooth, consistent operation. When new patients are accepted into the practice, they need to become aware of the specifics of each policy. Examples include night or weekend emergencies, appointment cancellation and failures, and financial arrangements. Policies need to be presented in an objective, nonthreatening manner so that the patient gains a good understanding of essential office procedures without becoming offended. Failure to mention office policies often results in misunderstandings and bad feelings in the future.

Conclusions

After the case has been presented and policies explained, it is very important for the dentist to summarize the mutual goals that were developed and to thank the patient for his interest and willingness to participate in the establishment of his treatment plan.

In closing it is always a thoughtful gesture to remind the patient to contact the dentist if there are questions or concerns. The dentist should be very sure that the doors of communication are left open when the case presentation is concluded.

CONSIDERATIONS TO INCREASE EFFECTIVENESS

There are numerous things a dentist should consider if he or she desires to maximize personal effectiveness with patients. The following section will include various techniques that can be utilized.

Treatment-plan summary letter
INTRODUCTION

Following the initial examination, one technique of improving communication is to write the patient a letter that *summarizes* the future case presentation. At first glance this repetition of information might seem to be needless. However, there are certain advantages in using this system.

Increased patient involvement. By allowing the patient an opportunity to preview the proposed plan, the dentist is including the patient in the decision-making process. Though the majority of patients have little understanding of modern dental therapy, many still like to be involved in the development of the plan.

Efficient use of case presentation time. When individuals are presented with numerous new facts and concepts and not allowed adequate time for consideration, it is very difficult for them to ask meaningful questions. If the patient is familiar with your proposal before the case presentation, then he will be able to ask meaningful questions.

Concise explanation of new concepts and unusual modes of treatment. One amazing phenomenon that transpires in the minds of patients following many case presentations is the transformation of sound dental philosophy into unrecognizable misconceptions. It is often hard for the dentist to imagine how such clearly presented facts could become so scrambled. This whole process can be greatly reduced by utilizing a summary letter that clearly defines new concepts and unusual treatment. A letter has the advantage of being *rereadable.* The patient can refresh his memory by reading the definitions and plan as often as is necessary.

Magic of the printed word. Many individuals respond to a typed letter as though it were sacred. W*ell-typed* letters add a dimension of credibility to the message. The extra effort demonstrates the professional's concern, thoroughness, and high level of organization. There is something definite and absolute about this kind of personal communication that can help build patient trust.

Blueprint for future events. It is so easy for patients to become disoriented in the middle of treatment. They remember some specifics about stabilization, definitive periodontal surgery, and some inlay and temporaries, but are unable to picture where they are in relationship to the *total* plan. By including a thumbnail sketch of the *sequential* phases of treatment in the letter, the dentist can help alleviate future midtreatment confusion and misconceptions.

Special emphasis for certain patients. Many different problems hinder patients from actively pursuing comprehensive dental treatment. Fear, professional distrust, low dental priorities, financial inadequacies, and procrastination are but a few of a long list of reasons why patients avoid the dentist. The summary letter is another opportunity to aid in eliminating these problems.

The "tone" of a letter should be varied for each patient. The dentist must be receptive at the examination appointment for problems and must tailor the letter to accommodate these feelings and concerns.

TREATMENT-PLAN LETTER FORMAT

There are many possible ways to write a treatment-plan letter. Various personalities will feel comfortable with *different* letter styles and format. The primary focus in this section will be to discuss essential information that should be given to the patient. The secondary focus will be to present a simple letter format that will facilitate the organization of the essential information. The letter can be arbitrarily divided into three sections: introduction, body, conclusion.

Introduction. The dentist should mention the last meeting with the patient and state in a concise yet personal manner the purpose for the letter. A short sentence letting the patient know that thought and time has been spent analyzing the data is meaningful. The patient will be much more receptive if he believes the dentist really cares.

Following is an example of an introduction incorporating these suggestions: "Since October 13, 1976, when I had the opportunity of getting acquainted with you and performing a thorough examination, I have reevaluated our findings and studied your x-ray films. In this letter I would like to briefly mention the areas of concern and outline a possible solution for you to consider."

Body of information. The body of the letter will consist of the following categories of essential information: areas of concern (problems) and consequence of neglected treatment, plan of treatment, and estimate of cost and time involved.

Areas of concern (problems) and consequence of neglected treatment. This section of the letter is basically a summary of the problems identified at the examination that is rewritten in laymen's terminology. The patient will either be aware or not aware that he has a particular condition. The areas of concern can be handled in one of two ways:

1. *Conditions patient is aware of.* These problems generally will not require a lengthy definition or explanation; merely name the problem. The dentist must be sensitive to the patient's dental IQ so that he or she does not waste the patient's time by describing concepts the patient already understands. The receptive patient will usually want to know the level or extent of a condition. For example, the patient who has been aware of a periodontal condition for a number of years will want to know the current status. Occasionally patients will be aware of a specific condition but will not be concerned, so often they are unaware of the morbidity that will result if the disease process is not stopped. Often a brief description of the disease process with special emphasis on the end product (pain, swelling, loss of teeth, death) will help clarify

the need for treatment. Informing patients of the probable consequences of neglecting treatment should be handled as positive patient education and not as a scare tactic.

2. *Conditions patient is not aware of.* The dentist should give a clear and concise description for any disease process that the patient does not understand or was not aware he had. The dentist should also help the patient develop a perspective for the condition by describing the end result of the disease process. It is very important that the patient be given a good definition in the letter so that the dentist does not have to spend an inordinate amount of time at a case presentation describing the disease process for the first time. By describing the new conditions in a letter, the dentist allows the patient time to consider this development. In addition, he can *reread* the definition or description if there are any questions. Avoid describing each carious tooth. It is adequate to say "numerous decayed teeth."

Plan of treatment. The proposed treatment can be handled very easily by utilizing a simple numbered outline form. A sentence or two preceding the proposed plan can be used to explain that the treatment plan contains the proposed solution to each area of concern (problem). Each area of concern and its proposed solution will receive the same number.

The dentist must concisely describe the plan for each problem and attempt to avoid detailed descriptions of each plan. For instance, it is unnecessary to write out the tooth-by-tooth restorative treatment plan. It is adequate to explain that certain teeth will require gold restorations because so little tooth structure remains and that the remainder can be treated with silver fillings. For the procedures that are unusual or new to the patient (i.e., root canal filling), a concise description is in order.

The dentist must explain the three phases of treatment (stabilization, maintenance and monitoring, and rehabilitation) and tell the patient that the order of treatment should be determined primarily by the relative urgency of each condition. A separate column adjacent to the problem plan can be titled "sequence," and each plan can be given a sequential number to assist the patient in understanding the order in which treatment will be completed.

Estimation of cost and time involved. The expense of dentistry very often deters patients from seeking care. Consequently, if the dentist intends to mention finances in a letter, it must be handled properly. It is very important to listen closely to the patient at the examination appointment. Many times patients will offer comments like "Dentistry is sure expensive" or "Could we go slow with the treatment at first?" If the patient indicates that he is concerned, then deference must be exercised.

The dentist should never put up a financial hurdle that the patient cannot negotiate. If the patient demonstrates concern over finances, then it is advisable to estimate the cost of stabilization and emphasize the fact that the patient will be *stabilized.* It should be mentioned that rehabilitation treatment could be considered in the future. In this situation it might be wisest to avoid estimating the total treatment because it might discourage the patient from proceeding with the urgent treatment. If the patient does not seem to be overly concerned about finances, then the dentist should mention the cost of each phase of treatment and also give an estimate for the total treatment. As a general policy, it is best to tell what the total fee will be. However, if the patient is not interested in having complete treatment because of restrictions, then it is not worth mentioning. An estimate of the number of appointments and length of each appointment should also be included in this section of the letter.

Conclusion. In the concluding remarks the dentist should let the patient know that he or she is looking forward to helping resolve the patient's oral problems. The patient should be encouraged to bring questions to the case presentation and be reminded of the appointment date. An example might be: "I hope this letter will help clarify your current oral condition. Please consider seriously the treatment proposals I have made. I will answer any questions you might have at our next meeting, at 2:00 PM, October 17, 1976. If you have any dental problems, please contact me at (phone number)."

COMMUNICATION SKILLS

The purpose of a case presentation is information exchange between the dentist and the patient, and therefore it is essential that the dentist not only be ready to clearly present the facts and proposals, but that he or she do it in such a way that the patient becomes actively interested. Communication is more than just someone talking—another individual must be listening. Developing a style that causes the listener to become actively involved in the thought and discussion process is the key to communication. The following discussion is designed to point out helpful techniques in improving one's communication effectiveness. The communication skills can be divided into two categories: verbal and nonverbal.

Verbal communication skills

SPEAKING THE PATIENT'S OWN LANGUAGE

Communication involves speaking in the same language. It is never enjoyable to sit and listen to a foreign language that you do not understand. If the dentist uses terms that confuse the patient, a clear understanding of the status of oral health and the proposed treatment is completely lost. It does no good to tell a patient that subgingival curettage is necessary unless the patient knows what it is.

It is very important for the dentist to determine the patient's dental IQ, determine the level of patient sophistication, and speak to the level of the patient's understanding. Common terms, with their meanings, include the following:

1. Class 5 (gum line)
2. Class 3 (between the teeth)
3. Class 1 (biting surface of teeth)
4. Occlusal adjustment (adjust the bite or the way the teeth touch)
5. Alloy (filling)
6. MOD (three-surface)
7. RPD (removable partial dentures)
8. Osseous (bony)
9. Gingiva (gum)

10. Periodontal disease (gum disease)
11. Malocclusion (improper bite)

By utilizing the common lay terminology, the dentist can avoid unnecessary explanations of technical terms.

Some patients will be embarrassed by not knowing the meaning of various terms. An embarrassed patient will often withdraw from active participation in a conversation. Confusing technical terms often defeat the purpose of meeting.

GIVING SIMPLE ANSWERS

When patients ask questions, the dentist should respond with the simplest answer. The more words used, or the more technical the response, the more likely the answer will be misunderstood. A concept that dentists often explain is "occlusion." For the most part, patients do not want to know the advantages or disadvantages of bilateral posterior group function in working occlusal relationships. Instead, a simple answer such as "We want each tooth to share an equal portion of the biting force" would suffice.

So often dentists try to answer a patient's technical question with an even more complicated technical answer. An example might be the answer to a question involving root canal therapy. Rather than explaining the types of instruments used to clean the canal, or the specific technique used to condense the filling material, it would suffice to say that the root canal will be cleaned by using small hand instruments and later filled with a rubberlike material.

INVOLVING THE PATIENT

So often dentists become frustrated because the patient "does not respond." Often the reason is that the dentist programs the patient into a passive role by the manner of the presentation and the nature of the dentist's questions. Questions that allow the patient to answer with a "yes" or "no" do not cause the patient to become involved or personally committed to the plan. Questions should be designed to discover the *level* of patient understanding and the degree of patient interest so that the dentist can direct the conversation at the correct level.

SPEAKING WITH POSITIVE VOICE INFLECTION

Quite often the tone of voice will affect the patient as much as the content of the discussion. A boring monotone could be misinterpreted by the patient as the dentist's lack of interest in the patient's care. Excitement is contagious. Positive voice inflections can help the patient focus on the bright aspects of dental care such as the healthy mouth and preventing future problems, whereas a negative voice inflection will cause the patient to focus on the problems with treatment, finances, areas of questionable prognosis, and so on.

REDIRECTING AIMLESS CONVERSATIONS

Although one of the objectives in a case presentation is patient involvement, the dentist must still help guide the patient to respond to the correct issues. Open communication must not be mistaken for a verbal "free-for-all" where the subject matter is whatever comes to mind. Rather, it is an *honest* discussion about a specific topic. When the patient becomes sidetracked by inconsequential events in his past that disrupt the orderly development of ideas at a case presentation, the dentist must redirect the patient's thoughts; if this is not done, the patient may go from one story to another, wasting the dentist's time with irrelevant conversation. The dentist needs to be skilled at differentiating between the patient who genuinely needs to "get something off his chest" before he can intelligently discuss his dental problem and the patient who just likes to talk and finds the dentist a "captive" audience.

An effective method of changing the topic of conversation is by asking the patient a question that is related to the subject matter of the case presentation. This allows the patient who feels the need to verbalize to continue speaking, but in a fruitful manner.

Nonverbal communication

The adage "actions speak louder than words" is worth the dentist's consideration. Something as trivial as a passing mannerism can undo what took many sentences to build. Patients' attitudes are often greatly influenced by the impression or feeling they have after observing the dentist during a case presentation. The following nonverbals are a few examples of behavior that may affect the perception of the dentist.

INTERRUPTIONS

Every time an interruption occurs, this tells the patient that the dentist believes something else is more important than their appointed meeting. The patient deserves undivided attention because the plan designed to establish and maintain the patient's oral health is being discussed. In addition, the case presentation is a personal matter. Patient's problems, desires, and finances are being talked about, and this is a private subject. Inadvertent interruption will suggest to the patient that the dentist does not have a very high opinion regarding these personal issues.

In addition to the lack of respect for the patient, interruption will disorient a conversation. Often the content of a discussion is disrupted to such an extent that the patient ends up confused and frustrated rather than enlightened and motivated.

In order to avoid interruptions, the dentist should schedule adequate time with the patient and conduct the meeting in a room that can be closed off, ensuring a private atmosphere. Staff employees should respect the privacy of the meeting and avoid disturbances. Light and soft buzzer systems can be installed in inconspicuous locations to alert the dentist to specific office needs (such as a new patient's arrival and so on).

ORGANIZATION

Often the case presentation is the first opportunity the patient has to observe the dentist's abilities to organize. To many patients the dentist's complete understanding of the patient's case gives validity to the rationale behind the proposed plan to resolve the problems. Patients also equate current organization and preparation with future abilities to manage potential problems. It is very important to establish a good rapport at the case presentation. The dentist should spend a few minutes before the meeting to review the data obtained at the examination and to recall personal notes about the patient. Patients feel secure when they believe the dentist has an excellent understanding and a detailed plan for their particular situation. Disorganization demonstrates lack of prior planning and often a basic disinterest in the patient's well-being.

Patients like others to respect the value of their time. So often in busy private practices the patient's time is not valued. Tardiness for appointments usually means the dentist is not very organized in the management of the office activities or else the patient's time is not considered very valuable. After having to wait 45 minutes for a disorganized dentist, the first impression a patient has is usually unfavorable.

Dentist's professional attitude

Probably the most important signals that patients watch for are the nonverbals that reflect the dentist's attitude toward the patient as a human being. Does the dentist consider the patient special or just another case that requires treatment? Is the plan designed to best treat the needs of the patient within the patient's means? Or is it designed to help pay the office bills?

Patients are more likely to be receptive to the dentist's suggestion for treatment if they feel the dentist has listened to their concerns and understands their priorities. So often dentists fail to communicate with the patient because the dentist fails to listen. Patients who are thus unable to have input often feel that the plan meets the dentist's needs but might not be the best for their situation. It is very difficult to make a patient feel that he is special if the dentist does not take time to listen to him.

Patients will be affected by the composure of the dentist. It is much easier to concentrate on a topic of discussion with a relaxed individual than with a nervous, uptight individual. One item that causes dentists to be apprehensive is the daily schedule. When the dentist realizes that patients are waiting or if the case presentation is scheduled during the middle of another procedure, then it is difficult to concentrate. Case presentations should be scheduled at times when the fewest number of outside distractions are likely to occur.

Open lines of communication are less likely to be established if the dentist is dictatorial and feels threatened by the patient's expectations. Such dentists believe that they are the only ones capable of knowing what is best for the patient and so they assume a dictatorial position and put the patient in the position of agreeing with the proposed plan in order not to offend the dentist. This is a very unrealistic posture for the dentist to assume. It is much more effective to attempt to educate the patient to his needs, explain the advantages of the various treatment modalities, and suggest a plan compatible with the patient's life situation and desires. This places patients in a nonadversarial role because they realize that the dentist is sharing the responsibility of decision making with them rather than mandating cooperation.

Personal appearance and mannerisms

The dentist's dress, hygiene, and mannerisms are very important patient cues with regard to the dentist's work habits. It is very difficult to imagine that a dentist who is not interested in his or her own hygiene would be able to manage another person's hygiene. The basis for many patients' satisfaction with treatment often reflects their opinion of the dentist's personal neatness, cleanliness, and attention to detail. Consequently it is valuable for the dentist to examine personal apparel and hygiene prior to beginning a case presentation.

Numerous personal mannerisms can be distracting to the patient. Examples include poor eye contact, shaking one's foot, wringing one's hands, playing with paper, and drawing unusual designs on paper. Often these mannerisms result because the dentist is apprehensive or uncomfortable in the situation.

Visual aids

The use of visual aids in the case presentation can be very helpful to the dentist in the explanation of various disease processes and unusual treatment. Often a well-selected picture or model will greatly simplify the verbal explanation required to give the patient a good understanding of a confusing topic. In addition, the patient will have visual reinforcement to a verbal message. A number of criteria can be used in evaluating the use of visual aids.

SIMPLICITY

A visual aid should be selected that explains only one point. The visual aids that attempt to explain periodontal disease, endodontics, oral surgery, and major reconstruction will only serve to distract the patient from the individual point the dentist is trying to make.

SELECTIVE USE

Use a visual aid only if it is necessary to help clarify an issue. So often dentists use visual aids merely because they have them and not because it would greatly enhance the patient's understanding. An example is the use of roentgenograms. Many dentists will have the patient's roentgenograms on the view box whether they intend to utilize them or not. The roentgenogram will distract the patient and usually require the dentist to explain where the normal teeth and sound fillings are located.

USE MINIMAL NUMBER AT ONE TIME

It is much less confusing to allow the patient to see one visual aid at a time and return the visual aid to an inconspicuous location as soon as its use is completed. When visual aids are allowed to collect in front of the patient, the patient can be distracted from concentrating on what the dentist is saying.

PERSONALIZING VISUAL AIDS

When possible, use examples from the patient's own mouth, such as the patient's roentgenograms, study models, and intraoral photographs. The patient enjoys comparing his own mouth with ideal descriptive visual aids. An example is malocclusion. It is very easy to allow the patient to examine his own occlusal discrepancies when models have been correctly mounted on an adjustable articulator. A patient will relate more favorably to examples from his own mouth than from other patients' mouths.

COMMONLY USED VISUAL AIDS

Photographs. There are two types of photographs that can be valuable at a case presentation: pictures of the patient's intraoral condition and pictures of other individuals that demonstrate a specific condition or therapy.

Often pictures of the patient can be used to show periodontal inflammation, orthodontic malalignment, intraoral lesions, and deterioration of restorations. It is very revealing to compare the patient's intraoral disease and deterioration with the photographs of healthy, well-restored mouths. So often the patients do not have a frame of reference for what is healthy because they have never visually compared their own mouth with the ideal.

Photographs can be very helpful in educating patients about the subtle tissue changes that occur in periodontal disease. In addition, the use of tissue photographs with simple diagrams can effectively be utilized to explain the destructive process of periodontal disease.

Models. Dentiforms can be effectively used to explain the various types of restorations for teeth. Patients can easily visualize the difference between an onlay and an inlay by observing an example prepared on the dentiform.

Study models can be used effectively to demonstrate areas of occlusal wear, migration of teeth, malocclusion, and defective restorations. Study models can cause the patient to accept a more realistic view of the intraoral problems and cause him to be more personally concerned after he has examined the study models himself. It seems as though the patient becomes more accountable after seeing the facts. Study models can help the dentist communicate to the patient that the patient does have some real areas of concern.

Diagrams. Concise diagrams are very helpful in explaining complicated concepts or treatment. For example, a simple series of diagrams can very easily explain the process of root canal therapy or the destruction of periodontal structures with periodontal disease. Patients can associate more easily with diagrams when they are used conjointly with the patients' roentgenograms, study models, or personal intraoral photographs.

17

Maintenance

Randy L. Gates
Daniel G. Durchslag

Traditionally the concept of maintenance has implied that therapy has been completed and the patient is in a phase of observing the durability of completed procedures. As part of this concept, dentists and patients may have a tendency to feel that (1) the dental problems have been solved, the patient is completed and requires less attention; (2) new dental problems are not necessarily expected; and (3) if there is a chief complaint, that is the only problem. The patient may feel "that all of my work has been completed and I don't understand why I am having new problems." This may place the practitioner in a defensive position and possibly lead to a weakened doctor-patient relationship.

An alternative to this is a continuing care concept. It defines a patient as never being completed, which may eliminate many of the pitfalls mentioned above. The orientation to continuing care needs to be established *early*. The importance of ongoing care (maintenance), stated at the presentation of the treatment plan and at the completion of the outlined treatment, sets the stage for a positive approach to future evaluation. Elimination of the idea that patients are completed at the end of treatment may make them more receptive to a continuing care program. The goal is to develop an interrelationship between treatment plans, treatment, and ongoing care.

By replacing the concept of the traditional recall or maintenance program with a continuing care program, the practitioner is still faced with the time-frame questions of when, why, and how often should the patient be updated or evaluated. At present, other than the customary 6-month checkup, there has been no real attempt to provide the practitioner with guidelines from which to formulate individual maintenance review programs.

The evaluation of dental health needs to be assessed on an individual basis because each patient's resistance and exposure patterns are different. In addition, an individual's resistance to disease and exposure to harmful irritants may alter throughout life. Hence, ongoing review of dental treatment and an assessment of potential problems is of utmost importance. With this approach the dentist can become more successful in future treatment planning. As stated in Chapter 1, successful treatment brings satisfaction to dentists and their patients. Successful maintenance of the treatment essentially establishes the treatment as a success and assures continued satisfaction.

In this chapter our goal is to aid the practitioner in developing his own "game plan" for monitoring the patient's dental health. This consists of (1) providing the practitioner with some general principles from which to develop an individualized evaluation program and (2) presenting time intervals, philosophies, and guidelines for this evaluation. The intent of the following philosophies and guidelines is to encourage an integrated thought process so that each patient will have a systematic review of the various dental disciplines. Essentially we want to provide the dentist with the structure for a pragmatic minievaluation that will lead to consistent patient evaluations. On the other hand, the evaluation must be flexible enough to ensure that each patient will receive appropriate care.

MEDICAL EXAMINATION

The appropriate place to commence the assessment of a patient's dental status is with an evaluation of the medical profile. The medical evaluation not only reflects a concern for the total patient, but it also has a practical application for ensuring appropriate dental care. In addition, the dentist, as an important member of the health profession team, has a responsibility to help his or her patients detect the earliest symptoms of significant disease. In order to be able to fulfill this function, it is necessary that the dentist have a good working knowledge of various systematic disease entities. It is no longer acceptable for the dentist simply to be content to look for carious lesions. The dentist is often the health practitioner that sees the patient at the most regular intervals and consequently is in a position to evaluate and detect early changes in the medical profile.

It would be prudent to ask the patient the following three simple questions in the beginning of the evaluation: (1) Has there been any change in your health since your last appointment? (2) Are you taking any new medications? (3) Have you seen a physician since your last appointment? It is essential to have these questions asked at every recall or checkup appointment, and anything less than that could possibly be construed as poor dental practice. At first thought this may seem to be overcautious; however, the few seconds that these questions take will convey to the patient the dentist's concern for the patient's medical status. This also alerts the patient to think in terms of informing the dentist if there is any change in his medical history because he will be conditioned to answer these questions on a regular basis.

Whenever the patient's medical history has a particular characteristic, vis-à-vis diabetes, cardiovascular problems, nervous disorders, and so on, the practitioner should carefully evaluate these specific areas before instituting any dental therapy. In addition, these systems should be very carefully analyzed during the recall or maintenance appointments to help the patient assess his own medical status. For example, if a patient suffers from angina, the dentist might want to ask (1) What medications are you currently taking? (2) How often do you have an attack? (3) When did you have your last attack?

The dentist's role in the patient's medical evaluation has been given a lot of attention in the dental literature recently. One of the most discussed areas is the dentist's participation in monitoring the patient's vital signs. Should the dentist take them at every patient visit? Many practitioners feel that every time a patient is to receive a local anesthetic or be subjected to significant stress, the blood pressure and pulse should be established. Should the vital signs be monitored routinely during a continuing care or recall appointment? Pragmatically, it would be very simple for a practitioner to schedule his or her patients early so that prior to the dentist giving a local injection the patient can be seated in the operatory with the auxiliary monitoring the pulse and blood pressure in a few minutes. What a nice way for a dental office to tell its patients that it cares about them as individuals!

The practitioner who does not feel the need for monitoring the vital signs at every treatment appointment should give consideration to monitoring them at the maintenance appointment. In addition, it would be prudent to monitor the patient's vital signs prior to (1) long or stressful dental appointments, (2) surgical procedures, and (3) intravenous or nitrous oxide sedation procedures. As mentioned earlier, a certain percentage of the patient population should have their vital signs monitored every time they are in the dental office because of their precarious medical status.

Soft tissue examination

With the completion of the medical history, a logical sequence leads to an evaluation of extraoral and intraoral soft tissues. The necessity of thorough soft tissue review has been well established in dentistry. A thorough examination need only take 2 minutes. It should be performed in a consistent fashion so that no area is overlooked. Consequently a reasonable time frame for this exam could be from 6 months to a year. In addition, many oral pathologists recommend a pantomograph (Panorex) every 3 to 5 years to identify possible hard tissue (maxillary and mandibular) pathology. These roentgenograms should be retained for a minimum of 5 years for comparison purposes.

In addition to completing the soft tissue examination, the practitioner should, where possible, correlate the soft tissue evaluation and the medical examination. For example, a patient who has lichen planus may be more likely to have diabetes than the general population.[1]

What are the recommended guidelines for a continuing care philosophy relative to the patient with a past history of oral tumors? For this evaluation to be effective the practitioner needs a working knowledge of the following areas: (1) biology of the tumor, (2) history of the tumor, (3) type of treatment that has been received, (4) the primary therapist's opinion, and (5) reoccurrence probability. Although it is uncommon for the general dentist to be the primary therapist for a tumor patient, it behooves him or her to have an understanding of these five questions relative to the patient.

Temporomandibular joint evaluation

It is suggested that the temporomandibular joint (TMJ) be evaluated when completing the extraoral examination. The dental literature has been progressively expanding the definition of TMJ syndrome to include muscle symptoms of the shoulder and neck as well as chronic headaches.[3] The actual definition of TMJ syndrome will depend on the particular practitioner and can therefore vary tremendously. This area of dentistry is filled with intense controversy and dogma.[6] The proposed TMJ evaluation is not aligned with any particular "theory" but is orientated to maintaining a physiologically functional joint and orofacial musculature.

The objective of the TMJ evaluation is to identify as efficiently as possible those patients who demonstrate early signs of joint pathology or obvious TMJ symptoms. Simply stated, each patient should show a negative profile in each of the following diagnostic categories: (1) pain, specifically in the area of the TMJ; (2) noises in the TMJ—clicking, popping, crepitus;* and (3) muscle physiology—unlimited opening,†[7] freedom in all functional movements, and no significant muscle trigger points (muscle tenderness) in the head and neck region. The consistent correlation of "occlusal disease" and TMJ symptoms has not been documented and is therefore absent from this evaluation.

There are some patients who show a susceptibility to TMJ syndrome and should be evaluated very closely; these are roughly categorized as (1) patients who have completed extensive rehabilitative dentistry, (2) patients who have had their vertical dimension altered, (3) patients who have had extensive orthodontic therapy, and (4) patients with a previous history of TMJ syndrome. This group should have a TMJ evaluation at least every 6 months.

Periodontal evaluation

Since all dental therapies are supported by the periodontium, the monitoring of periodontal health is of obvious importance. As a continuation of the soft tissue examination, certain conditions of the intraoral structures to the periodontium should be evaluated for (1) pocket depth, (2) color, (3) texture, (4) form of the gingiva, (5) amount of attached gingiva, (6) vestibular depth, (7) frenum attachments, and (8) oral hygiene. This clinical data forms the basis from which the dentist begins to evaluate the patient's total periodontal health.

The major determinant in the periodontal evaluation is the level and architecture of the supporting osseous structures. The bone level can be determined by periodontal probing, roentgenographic examination, and direct observation (surgical exposure). When the clinical data supports the presence of periodontal disease, specific roentgenograms should then be ordered, which will provide the maximum diagnostic information with a minimum of x-ray exposure. The most efficient means of evaluating the overall bone level would be with bite-wing and anterior roentgenograms. The dentist can then correlate the clinical examination with these films to assess the severity of the periodontal disease. At that point the dentist can intelligently decide whether a full-mouth series is required in order to help formulate a treatment program for the patient.

Let us define two patient types: nonperiodontal and periodontal. The nonperiodontal patient is defined as showing no sign of active disease (clinical data is negative). This patient is evaluated during his cleaning appointments,

---

*Joint noises in the absence of other symptoms may not be indications for treatment.
†Normal mean opening from maxillary incisors to mandibular incisors is approximately 47 mm and is slightly larger for men than women.

which would be done on a periodic basis with intervals anywhere from 3 months to a year. Generally the extent of periodontal problems can be controlled by the hygienist.

The dentist has always been plagued with questions like (1) Should all patients be evaluated at the same interval? (2) Will evaluation intervals vary within a patient's life span? (3) How often should the dentist completely probe or evaluate each patient? Some practitioners have recommended that since it only takes 10 minutes to record full-mouth probings, it should be done at each recall appointment. This time can be reduced to 3 minutes, however, if the clinician is skilled and only pockets in excess of 5 mm are recorded. One alternative might be to probe the mesiopalatal aspect of the maxillary first molars and the mesiobuccal aspect of the mandibular first molars. If any of these areas are in excess of 5 mm, there is some correlation to periodontal disease.[5] This may indicate that full-mouth probing would be appropriate. The following factors should influence the frequency and extent of periodontal probing: (1) clinical findings—form, texture, bleeding upon probing, and oral hygiene; (2) age; and (3) past history of periodontal disease.

There is a tendency for the dentist to perform a "quick dental checkup" on the nonperiodontal patient after the prophylaxis is completed. As discussed earlier, this type of behavior should be avoided because it may reinforce indifferent patient attitudes. Consequently the significance of continuing care to the patient will be minimized.

The periodontal patient is defined as one who has received some type of surgical procedure. After surgery, these patients should be seen every 2 months until the patient can become nonperiodontal. The same factors should be assessed as they are for a new patient. Some periodontal patients reach this stage in 8 to 12 months. However, a significant group of patients may take approximately 2½ to 3 years to reach the nonperiodontal category. This can be because these patients are changing a behavioral (habit) pattern that they have had for many years. Under these circumstances it may take that long to develop an acceptable plaque control regimen. Unfortunately a third group never does attain nonperidontal status.

RESTORATIVE DENTISTRY

At this point in the patient review the dentist can now evaluate the dentition. The previous information has provided the dentist with the necessary background data for him or her to be able to propose personalized treatment recommendations. Not all patients have the same needs, nor are the objectives of treatment the same for all patients. The concept of continuing care not only represents the notion of perpetual evaluation, but also will allow for the objectives of treatment to be flexible. Should the 60-year-old man with a recently placed cardiac prosthesis be approached differently than the 35-year-old in good health?

Endodontics

As the dentist begins to focus specifically on the dentition, the first area to be covered is an assessment of the endodontically treated teeth. Those teeth that have been successfully treated should be indistinguishable from the patient's vital teeth. The patient should be queried as to "How does the tooth feel? Is it comfortable?" In addition to the patient's own evaluation, the dentist should employ diagnostic procedures to confirm the health of the tooth. The salient feature of this evaluation is the presence of pain. Since the presence of pain is intimately associated with failure, the characteristics of the pain are important. The dentist should know if the pain (1) is present when chewing or biting, (2) varies during the course of the day, and (3) is constant or intermittent. In addition to pain, the presence of swelling or mobility is significant. The frequency and severity of these symptoms should be noted and the area carefully examined. A periapical roentgenogram should be taken in order to assess the healing in the surrounding bone. Without the presence of specific symptoms, it is generally recommended that the postoperative roentgenogram be taken 1 year after the treatment is completed. It is believed that the 6-month postoperative roentgenogram is of diminished value because there has not been sufficient time for tissue responses to manifest on a film.

Fixed and operative evaluations

We have placed the routine or typical dental problems last because we feel they are least likely to be overlooked. In addition, when the practitioner begins to evaluate the dental structures, he or she should have developed a "sense of the patient." How is the patient feeling generally? Is the patient in an extremely stressful period of his personal life? Does he feel he has serious dental problems? This additional input will be more useful to the dentist prior to discussing dental problems with the patient.

The continuing-care philosophies of fixed and operative dentistry are rather simplistic. As dentists we want to evaluate the durability of previous dental restorations as well as detect new decay. A valuable concept to keep in mind is the realization that restorative dentistry is not the "breadth and width" of dentistry, but it is only *one* of the elements that contribute to dental health. The frequency of observation intervals will depend partly on the patient's past DMF rate and the estimated future susceptibility. In general, a patient in his high-caries-prone years should be seen at more regular periods than those patients whose decay rate has leveled off.

In evaluating the restorative patient, the existing dental treatment should be evaluated for (1) good marginal adaptation, (2) the intactness and solidity of existing restorations, (3) evidence of recurring decay, (4) tolerance of existing restorations by the periodontal tissues, and (5) the patient's ability to chew comfortably on the restoration. In addition, the practitioner should be scrutinizing the restorations for areas of plaque buildup, which would indicate that the hygiene should be reinforced.

An important consideration is how the previous dental work blends with the masticatory apparatus. One good index is to carefully examine the occlusal surfaces of the existing restorations and the natural teeth for the presence of wear facets. These wear facets can indicate the presence of occlusal instability and the necessity for additional evaluation. The patient should be monitored carefully in order to determine if additional symptoms begin to appear.

A patient who has had fixed bridges completed should have them carefully examined. A great deal of time and money goes into the delivery of a bridge, particularly one that has a long span. It would be wise for all of the bridgework to be pulled in an occlusal direction. The purpose of this would be to identify previously undetected mobile abutments. Also, the cement seal on the abutments can be checked to see if they are intact. This is an easy step to overlook, but it can save both the patient and the practitioner a great deal of future problems.

Inherent in the continuing-care philosophy is the ongoing opportunity to advise the patient of methods of improving his dental health. This might take the form of recommending replacement of the old alloys with castings. It might be reaffirming that a missing lower first molar should be replaced. When the patient realizes his dental health is always being upgraded, he may be more receptive to these recommendations.

Removable prosthodontics evaluations

Of the restorative disciplines, removable prosthodontics requires more frequent assessment than does operative or fixed prosthodontics. Considerations such as patient comfort, adaptation, and manipulation of the appliance contribute to this. This assessment generally should consist of the following: (1) educating the patient, (2) checking the occlusion, (3) evaluating the soft tissue response to denture coverage, (4) looking for oral lesions associated with the denture, (5) checking the denture for sharp edges possibly caused by chipping or wearing, and (6) reinforcing oral hygiene.

With complete and partial denture patients this assessment generally will occur every 6 months. Immediate denture patients are also usually seen every 6 months *after* the first year. During the first year they are seen every 3 months because of the extent of tissue and bone changes during that period. With overdentures it is best if the dentist uses the patient's dental hygiene as a barometer of the frequency of recall. These teeth are not cleaned by "natural" means, as they are covered by the denture and need careful monitoring. The maintenance guidelines mentioned earlier for endodontics should also be a consideration.

The partial denture patient requires specific observations. This is especially true of distal extension (class 2 and 3) partial dentures. The dentist needs to check for tissue support. If it is lessened or absent, it would create torque on the framework, which would be transferred to the supporting dentition. The dentist should make sure the framework (i.e., lingual bar) is not bent because this can also cause torque. The dentist also should inspect the clasps, making sure they are not too tight. In general, tight clasps cause more problems than ones that are loose.

Natural dentition in association with a removable prosthesis certainly plays a significant role in determining recall timetables. Natural dentition generates more force to an opposing prosthesis and the supporting structures. This would necessitate more frequent observations. This is particularly true in the patient presenting with a complete upper denture over a lower partial where the only remaining teeth are the six anterior teeth. This situation appears to concentrate the forces in the anterior area. Kelly states that almost total loss of bone in the anterior portion of the maxilla is very common because only natural anterior teeth remain in the mandible, which occlude with a complete upper denture. He also states that the "anterior part of the maxilla is the weakest part of the upper arch to resist stress."[2]

ROENTGENOLOGY

It may be surprising to have the roentgenology discussion located at the end instead of the beginning of the patient review. The philosophy we would like to present is that films should be taken when there is a clinical need for further diagnostic information that only a roentgenogram can provide. When such films are required, the maximum information should be retrieved using the least possible number of films. It follows that the need for further diagnostic information can only be determined by a clinical examination. The clinical review precedes and dictates which roentgenograms are to be taken. This is followed by roentgenographic examination and correlation with the clinical findings in order to arrive at a diagnosis.

Specifically, the patient who has completed a significant amount of treatment and is under observation will need certain films at later times, depending on the type and extent of the work that has been completed. For example, after extensive periodontal therapy, posterior bite-wing and anterior periapical films may be all that is needed in the first year in order to determine the success and long-term prognosis of the therapy. A patient with endodontic therapy will need 12-month follow-up films to determine the presence or lack of resolution of periapical lesions. Most patients, particularly those with high caries indexes and at caries-prone ages, will need bite-wing films taken at regular intervals to evaluate new or recurrent caries. Bite-wing films are frequently rich sources of information for the periodontal and caries status of patients with little radiation burden or cost (0.5 rads for two bite-wing films).

A *routine* follow-up full-mouth series is probably unnecessary under any circumstances having to do with dental treatment. If a full-mouth series has been taken within the last few years, the information on trabecular bone will not have significantly changed unless disease is present, in which case there would be a clinical indication for the films. Without this indication they should not be taken.

The disease-free patient would be approached in the same general manner, although the frequency and number of roentgenograms would certainly be reduced—18- to 24-month bite-wing films in an adult with a very low caries index and in the absence of peridontal disease, and single periapical films as dictated by any positive disease signs revealed during the continuing-care examination.

Panoramic roentgenograms for routine examinations have no significant contributions to follow-up care. Their use should be confined to special cases where their unusual projection geometry and technique renders them useful, for example, patients in intermaxillary fixation and trauma patients who cannot be adequately positioned for conventional skull roentgenology because of their injuries.

Occasionally dentists are called upon to follow patients who have received extensive restorative or surgical treatment for TMJ problems. There have been questions raised as to the appropriateness of conventional roentgenograms in the management of the TMJ patient. Plane and tomographic films have demonstrated themselves to be the only films that adequately demonstrate the TMJ anatomy.[4] The examination of the TMJ region offers a good example of where specific clinical signs and symptoms dictate the need for a roentgenographic examination of the joint. Conversely, the use of TMJ roentgenograms as a *primary* diagnostic tool should be viewed with skepticism.

REFERENCES

1. Howell, F. V., and Rick, G. M.: Oral lichen planus and diabetes: a potential syndrome, J. Calif. Dent. Assoc. **1**:58, 1973.
2. Kelly, E.: Changes caused by a mandibular removable partial denture opposing a maxillary complete denture, J. Prosthet. Dent. **27**:140, 1972.
3. Laskin, D. M.: Etiology of the pain-dysfunction syndrome, J.A.D.A. **79**:147-153, 1969.
4. Lurie, Alan G.: Personal communication, 1977.
5. Oliver, R.: Odontic seminar, University of Southern California School of Dentistry, December 8, 1976.
6. Schwartz, L.: Disorders of the temporomandibular joint, Philadelphia, 1957, W. B. Saunders Co.
7. Sheppard, I., and Sheppard, S.: Characteristics of TMJ problem, J. Prosthet. Dent. **38**:180-191, 1977.

18

Pitfalls in treatment planning and patient management

Charles Olivieri Munroe

This chapter arrives near the end of a whole text devoted to treatment planning and patient management. Inevitably, a large number of pitfalls or problems encountered in this area have already received consideration in previous chapters. The following pages will try to summarize and bring into some order the main areas of difficulty encountered in general practice when managing and planning treatment for a patient.

Pitfalls lurk along the entire process of patient management. It is therefore logical to review the steps that are followed in receiving a patient, obtaining data about his problem, analyzing this information, making a provisional diagnosis, formulating a treatment plan, and then carrying it out. Following are these steps:

1. Patient reception
2. History taking
3. Examination
    a. Extraoral
    b. Intraoral
4. Special investigations (where necessary)
5. Consultations with specialists (where necessary)
6. Diagnosis
7. Treatment plan
8. Prognosis
9. Actual treatment
10. Recall or follow-up examinations or assessments

Pitfalls lie in wait for the unwary all along the route to successful treatment of a patient's problems. It is only by a logical and systematic approach, together with a conscious effort to learn from inevitable mistakes, that these can be avoided. It is therefore proposed that each stage in patient management and some of the major pitfalls encountered at each step be considered in turn.

PATIENT RECEPTION

Patients who come to see a dentist generally have problems. The only exception to this is the routine patient who attends for periodic checkups. Many of the subsequent problems in patient management may be avoided by a courteous and careful reception of the patient. This will allow a complete and systematic collection of all the routine personal information required at this stage. It will also often identify the patient with special problems such as personality or other handicaps and forewarn the dentist, who can then take adequate and individual measures to deal with these when he or she sees the patient.

The first pitfalls in patient management are therefore encountered here. To achieve satisfactory results in this area, considerable care must be given to the selection of a receptionist. It is a mistake to equate patient reception with good looks and expensive surroundings. Courtesy means that the patient feels that the person receiving him is taking a genuine, unforced interest in his problem and in his presence in the office. This cannot be forced out of a receptionist. Patients are quick to sense a forced smile or automatic tone of welcome, and the antagonisms or dissatisfactions born at this stage may only come to light later with disastrous results.

HISTORY TAKING

The pitfalls that await the practitioner in the history-taking stage of patient management are numerous and potentially extremely serious. They are serious for the patient who may receive treatment that may be dangerous in view of a complicating medical history, and they may be serious for dentists who may one day face litigation for malpractice or negligence.

The pitfall to be avoided here is the incomplete history. Dentistry today does not allow any safe compromise in this area. The dentist is expected to take a complete and full history similar to one taken by a physician. It is a mistake to allow a history to be taken by a nurse or assistant. In taking a history personally, the dentist is achieving many goals. He or she is becoming personally acquainted with the patient and with the patient's problems and desires. He or she will be able to assess the personality and background of the patient and his suitability for the various treatment plans that may all be possible but not necessarily indicated for this person. This will enable the dentist to avoid the possibility of merely assessing and diagnosing the condition of the oral cavity and ignoring completely the personality that is carrying the condition about. For example, the same basic set of intraoral findings may be present in one patient in whom complete extractions and full dentures may be indicated, in yet another patient for whom selective extractions and removable partial dentures may be indicated, and in another individual for whom extractions may be avoided with aggressive periodontal therapy and patient cooperation followed by fixed bridgework. In these widely differing treatment plans, the difference would be not in the oral cavity but in the personality of the patient, his educational background, his desire to retain his dentition and cooperate in preventive measures, his financial resources, and even his home locality and availability for numerous appointments.

This brings one naturally to a consideration of the pitfalls encountered in the taking of a history solely with the use of questionnaires or personally without the help of any lists or prepared questions. The pitfalls in the use of a questionnaire are numerous, even if its advantages of timesaving and so-called "efficiency" are obvious. The filling out of a questionnaire about a health background presupposes a good command of the language and of the terms used in the questionnaire. The question "Have you ever had rheumatic fever?" may sound simple enough. However, many patients do not have any idea of the nature of rheumatic fever at all. They may link it wrongfully to arthritic diseases and reply inaccurately. The answer "yes" or "no" is not enough for this purpose. Even when a patient in a personal interview says he has never had rheumatic fever, the examiner should still pursue the matter further by asking questions about the patient losing time from school when young or suffering from any illness that will have restrained him to bed or home for weeks or months. A positive answer at this stage may reopen the whole investigation. Similarly, if the concerned patient replies that he does not know the nature of rheumatic fever, the examiner is at hand to give more details, a process which in the questionnaire is not possible. The use of prepared questions depends on a clear understanding of the language, of a certain basic intellectual capability, a knowledge of the terms used, and a willingness to cooperate in giving the information accurately. All or some of these factors may be absent in recent immigrants or people not proficient in the use of English, in poorly educated or mentally handicapped persons, in the very young, and in those persons who unfortunately think they can and should decide what medical information is relevant to dental treatment. All these potential problems make the use of questionnaires as a routine procedure unsafe. The only certain method of obtaining all the available facts is the personal interview.

The personal history allows the dentist to analyze the person that he or she is interviewing while talking and listening. The dentist can draw conclusions about the patient's knowledge of the language and adjust questions accordingly. He or she can sense an uncooperative attitude and try and overcome this by calm explanation of the reasons for a thorough medical history. The dentist can feel that a patient is censoring or adjusting his information for what he regards as sufficient for dentistry and again become more searching in his or her questions or explain the reasons for completeness.

The pitfalls, therefore, in the process of collecting a history usually result in incomplete or wrong information. If this incompleteness is in the description of the chief complaint, then the dentist may be misled and actually reach a wrong diagnosis and therefore a wrong treatment plan. A lesser evil would be for the dentist merely to be temporarily misled and realize during the procedure or later that he or she has been misled and to retrace his or her steps and possibly conclusions. This pitfall is most often encountered when interviewing patients who are very definite about the reasons for their problems, even though these may be wrong. These patients can become the victims of their own misjudgments and of the dentists whom they lead forcibly to wrong conclusions. A good example of this is the patient suffering from trigeminal neuralgia who insists that the pain is coming from his teeth and who eventually presents with an edentulous quadrant after all his teeth are vainly extracted one after the other in an effort to alleviate the neuralgia. Another more common example is the patient who undergoes root canal therapy on tooth after tooth for an unlocalized and poorly diagnosed pain in the mouth. The only way to avoid this pitfall with its drastic consequences is to collect the information in the history firmly and refuse to be led astray.

One of the most dangerous pitfalls to be encountered in history taking is in assessing the medical history. It is a mistake to allow all this information to be collected without some order or method. One such method is to separate the *present state of health* of the patient from the *past medical history*. The dentist faces two tasks in recording the medical history. The first is to assess the present state of the patient in relation to the procedures that he is going to be subjected to. The second is to find out whether in the past history of the patient any disease or condition existed that may affect him now and his projected treatment plan.

The "present state of health," or as some clinicians call it, the "functional inquiry," is an assessment of the condition of the patient as he sits in the dental chair. This assessment must be complete. An incomplete inquiry into the state of health may lead the dentist into treating a sick patient blindly with potentially disastrous consequences. In this inquiry the dentist faces two types of patient. The first knows about his health problems and on questioning gives this information to the interviewer. An example is the patient who knows that he is suffering from diabetes mellitus and upon questioning volunteers this information. The second type of patient is unaware of the presence of a health problem such as diabetes and therefore cannot answer affirmatively to direct questioning about such potential disease states. Simple questioning about present diseases and being under medical care or taking medications usually isolates patients of the first type; however, the other group can only be brought to light by questioning about the signs or symptoms of the present but undiagnosed disease. Thus a patient on the brink of cardiac failure may be unaware of his condition and therefore answer negatively to questions about cardiovascular disease; however, if further questions are put to him regarding the functions of this system, they may lead to conclusions that will put the dentist on guard about this possibility. For example, such a patient upon questioning may inform the interviewer that he gets tired easily, can no longer tackle the same physical exertions that he did a year ago, that his ankles swell, and that he can no longer sleep in the horizontal position but requires pillows to be comfortable. All these point to the possibility of heart failure and may either delay dental treatment until a firm medical opinion is available or may force a change in the various possible treatment plans for this patient. It would be a serious pitfall to fail to inquire into the general state of the patient even if he replies firmly that there is nothing wrong with him. Therefore general questioning about the functioning of the various systems of the body is necessary to eliminate the possibility of hidden disease that should be investigated further. Failure to make a complete inquiry in respect to present illness cannot be accepted. The patient's own ignorance may not be taken as an excuse in a court of law. The dentist is obliged to take all reasonable steps to ascertain the condition of the patient prior to commencing treatment.

The past medical history can also present pitfalls for the unwary. One most common error is to ask the patient whether he has ever suffered from any serious illness. This throws the decision as to what is or is not serious onto the patient who is usually not competent to do so. It is too easy for the patient who believes he is going to undergo a minor procedure in the mouth of little relevance to his general health to think that his past medical experiences are probably of no concern to the dentist. The reply is too often negative. Further questioning often reveals that in fact the patient may in the past have had serious illnesses or surgical procedures performed. Again, in a court of law, failure to have found out that a patient had suffered in the past from a disease that now remains highly relevant to dental treatment because the patient chose not to speak up will not be a strong defense against negligence. An example of this could be the patient who has been on steroid therapy but stopped a few months ago. This fact remains hidden during history taking. Oral surgery is performed in the dental office under some form of general anesthesia and, for example, the patient goes into shock because his circulating levels of corticosteroids are insufficient for the stressing situation he is undergoing. The dentist should have discovered this item of history and taken adequate steps to prevent the complication that occurred, perhaps in conjunction with the patient's physician.

The past dental history is often neglected. The information that can be gained here is extremely useful in assessing the type of treatment the patient has undergone in the past and his reaction to this treatment. This reaction may be physical, giving the dentist an idea about problems such as excessive bleeding following extraction, true allergies, anesthetic problems, and so on. However, the reaction of a patient to treatment is also mental. It is very useful and indeed essential for the practitioner to assess the patient's satisfaction or otherwise with the treatment he has received in the past. If the patient shows clear dissatisfaction with the standard or type of care that is evident in the mouth, it is wise to pause and consider carefully whether one can do better. The attitude of the patient is a valuable indicator of his appreciation of dentistry. For these reasons and their relevance in the formulation of a correct treatment plan at the end of the assessment, a clear understanding of the past dental history is extremely important.

Similarly, the social history of the patient may contain much useful information. It would be a pitfall of some consequence to fail to find out the relevant details about the patient's background, occupation, interests, social habits, and other facets that make up the picture of the person who is in the dental chair. All may have a bearing on the treatment plan. The needs and the desires of the first generation European immigrant will differ from those of an employee of a bank whose family has been in the country for generations. The differences may be more sharply outlined in the person whose occupation brings him in daily contact with the public, such as the stage or television personality, teacher, public speaker, or anyone in whom aesthetics are going to be of primary importance.

The social habits are also not to be ignored. The heavy smoker or heavy drinker may not only present the dentist with potential hazards, especially in general anesthesia, but may often indicate a type of person in whom a high standard of oral hygiene may not be attained easily, and this may have a bearing on the choice of treatment plan.

It is too easy for the dentist, tired after a day's work, to take a superficial history or to rely on a questionnaire. The medical history is too important to be dealt with lightly. Today the incredible advances of medicine have made it possible for many patients to be alive and walking into dental offices where one generation ago they would either have been chronic patients in an institution or would not have survived. The onus is on the dentist to be better trained and prepared for these patients than in the past. The pitfalls related to the various diseases, drug complications, and preventive measures necessary for such patients are too numerous to discuss here. There is only one way to avoid these. The dentist must have an adequate knowledge of general medicine to appreciate the significance of these conditions, and he or she must consistently take a full medical history and leave no doubt in his or her mind that he or she has exhausted all avenues in his or her inquiry.

EXAMINATION

So far in this chapter, emphasis has been placed on the logical approach to patient management. This applies to the method of examination as well. Any departure from a systemic and logical approach to the examination of a patient may lead to errors, omissions, or faulty conclusions. The examination should always proceed from the simple to the complex. That is to say, the examiner should first make use of simple methods before having recourse to more complex systems utilizing intricate equipment or laboratory methods. Why is this? By first proceeding through the simple method of examination using one's eyes and fingers *(inspection* and *palpation)*, nothing will be missed at this early stage. It is, for example, poor dentistry to return to the patient to reexamine the mouth for a large cavity that has now become clearly obvious in roentgenograms. It should have been detected originally during the clinical examination.

Another firm principle in examination should be that the *extraoral* examination should always precede the *intraoral* examination. In fact, the extraoral examination must never be omitted. To go straight to the mouth generally means the extraoral findings will be forgotten or neglected. They should be assessed first before the mouth is opened. Again, this may have to be explained to the patient calmly and clearly. There are numerous signs of disease to be found in an extraoral examination. There are changes in the limbs or head and neck that may be vital to supplement the assessment of the patient's present state of health made during the history. It is possible to examine the patient's pulse and blood pressure. Failure to do so may mean neglecting to discover an obvious cardiovascular anomaly. Failure to make a thorough examination of the lymphatic drainage area of the head and neck may mean a tragic delay in the discovery of a hidden malignancy in this area.

The extraoral examination commences as soon as the patient walks into the office and sits in the dental chair. These highly useful few seconds of inspection of the patient as he walks across the room and sits down are lost if the patient is received by an assistant and the dentist, busy in a second room, walks in later to find the patient already seated. There is much in the patient's passage from door to chair that can contribute to the assessment of his physical and indeed psychologic condition. The patient who crosses the room calmly and seats himself without fuss is going to present differing problems in management to the person who starts talking to the dentist volubly about his ailments before he is even halfway across the room.

These are days of speed and efficiency, and both as undergraduate students and practitioners, dentists are inundated with information, courses, and other pressures to improve efficiency and earning capacity in practice management. Let me remind them that in the dental office the object under scrutiny is a human being, often in some distress. This human being is the prime reason for the existence of the office. To have the dentist waiting courteously as the patient enters the clinicial area is comforting and builds up confidence. It is yet another pitfall to believe that the patient will be impressed by the highly efficient but impersonal organization where he is received by an assistant, works through a history questionnaire, and eventually sees a harassed dentist dart out of a second or third office to ask the assistant whom he or she is going to see next.

The extraoral examination should be thoroughly documented as indeed are all other areas of patient management. It is a common occurrence for a practitioner to find himself or herself in a court of law and find that his or her evidence is not substantiated by written records of what happened at the time in question. These records must be clear and not written in some code that is only intelligible to the dentist.

The extraoral assessment of the patient is followed by the intraoral examination. Again, as throughout the examination, it is to follow a logical system to avoid forgetting something. There should be a systematic progression through the areas of the mouth always commencing with the soft tissues and ending with the examination of the dentition. This order should be adhered to meticulously. To go straight to an assessment of the teeth usually leads to an omission of a proper examination of the rest of the mouth. Discharging sinuses, swellings, ulcerations, or other pathology may be overlooked. If such a lesion is an early malignancy, this could be tragic for the patient. Even in a less disastrous example, such as draining sinus, the consequences may be a wrong or delayed diagnosis. The pitfalls awaiting the examiner are numerous and affect even the most experienced clinician from time to time. There is only one foolproof method to avoid them, and this is to carry out the examination in the same meticulous way for each patient. One way is to proceed from lips to a complete examination of the buccal sulcus, proceeding then to the floor of the mouth, tongue, posterior aspects of this organ, the tonsillar area and oropharynx, then back to the mouth proper with the soft and hard palates. Then the dental structures can be given the examiner's full attention. In this way, any unsuspected lesion of the mouth or oropharynx can be discovered before the dentist's major attention is focused on the teeth. In a similar fashion, even when a patient attends with a clear history of an obviously localized problem such as a broken tooth, this full step-by-step examination should still be carried out. The complete examination and assessment of the condition of the oral cavity is the responsibility of the dentist and not necessarily of the specialist in oral medicine and should never be neglected.

SPECIAL INVESTIGATIONS

After the information obtained during the history and during the examination is collected and analyzed in the mind of the practitioner, it is often possible to come to an accurate diagnosis without the help of any further investigations. Some problems such as toothache caused by an obvious cavity are possible to diagnose by simple means. However, very often further investigations are necessary. These may be required to supplement the diagnosis even if this is quite certain, in order to finalize some potential treatment plan. For example, the obvious cavity may be the cause of the patient's discomfort; however, roentgenograms should now be taken to ascertain whether simple conservative measures will be enough to treat the tooth or whether changes will be found that indicate the necessity for root canal treatment or even extraction. This type of special investigation or test is required to supplement the information already obtained.

Other reasons for the special tests are to supplement the information already collected because this has so far not led to a firm diagnosis and more is required. The clinical findings may not show a reason for a patient's pain; however, roentgenograms and other tests may then demonstrate the presence of a necrotic tooth with apical pathology. There is a large range of supplementary investigations employing more complex means of examination that are available to the dentist. Some are possible to carry out in the dental office, some in the specialist's office upon request, such as special roentgenograms, and some only in a more highly complex environment such as the hospital laboratory.

What pitfalls await the dentist in this area? First, the pitfall of breaking the rule to use simple means before complex ones. For example, it is usually a mistake to take and examine roentgenograms of a patient before having made a complete clinical examination. Roentgenograms are of considerable assistance but should never be the sole basis for a diagnosis. On their own, they may be misleading. It should be the simplest method available that leads to a diagnosis of a problem.

The other obvious pitfall is, on the other hand, not to make proper use of the further methods of investigation available to us. Thus not to make use of roentgeographic examination when indicated may lead to serious errors of omission. Cases of trauma that do not have the necessary roentgenographic views taken from differing angles may result in the overlooking of a fracture of the jaws or alveolar ridges. To utilize a bite-wing view alone in the diagnosis of dental caries may result in conservative restorations being placed in teeth whose pulps are really necrotic and that on full periapical x-ray examination would be shown to possess apical pathology as well.

Omission of the use of an electric pulp tester, omission of the use of study models, or proper articulation to analyze the occlusion—these are all examples of failure to make proper use of diagnostic tests that are available in the dental office. Others may be available at specialists' offices or in hospital laboratories. The specialist radiologist will be able to carry out x-ray examinations of patients that are impossible in the general practice. These may include fuller examination of the jaws and skull, the temporomandibular joint, or the salivary glands. The laboratory may carry out more complex tests in many areas such as hematology, urinalysis, bacteriology, histopathology, and so on.

CONSULTATIONS WITH SPECIALISTS

More potential pitfalls await the unwary when consulting with specialists. The dentist must first decide that such consultation is required and then must select the correct specialist to refer the patient to. Consultations are usually required for the same basic reasons: the dentist is unsure of a diagnosis and requires assistance from someone more experienced or better trained in a particular area of dentistry or medicine; at other times, he or she may require a confirmation of a diagnosis either for his or her own benefit or because of a wish of the patient. Consultations are also sometimes requested because a dentist feels that the treatment of the patient is best done in a special environment such as the dental department of a hospital or a specialist's office rather than in general practice. Finally, there are those consultations requested to give a report on the condition of a patient. These are often required during litigation or by dental societies to whom a patient has complained about treatment.

The dentist is rarely on unsafe ground when he or she requests a consultation for the first of these reasons. If the diagnosis is uncertain, he or she will never adversely impress the patient if the reason for the referral is clearly explained. On the contrary, failure to do so and to proceed with an uncertain treatment plan in the face of an uncertain diagnosis is courting disaster. In this area a further pitfall to avoid is to refer the patient to the wrong type of specialist or to one in whom the dentist does not have full confidence. The dentist in practice should be aware of the specialist services available to his or her patients in the area and to use them correctly. The patient should be referred with a clear letter of introduction containing all the relevant history and clinical findings. It is highly frustrating to the specialist to receive a patient with no such information, and it is not very satisfactory for the patient either.

The second type of consultation is required to confirm a diagnosis already made. This is sometimes necessary because the patient is not contented with this diagnosis or is frankly dubious about it. To persevere with treatment in the face of such lack of confidence would be an error of judgment, one that would probably make for difficult relationships throughout the treatment. It would be far safer and ultimately more satisfactory to suggest that the patient obtain a further opinion. The patient would appreciate this, form a better opinion of the dentist, and subsequently, after the confirmation of the diagnosis, cooperate with the practitioner in a far more positive way.

Consultations for patients who require treatment in a specialized environment are often required in practice. Again it would be an error to persevere in the treatment of such patients when the personal experience of the dentist or his or her expertise is beyond what is required. This may be in an area of dentistry where the dentist has not sufficient training such as orthodontics, periodontics, or other specialty. Or it may be that the facilities offered by the dental office are insufficient to meet the needs of the case in question. Such patients are those with special medical problems that render them unsafe to undergo dental treatment in an ordinary office. For these the dental department in a hospital may be the safer environment, containing facilities to deal with medical emergencies and staff who are experienced to handle them. For these patients it could be a tragic error to persist in treatment in the dental office. The patient with severe cardiovascular disease, with bleeding abnormalities, or other potentially serious problems is best treated in a specialized environment, and for these a consultation is mandatory.

In cases of doubt with patients who have medical histories that cause concern, the consultation may take the form of a telephone call to the physician or perhaps a written letter requesting information or advice. Having received this advice, it would be a very grave pitfall to ignore or deviate from it in any way.

The consultations for patients who are the subject of litigation or who have themselves requested a further examination because they have become dissatisfied with some dental experience are often the result of pitfalls that we have already considered. However, more pitfalls lie in wait for the person who is now carrying out the consultation. No matter how correct the patient may be with his dissatisfaction or, on the other hand, how incorrect he may be found to be by the consultant dentist, it would be a profound error for the latter to allow his or her personal feelings to find their way onto the report or indeed to express these feelings to the patient. In contradistinction to all other areas of dental patient management, it is here important to remain aloof from the problems that are brought to light and to view these without emotion and to report on them objectively, that is to say, clearly, calmly, and without taking sides. All information that is given by the patient should be reported using words similar to "the patient reported that . . . ." All clinical findings should be clear and understandable and not subject to alternative interpretations. It is necessary to avoid pitfalls such as these because the consultant here may find himself or herself in court explaining his or her report and being subjected to questioning by both sides in the case.

For the dentist who is the subject of the litigation, many pitfalls would have been avoided if he or she kept the patient fully informed about the procedures to be carried out and their risks, if any, or their chances of success. He or she would also have avoided problems if this was all thoroughly documented. It should almost be a reflex action for the practicing dentist to turn to the patient's records to describe there in full what occurred in the office on that occasion. To omit to keep full and clear records of everything that has been done to a patient is today unacceptable. These records should include everything from a summary of a conversation between patient and dentist, for example, about the prognosis of a treatment plan, to an actual record of treatment carried out with all details of anesthetic used, procedure, postoperative instructions, prescribed drugs, and so on.

DIAGNOSIS

The diagnosis follows as the next step. The obvious error here is to make a mistaken diagnosis. There are times when this cannot be avoided; however, the error will never be very great if the principles already mentioned are adhered to and if assistance is sought whenever in doubt. The diagnosis is the identification of the cause of the patient's problems or complaint. The saddest pitfall to occur in formulating a diagnosis is not to make a wrong one but to be reluctant to admit to the patient or oneself that it has not been possible to reach one. This can lead to serious consequences. The patient with a pain can suffer needless treatment such as root canal therapy, extractions, or other procedures because the dentist will not admit, perhaps, even to himself or herself, that he or she is not sure of the cause of the pain. The pain may be caused by an unsuspected more serious lesion such as a malignant neoplasm, or may be totally nondental in origin, and the delay may be tragic for the patient who would be more confident of his dentist if he were sure that the latter knew his or her own limitations and would seek assistance from others when in doubt.

A further pitfall to avoid in this connection is in not informing the patient of the nature of the diagnosis. It is a mistake to make a diagnosis, proceed to a treatment plan, and then begin to treat the patient without his having a clear understanding as to the nature of his problem and what is going to be done about it. Once the various steps have been completed and the dentist has a clear idea in his or her own mind as to the nature and severity of the patient's problems, then he or she should explain it in layman's language. The patient will now be prepared for the next stage, which is the treatment plan.

TREATMENT PLAN

The most serious pitfall in the treatment plan stage of patient management is to omit it altogether. That is to say that the dentist will commence treatment in an automatic manner, depending on the clinical findings, and will make no effort to plan this in a systematic way that is in the best interest of his or her patient and of the final prognosis. The treatment plan should be formulated and explained to the patient. It should be a step-by-step procedure with the various stages in the best order possible for the final result.

The order of the various items on the treatment plan can be worked out in a logical fashion in most cases. This aspect has been discussed in detail in Chapter 10.

The selection of the *right* treatment plan is a more subtle and difficult task for the dentist to accomplish without falling into more pitfalls. This is where all the information that he or she has gathered is going to be so useful. This is where the impressions he or she gained when taking the history personally and learning all about the personality of the patient will bear its fruit. At this stage a treatment plan that does not take into consideration the personality, age, health, and makeup of the patient, his educational background, his financial resources, his interest in his oral health, his actual intellectual level, and even his home address or distance from the practice may subsequently find itself in difficulties. This type of patient will influence the treatment plan in many ways, for example, one patient will find thoroughly acceptable an acid-etch restoration for an anterior class 4 cavity; however, to another more conscious of his or her aesthetic appearance, only a porcelain crown will suffice. The treatment must not only be dictated by aesthetic requirements it is true; however, it is rarely possible to attain a successful end of treatment with a satisfied patient without obtaining his approval for all that has been done.

With the difficult or demanding patient it is even more vital that this approval for all stages of the treatment plan be obtained ahead of time. With the patient who does not fully approve of what is being done but for various reasons would go through with it, disaster lies ahead. The dentist is well advised not to persevere with treatment of a patient who shows obvious signs of dissatisfaction and who is sitting sullenly through the procedure. It would be best here to attempt a clear and polite discussion to try and ascertain the reasons behind the lack of cooperation, and if this is not possible, to desist from further attempts to push the treatment to a final conclusion.

A further important aspect to formulating treatment plans is a consideration of the age and potential length of life of the patient. An elderly patient with a poor prognosis with regard to length of life, often with serious medical complications, is not a candidate for complex dental procedures. Such a patient, for example, who suffers from advanced periodontal disease accompanied by grade 3 loosening of many teeth, may be worse off with extractions and provisions of dentures than by some simple form of splinting using perhaps wires and acrylic cement. This method may be condemned in a younger patient where either active periodontal treatment or extractions may be the obvious choice. However, in this case the patient who may only have about a year to live will retain his teeth to the end and not go through surgery and then have to become accustomed to partial or full dentures. This type of modification to a treatment plan is particularly necessary in cases of advanced age, debility, and serious medical problems.

Another serious error in treatment planning is in connection with mentally handicapped patients whose neurologic capability will not allow them to understand what treatment is needed to achieve suitable oral health or what home procedures will be necessary to maintain the treatment after completion. To give an example, a young patient with severe mental retardation also suffered from recurrent seizures of such severity that, though institutionalized, complete control of these attacks was not possible. In the course of these seizures she traumatized her anterior teeth and the adjacent soft tissues by falling against hard surfaces or by biting herself unconsciously. This patient's handicap made her totally unable to understand or respond to her environment. To look at, she was a young person of about 20 years of age. An initial treatment plan was made at the request of her physician, whose main concern was the recurrent trauma to the lips by her fractured teeth. This treatment plan was for the patient, under general anesthesia, to have a thorough scaling of the teeth, restorations in those teeth that were decayed, immediate root canal therapy for one central incisor whose pulp was exposed in a fracture, plus crowning of a total of four anterior teeth. Any standard book could have produced an identical plan. What would have been the result of this treatment? For a time, the young 20-year-old woman would indeed have looked aesthetically acceptable, it is true, and her eating may have been improved; however, all that the dentist who made the plan was seeing was a young patient with dental disease, and he had applied standard textbook treatment plan techniques to this condition. The patient was neither aware that her traumatized teeth looked unsightly nor was she aware of any masticatory discomfort because her mental handicap prevented any such appreciation. After an epileptic seizure or two, her beautiful anterior crowns would be fractured again, and as time passed, her complete lack of oral hygiene would produce another wave of rampant decay and calculus and plaque accumulation. In such a mouth, multiple extractions were indicated even if no replacement with dentures or bridges was possible. The patient would then not traumatize herself anymore and throughout her life would never feel the slightest regret for the loss of her front teeth. This case has been discussed in more detail because it is illustrative of a frequent and major fault especially common in the recent graduate, namely, that it is not possible to take textbook recommendations and apply them to the mouth of a patient as though he were a mannequin. This textbook ideal may have to be modified out of all recognition when the factors outside the mouth are taken into consideration.

The educational background of the patient and his knowledge of what dentistry can offer is also important in formulating a treatment plan. A recent immigrant from a country where the level of sophistication in oral rehabilitation that is available on this continent is unknown or not possible for other reasons is unlikely to appreciate the necessity for the more complex procedures possible to restore the dentition to its maximum possible function. However, a reasonably educated person brought up in an area where such levels of dentistry are routinely practiced and available will be far more receptive to a treatment plan that will restore and maintain his dentition despite its length or complexity. His background educationally will help in understanding the explanations as to the reasons for the various stages and types of treatment.

The financial resources of the patient also influence the treatment plan. While it is regrettable that not all patients can afford the ideal textbook treatment, it should also be remembered that many of these patients also will not desire the complexity and length of such treatment and moreover will often not be the type of person that will be able to maintain the health of the mouth adequately after completion of the treatment. The question that should be asked for each treatment plan should be "What is the most practical and best treatment that I can give to *this* patient?" Every individual patient will need some modification in plan even if the clinical findings were identical for all. Thus the patient with weaker financial resources may often be better off with selected extraction of teeth that in another patient might have been saved with considerable effort, and then followed by the provision of partial removable dentures, again which in another person might have been replaced by fixed bridgework. This is not always a compromise dictated by financial resources but by an overall analysis of the best interests of the patient, who may maintain his remaining teeth and partial dentures far better than he would complex bridgework. In these cases it would be a serious error to insist on the wrong treatment plan in the face of these indications and perhaps force the patient into a treatment he cannot afford and which he may not have desired.

Coupled with all these factors affecting the choice of treatment plan, inevitably to be considered is the actual interest of the patient in what the dentist is suggesting. To force him to accept a treatment plan that does not interest him is a major pitfall. The result is never satisfactory. The patient regrets the time, expense, and even the result, and resents the part that the dentist has played in getting him involved in the treatment. The dentist ultimately will regret it too, as poor patient cooperation will inevitably result and will be followed by poor maintenance of the work that has been done.

Once all these factors have been sifted and weighed against what are the basic needs of the patient, a treatment plan that the dentist considers in the best interest of that individual patient is proposed. It should be clearly explained to the patient so that he will attend the various appointments, know what is going to be done, accept this, and indeed approve it. If additions or changes in the basic plan become necessary, they should be explained further and the reasons for the changes made clear. It is dangerous to make changes and carry them out without informing the patient and obtaining his consent. Subsequent dissatisfaction about some issue connected with the treatment could then find concrete ground and end up in court.

In the treatment plan it can be seen by a consideration of what has been said in these pages that the choice of which procedure to carry out will be the crucial factor in success in many instances. The operator may be a splendid endodontist, but to perform root canal therapy on a solid and intact molar when virtually the entire remainder of the dentition is affected by advanced periodontal disease with a poor general prognosis would be a poor choice.

To construct a removable full denture, occluding with six remaining anterior teeth may also in many cases be a poor choice as the heavy strain on the edentulous area opposite the natural teeth may cause deterioration and show swift resorption of the alveolar bone.

In other words, the technical skill of the dentist may be of the highest caliber; however, the best interests of the patients and ultimately of the dentist are achieved by care in choosing where to apply this high degree of ability. The endodontist may forego root-treating the molar in question in the above case, reluctantly going to extractions in view of the general poor prognosis of the whole mouth, while the dentist in the second case may do likewise in the long-term interest of the patient or consider another alternative.

PROGNOSIS

The treatment plan and its frank discussion with the patient should be accompanied by an equally frank discussion of the prognosis, or the chances of success in achieving the aims of the treatment. This should never be omitted in patient management. Any limitations in treatment or in attaining the ultimate goal should be clear to the patient and should be documented in the records. This will serve to avoid discussions later on what was promised and what was achieved.

This chapter will not proceed to discuss the pitfalls that may await the dentist during actual treatment; however, if the principles that have been discussed previously are applied in the actual treatment, many potential pitfalls will be avoided.

Avoidance of problems throughout the management of patients can be described as a type of preventive dentistry. It is the use of common sense and logical thought throughout. If something appears a trifle illogical, then it probably will lead to a pitfall. Cultivation of a systematic approach to patient care together with an understanding and compassionate attitude will go far in avoiding these errors. The patient is not an automobile going for service. He is a person with emotions and desires who will rarely react with anger or resentment at unavoidable mistakes by his dentist or ultimate failure to reach complete success with a treatment plan if he feels that he is being treated as a human being with interest and care. This reserve of good will on the part of patients, which serves to make up for the smaller pitfalls the dentist still encounters from time to time, has to be earned. It is wise to set about earning it from the start by treating patients in a manner that would be acceptable to oneself if receiving treatment and by avoiding the pitfalls discussed in these few pages.

PART V

Records

19

Problem-oriented dental record system—an alternative

Roger G. Sanger
Malcolm E. Boone II

Dental educators have for years, both in revered journals and in clandestine meetings, eluded to and discussed with frustrating fervor the "silent curriculum" that has been firmly entrenched in dental schools. The silent curriculum refers to those student educational experiences that are never officially listed by the school's registrar, yet which have considerable impact on dental education and dental practice. Educators attempting to formalize this silent curriculum have met with failure, and so it continues to perplex the profession. The core of any school's silent curriculum is always the dental health care delivery system. The theoretical aspects and concepts of such a system may be presented with classroom formality, but certainly practical aspects and applications must be derived from actual clinical experiences. The record system previously thought to be incidental in dental education and dental practice is now being rapidly advanced to accountable status because of its present ethical, legal, and financial importance. A review of the literature on record systems reveals very little, obviously reflecting its past sedentary existence in the silent curriculum.

CONVENTIONAL DENTAL RECORD SYSTEM—A TREATMENT-ORIENTED SYSTEM

The record system taught to most of us in dental schools was probably the conventional dental record system that was almost certainly changed once we were in private practice. Why? First, the conventional system is typically a *treatment-oriented system*. In most dental schools treatment is centered around academic departments or disciplines instead of being oriented around patient problems. Patients do not present themselves *for* endodontic treatment, they present themselves *with* a pulpal problem. Departments or disciplines of dentistry exist only in dental education and not in the general practice of dentistry. Hence the dental graduate finds it necessary to restructure the dental school record system so that it will be suitable for dental practice.

Second, the conventional system is typically an extrinsic patient comparison system. When a structure or physical finding of a patient is examined, it is usually compared with some other extrinsic patient structure or physical finding that was defined as within normal limits (WNL) by human clinical studies. Therefore when the gingiva of a patient is examined, it is compared not with the total patient, but with some WNL definition derived from numerous human clinical studies. In other words, the gingiva of one patient is compared with the gingiva of some unknown groups of patients whose gingiva was within normal limits—an extrinsic comparison.

A physical finding such as the blood pressure value of a patient is another good example. The World Health Organization has defined the WNL for blood pressure as being 120/80, and 140/95 as being excessive. However, caution is always mentioned when comparing a patient with these values, since they reflect statistical values and do not take into consideration the intrinsic determinants of blood pressure in a particular individual (i.e., race, age, occupation, systemic disease, familial background, and so on). The WNL should serve as a baseline of initial comparison, but the final comparison of the structure or the physical finding of a patient should be an evaluation based on the intrinsic totality of that patient, not on the extrinsic totality of a group.

Hence the dental graduate must change the record system for a second reason: to represent a more individual intrinsic examination and evaluation system instead of the conventional group extrinsic examination and comparison system. The discovery that patients do not wish to be examined and compared with other nondescript groups of people who are supposedly WNL is quickly determined. Rather, patients wish to be examined and evaluated as individuals with intrinsically related problems, not with extrinsic discrepancies.

Because of these two deficiencies in the conventional dental record system, many dental educators with the help of dental practitioners are producing an alternative dental record system. This system is by no means a new and unproven system that was established in hasty response to these disparities and with a need for a more accountable dental record system.

PROBLEM-ORIENTED DENTAL RECORD SYSTEM—AN ALTERNATIVE

This alternative system is the problem-oriented dental record. As was mentioned, this is not a new or unproven system. It is an extension of the problem-oriented record system that was introduced in medicine by Weed, a medical educator in the late 1960s. Shortly thereafter, two medical practitioners, Bjorn and Cross, developed the system further, and finally the Hurst and Walker team evaluated and refined it during the early 1970s.[2, 5, 10, 11] The system has had so much attention in the literature that the Veterans Administration now publishes a 42-page source bibliography on the system.[8]

The problem-oriented dental record system was introduced in the mid-1970s as a few dental schools sought to advance the quality of clinical education in their silent curriculum. Now approximately ten schools and their affiliate hospitals and clinics have instituted the system, with many more schools contemplating adoption. The dental services of the Veterans Administration hospitals have fully implemented the system nationally also, and the list of private hospitals may go on ad infinitum. Already the problem-oriented dental record system is appearing in the dental literature with discussions on its theoretical and practical application.[3, 4, 6, 7, 9] The system has even been manufactured and marketed by a private printing company in hopes of attracting the dental practitioner.[1]

The problem-oriented dental record system is, as the name implies, oriented primarily around the problems of the patient and secondarily around the dental health care necessary to resolve these problems. It is not specifically or primarily oriented to the treatment of problems based upon academic dental departments or disciplines, as is the conventional dental record system. It is based upon the fact that patients seek dental care because of some known or unknown problems that need identification, evaluation, planning, and treatment. To use our previous example, a patient presents with oral pain (known problem), is identified as having an abscessed tooth (unknown problem), has evaluation and planning for possible endodontic therapy, and finally, has specified treatment rendered. Sometimes during treatment further unknown problems may be identified that require evaluation, planning, and treatment. In our example patient, the tooth may have a root fracture (another unknown problem) after endodontic therapy commences, which necessitates new evaluation, planning, and treatment (routine endodontic therapy continued, hemisection, extraction with subsequent prosthesis, and so on). Since the system is problem oriented with identification, evaluation, and planning for these problems, the system is always cyclic and ongoing and never tangential and fragmented, which may be the case with systems that are treatment oriented, where treatment is usually considered definite and final.

Second, the problem-oriented dental record system is basically an intrinsic evaluation system. Its motto might well be: "What is a problem for one patient may not be a problem for another patient." Intrinsic evaluation implies the collection of data in the usual manner, but then the evaluation of that data with the individual as a whole, not the comparison of that data with an extrinsic WNL value. Again, to use a previous example, data collection reveals a blood pressure value of 140/95 on a patient. If we empirically compare that value with our WNL, we might ascertain that this patient has a medical problem. But if we, in communication with the physician, evaluate this value in contrast to the patient's age, race, physical status, emotional status, systemic health status, familial background, occupation, medications, and so on, we might well ascertain that there is no problem with this patient even though the WNL value has been disturbed. Again the system became a cyclic and ongoing system since, as the patient represents a constantly changing organism, the intrinsic evaluation and problem identification must be ongoing and repetitious and not definite and final. Extrinsic comparison is both cyclic and definite since the organism is constantly changing, but the WNL is always constant. Intrinsic evaluation is totally cyclic since any particular part of an organism is changing even as it is evaluated with the whole organism, which is constantly changing. Obviously, then, the problem-oriented system provides a more complete and dynamic approach to comprehensive health care (see boxed material).

Dental health care is a multiphasic operation that should involve (1) collection of data pertinent to the orofacial organ system in function and balance with the whole person; (2) transformation of this data into a meaningful, coordinated body of information from which a rational problem-oriented diagnosis can be established; (3) generation of a therapeutic plan for this problem-oriented diagnosis; (4) skillful execution of these plans; and (5) careful maintenance, surveillance, and reassessment of the patient in the dental health care system.[10]

To expand further, a good dental health data collection and recording system should accomplish the following:

1. It should integrate the patient examination data.
2. It should provide a means of assessing patient problems and needs.
3. It should help establish the plans and sequential listing of projected treatment for these plans.
4. It should provide for a record of patient treatment, maintenance, surveillance, and assessment of the patient.
5. It should provide an objective evaluation of the performance of the dentist and the other members of the dental team.
6. It should provide a means for communication between all health care professionals and auxiliary personnel to function.
7. It should provide education and motivation for the patient.
8. It should provide for the means of auditing patient care.
9. It should be able to be used as an educational tool for the training of the health care student in a clinical environment.
10. It should be in an organized format to allow for meaningful usage over

CONVENTIONAL RECORD SYSTEM	PROBLEM-ORIENTED RECORD SYSTEM
Treatment oriented Extrinsic comparison	Problem oriented Intrinsic evaluation

---

PROBLEM-ORIENTED RECORD SYSTEM

1. Educational system
2. Health care delivery system
3. Audit system
    a. Educational component
    b. Health care delivery component
    c. Practice profile component

a period of years and for transferring between different health care professions and institutions if necessary.

11. It should provide statistical information for research purposes if needed.[1,9,10]

The problem-oriented dental record system has been designed as a vehicle for achieving both the goals of dental health care and the goals of a dental health data collection and recording system, since it is an *educational system*, a *health care delivery system*, and an *audit system* (see boxed material on bottom of opposite page). It is an educational system since it trains and aids the health care professional to be a comprehensive and evaluative diagnostician viewing the patient's dental health care problems and needs as they relate to the total patient. It is a health care delivery system since it delivers modern dental health care to patients as dictated by the problems of that patient on the priority basis established by the patient and the diagnostician. Therefore problem identification as well as problem prioritization is essential for the system. It is an audit system since it will audit the educational component, the health care delivery component, and the practice profile component. As an educational audit it allows the professional or a peer organization to audit the proficiency of comprehensive diagnosis. As a health care delivery audit it allows the professional or a peer organization to audit the problems of the patient according to the diagnosis, treatment plan, and rendered treatment. As a practice profile audit it enables the professional or a peer organization to establish a practice profile according to identified patient problems, established treatment plans, and rendered treatment.

Components of the system

The components of the problem-oriented dental record system are the data base, problem list, diagnostic and therapeutic plans, and progress notes (see boxed material). This is in contrast to the treatment-oriented system with its components being diagnosis, proposed treatment, and treatment notes (see boxed material).

PROBLEM-ORIENTED SYSTEM

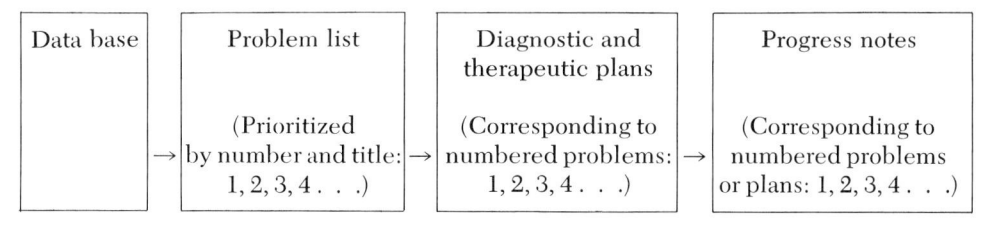

Data base	Problem list	Diagnostic and therapeutic plans	Progress notes
	(Prioritized by number and title: 1, 2, 3, 4 . . .)	(Corresponding to numbered problems: 1, 2, 3, 4 . . .)	(Corresponding to numbered problems or plans: 1, 2, 3, 4 . . .)

TREATMENT-ORIENTED SYSTEM

Diagnosis	→	Proposed treatment	→	Treatment notes

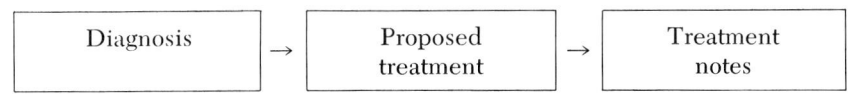

Data base

The data base can be discussed from both a theoretical and a practical aspect. In the theoretical aspect the data base is that information resulting from the initial collection of health care–related facts that an environment defines as sufficient for the identification or recognition of patient-related health problems or difficulties. The collection of the data must then be controlled, systematic, accurate, and uniform for this environment. In dentistry there appears to be an absence of an adequately defined data base. There is little standardization in dental education or dental practice in the collection of health data, which further complicates the matter. The data base can be divided into three major categories: historical data, physical and physiologic data, and laboratory data.

In the practical aspect the data base is that physical location within the problem-oriented dental record where the initial health data is recorded. It is separate and distinct from the other sections of the record.

Problem list

The problem list consists of all significant health care–related problems of the patient defined at the level of understanding of those problems by the recording clinician. The term "problem" in the literal sense refers to questions raised for inquiry, observation, or intervention, but in health care it best refers to a situation in need of improvement. The term "significant" must be used in the context that this is ultimately a matter of clinical judgment that includes a clinician-patient negotiation. The phrase "level of understanding of those problems by the recording clinician" may refer to the degree of clinical competence in diagnosis, but in the true sense it refers to the "time factor" in gathering information to adequately define the problem. Some problems require less time and less data gathering than other problems to identify and recognize. Therefore there is definitely a time factor in the evolution of this level of understanding of the patient's problem.

Problem identification and recognition should not be confused with the establishment of a diagnosis. Diagnosis is the act of determining the nature of a

Table 6. Problem identification versus diagnosis

Problem identification	Differential diagnosis	Prognostic and therapeutic plans	Definitive diagnosis
A well-delineated and circumscribed 3×3 mm ulcerative lesion on the lateral border of the tongue that has been present for 2 weeks	Traumatic ulcer Herpesviral ulcer Aphthous ulcer Squamous cell carcinoma	Initial manipulation and observation Subsequent excisional biopsy	Squamous cell carcinoma

disease condition. It is possible to identify a problem without establishing a diagnosis. Oftentimes a definitive diagnosis is not established until treatment of a problem is instituted (Table 6).

A problem may be identified using multiple data collection. For example, an occlusal problem may well be identified only after collecting data pertinent to static occlusal classification, functional occlusal classification, tooth structure status, periodontal status, temporomandibular joint status, and so on. Many times one general problem represents the accumulation and synthesis of many possible problems. However, it is not until all other possible problems are accumulated and synthesized that a general problem will materialize and be identified (see boxed material).

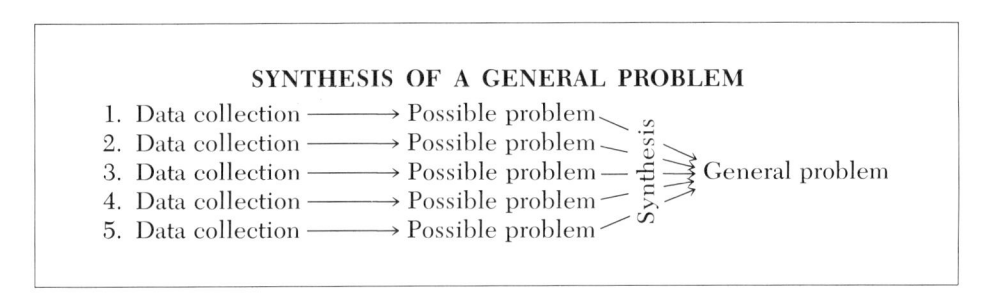

SYNTHESIS OF A GENERAL PROBLEM

1. Data collection ⟶ Possible problem
2. Data collection ⟶ Possible problem
3. Data collection ⟶ Possible problem — Synthesis ⟶ General problem
4. Data collection ⟶ Possible problem
5. Data collection ⟶ Possible problem

The complete problem list consists of all of the patients general problems that can be identified from synthesis of the possible problems accumulated during initial data collection. They are prioritized using the numbering system "1" to indicate the highest priority, "2" to indicate priority ranking after "1," and so on.

The shorter the title for identifying the problem without sacrificing the meaning the better, since each time the problem is written about, its number and title must be written. In dentistry it is best to use general, one-word titles that reflect organ subsystems (i.e., pulpal, periodontal, occlusal, and so on) or situations (i.e., emergency, psychologic, medical, pathology, and so on). Titles should be pragmatic, operational, or observational where possible. Since the treatment plan will be specific for the problem, where possible the title should reflect this reciprocity. The length of the problem list will also be kept to a reasonable minimum if appropriate synthesis of possible problems into general problems is accomplished (see boxed material). Therefore instead of listing caries or hypoplasia of specific teeth as problems, they should be synthesized into a more general dental problem. In general, the problem list should serve both the clinician and the patient by being the appropriate length, unambiguous, pragmatic, and showing ample evidence that the critical thinking process of the clinician is evolving. Judgment must be exercised, since each numbered and titled problem will require a correspondingly numbered and titled plan for its resolution or inactivation.

Diagnostic and therapeutic plans

When the problem list has been formulated, it is necessary to establish *diagnostic and therapeutic plans* that consist of diagnostic tests or proposed treatment for the resolution or inactivation of the corresponding problem. Diagnostic or laboratory tests might be necessary to clarify and further define a particular listed problem before definitive diagnostic and therapeutic plans can be delineated. Each plan must include (1) a *goal* of diagnosis or treatment, (2) *diagnostic criteria* logically sequenced that may be needed to complete a differential diagnosis or definitive diagnosis, (3) *therapeutic procedures* with means to achieve them, and (4) *patient education* methods regarding any instructions, treatment limitation or expectations, and prognosis of the problem. Plans are always established in consultation with the patient. The plans become the working outline for patient care. A date is attached to all problems or plans for purposes of auditing the resolution of a problem by time. After all additional data listed has been collected, so as to establish a definitive diagnosis, a final plan can be developed. The plan should contain an integrated and sequential outline of treatment. This should contain a temporary sequence of treatment by appointment and, if desired, the appropriate estimated professional fees. Finally, a master treatment plan can be constructed for all problems.

Progress notes

The final component of the problem-oriented dental record system is *progress notes*. It is probably the most dynamic and vivid component of the system. In essence it contains a narrative of the resolution procedures performed according to the master treatment plan. In the conventional systems the progress notes are usually very simple yet descriptive. If they are detailed they usually do not follow any logical format. In the problem-oriented dental record system, progress notes for each problem should be recorded and identified by referring to the numbered and titled problem for which that progress note is being entered. In this manner, auditing of progress notes can be accomplished not only for chronologic events, but also for specific problem resolution development. The progress notes may contain any or all of the following elements dependent upon the needs of both clinician and patient: (1) the *subjective* reactions or feelings of the patient toward the situation or treatment; (2) the *objective* statement of procedures that were attempted during the situation or treatment; (3) *assessment* of the problem at this particular date as to any changes in the status of the problem; and (4) a record of the procedures actually performed during the appointment or a *plan* for subsequent problem resolution procedures. This format is known as the SOAP format. On many occasions, only the "O" and "P" sections of the SOAP format are used when treatment is repetitive for a static problem. Of paramount concern to the clinician should be the development of professional communicative skills in the SOAP format so as to promote interdisciplinary and interprofessional communication.

PROBLEM-ORIENTED DENTAL RECORD—A MODEL

Hopefully, sufficient information has been presented regarding the problem-oriented record system in review, introduction, and definition for conceptualization of the system. Next, it seems appropriate to review an actual model record of a problem-oriented dental record system. The actual record itself may vary from system to system, depending upon individual and institutional determinants.

A model record for a problem-oriented dental record system should include the following: first, the record should be housed in a substantial, physical *chart* document so as to include all of the components of the problem-oriented dental record system. In most models this chart is a 9- by 12-inch file that has a computerized patient alphabet or color identification code present on one side of the chart and a medical alerting area on the front cover. The medical alerting area should be an isolated area where appropriate alerting symbols or designation may be placed. The medical alert usually reflects the medical problem or problems of the patient that may influence patient management or dental therapy (see boxed material). If no medical problem exists or if one exists that is unremarkable, then the word "unremarkable" should be placed in this area.

MEDICAL ALERT
DIABETIC

The inside of the chart should afford adequate access to the data base, problem list, diagnostic and therapeutic plans, and progress notes.

Second, the *data-base* component of the problem-oriented dental record system should be a separate and distinct section of the chart. It should be organized as follows:

1. Data base
    a. Patient background data base
        (1) Patient background data
        (2) Social-family data
        (3) Health questionnaire
        (4) Chief complaint
        (5) Medication regimen
        (6) Patient resumé
    b. Patient physical/physiologic laboratory data base
        (1) Review of systems
        (2) Physical examination of systems and laboratory studies
        (3) Roentgenographic examination
        (4) Intraoral examination

(5) Periodontal examination
   (6) Dental examination
   (7) Pulpal examination
   (8) Pathology description
   (9) Occlusal examination and malocclusion assessment
   (10) Prosthetic examination
   (11) Dental charting (as appropriate for 3 through 9)

A signed, witnessed, and dated informed patient consent form should precede the data-base section.

Third, the *problem list* component of the problem-oriented dental record system should be a separate and distinct section of the chart. It should be organized as follows:

2. Problem list
   a. Problem number
   b. Problem title
   c. Date problem activated or entered
   d. Date problem inactivated or resolved

Fourth, the *diagnostic* and *therapeutic plans* component of the problem-oriented dental record system should be a separate and distinct section of the chart. It should be organized as follows:

3. Diagnostic and therapeutic plans
   a. Problem number
   b. Problem title
   c. Plan
      (1) Goal of treatment
      (2) Diagnostic criteria
      (3) Therapeutic procedures
      (4) Patient education

Fifth, a *master treatment plan* should be included as a separate and distinct section of the chart. It should include all proper sequenced diagnostic or therapeutic procedures for all of the numbered and titled problems or plans listed in the problem list section and the diagnostic and therapeutic plans section. Each line addition in this master treatment plan should include the following:

4. Master treatment plan
   a. Line number
   b. Problem or plan number
   c. Problem or plan title
   d. Procedure number
   e. Procedure description
   f. Procedure fee
   g. Starting date
   h. Completion date

Following the master treatment plan should be a final signed, witnessed, and dated informed patient consent form.

5. Progress notes

Finally, the *progress notes* component of the problem-oriented dental rec-

ord system should be a separate and distinct section of the chart. It should be organized as follows:
  a. Date
  b. Master treatment plan line number
  c. Problem or plan number
  d. Problem or plan title
  e. Procedure
     S = Subjective reactions
     O = Objective statement
     A = Assessment of problem
     P = Plan for subsequent appointment
  f. Signature of professional

CONCLUSION

The problem-oriented dental record system has been presented as an alternative to the more traditional and conventional treatment-oriented dental record system. The problem-oriented dental record system can be an educational health care delivery and audit system that is highly communicative and accountable. Obviously for those professionals that were trained with the conventional dental record system during their silent curriculum education, this alternative dental record system may seem different, but certainly it is sound in principle. With more dental schools, hospital dental services, public health dental clinics, and private practices using a modification of Weed's problem-oriented record system, the problem-oriented dental record system is proving that it has more advantages than other conventional dental record systems and is an invaluable tool in dental education and dental practice.

REFERENCES

1. Berg, G. R.: Personal communication, Salt Lake City, Recordofax, Inc., 1977.
2. Bjorn, J. C., and Cross, H. D.: Problem-oriented practice, Chicago, 1970, Modern Hospital Press, McGraw-Hill, Inc.
3. Boone II, M. E., and Sanger, R. G.: Problem-oriented dental record manual, Denver, 1977, University of Colorado Medical Center Press.
4. Coleman, H. L.: The problem-oriented dental record, J. Calif. Dent. Assoc. 4(2):51-54, 1976.
5. Hurst, J. W., and Walker, H. K.: The problem-oriented system, New York, 1972, Medcom Press, Inc.
6. Ingber, J. S., and Rose, L. F.: The problem-oriented record: clinical application in a teaching hospital, J. Dent. Educ. 29(7):472-482, 1975.
7. Ingber, J. S., and Rose, L. F.: The problem-oriented system, Dent. Clin. North Am. 19(4): 703-715, 1975.
8. Pfifferling, J. H.: The problem-oriented medical record—a source bibliography, Togus, Me., 1974, Veterans Administration Center Press.
9. Tryon, A. F., Mann, W. V., and DeJong, N.: Use of a problem-oriented dental record in undergraduate dental education, J. Dent. Educ. 40(9):601-608, 1976.
10. Weed, L. L.: Medical records, medical education, and patient care: the problem-oriented record as a basic tool, Cleveland, 1969, Case Western Reserve University Press.
11. Weed, L. L.: Medical records that guide and teach, N. Engl. J. Med. 278:593-599 and 652-657, 1968.

20

Problem-oriented record system—case example

Malcolm E. Boone II
Roger G. Sanger

The previous chapters on the problem-oriented record system and treatment sequencing have explained the theoretical aspects of the problem-oriented record system and treatment sequencing. In this chapter the case of a patient presenting with relatively simple dental health care problems or needs will be utilized for the purpose of illustrating the problem-oriented record system.

The administration of the patient background data base and health questionnaire (Forms 1 and 2) must be completed as soon as possible and may be done in one of the following ways:
1. While the patient's roentgenograms are being processed
2. Can be mailed to the patient after explaining by telephone that it should be completed and brought to the first appointment
3. Have the patient arrive for his first appointment early enough so he will have ample time to complete the health questionnaire prior to seeing the dentist

DATA COLLECTION
Health questionnaire

The first procedure to complete in a thorough patient workup is the patient background data base (Form 1). Upon reviewing the health questionnaire (Form 2), it was found that James was a 19-year-old student. Responses to the health questionnaire included:
1. Have you ever been seriously ill? *Yes*
2. Have you ever been hospitalized? *Yes*
3. Have you ever had surgery (an operation)? *Yes*
4. Have you ever had any of the following:
    a. Measles? *Yes*
    b. Chickenpox? *Yes*

Text continued on p. 340.

PATIENT BACKGROUND DATA BASE

Name of patient
Jones   James   —
LAST   FIRST   MIDDLE

Birthdate
4-3-59

Social security number
XO-1-77

Address
4200 ABCD Ninth Avenue   Denver   80262
STREET   CITY   (ZIP)

Telephone number (if no phone, neighbor's phone)
306-4781

Occupation (if patient is child, give occupation of parent)
Student

Employer's phone
—

Employer's name and address
—
NAME   STREET   CITY   (ZIP)

Yearly family income
$10,000

Spouse's occupation (if patient is child, father [x] or mother [ ])

Employer's name and address
Univ. of Colorado Medical Center
4200 East Ninth Avenue, Denver 80262
NAME   STREET   CITY   (ZIP)

Employer's phone
306-5211

Name of person to contact in emergency
Jones   William   —   Father
LAST   FIRST   MIDDLE   RELATIONSHIP

Home phone
306-4781

Business phone
306-5211

Name of person financially responsible
Jones   William   —   Father
LAST   FIRST   MIDDLE   RELATIONSHIP

Name of dental insurance

Policy number

Other financial plan (Check one or more)
[ ] Bank Americard # _____   [ ] Master Charge # _____
[x] Cash   [ ] Check   [ ] Other _____

Continued.

Form 1

SOCIAL-FAMILY DATA

Person to contact in case of emergency

William Jones	_306-4781_	_306-5211_
NAME	HOME TELEPHONE NO.	WORK TELEPHONE NO.

Please check the appropriate response to the following questions:

1. What is your current marital status?
   _x_ Single   __ Married   __ Separated   __ Divorced   __ Widowed
2. Do you fear receiving dental care?
   _x_ Not at all afraid   __ Somewhat afraid   __ Very much afraid
3. How often have you delayed going to the dentist because you expected pain or discomfort?
   _x_ Never   __ Occasionally   __ Frequently
4. How often have you had an unpleasant experience in a dental office?
   _x_ Never   __ Occasionally   __ Frequently
5. When you go to the dentist, what kind of experience do you generally expect?
   __ Good   _x_ Indifferent   __ Unpleasant
6. How satisfied have you been with your dentist(s)?
   _x_ Satisfied   __ Indifferent   __ Unsatisfied
7. How important to you is the way your teeth look?
   _x_ Very important   __ Somewhat important   __ Unimportant
8. Do you think that your oral health is important to your general health?
   __ Very important   _x_ Somewhat important   __ Unimportant
9. How concerned are you about the way your teeth and jaw affect your general facial appearance?
   _x_ Very concerned   __ Somewhat concerned   __ Unconcerned

Please write the answers to the following questions:
10. How many years of school have you completed? ____10____
11. How many people live in your household? ____4____
12. If any of these people have special health problems, please identify the person(s) and the problem(s): _____

13. Who is your physician or clinic?

Medical "B"	_4200 E. 9th Ave., Denver_	_306-8207_
NAME	ADDRESS	TELEPHONE NO.

Form 1, cont'd

HEALTH QUESTIONNAIRE

Answers to these questions will aid your dentist in your proper treatment. They will be considered confidential. Please check the appropriate response.

1. Have you ever had any of the following diseases or conditions?

Jaundice (yellow skin and eyes) ○ Yes ● No	Diabetes (sugar disease)	○ Yes ● No
Hepatitis ○ Yes ● No	Measles	● Yes ○ No
Tuberculosis ○ Yes ● No	Chickenpox	● Yes ○ No
Venereal disease ● Yes ○ No	Mumps	● Yes ○ No
Heart attack ○ Yes ● No	Polio	○ Yes ● No
Congenital heart lesions ○ Yes ● No	Rheumatic fever	○ Yes ● No
Stroke ○ Yes ● No	Scarlet fever	○ Yes ● No
Ulcers ○ Yes ● No	Arthritis	○ Yes ● No
Epilepsy ○ Yes ● No	Glaucoma	○ Yes ● No
Emphysema ○ Yes ● No		

2. Have you ever experienced an unusual reaction to any of the following drugs?

Penicillin ○ Yes ● No	Iodine	○ Yes ● No
Barbiturates (sleeping pills) ○ Yes ● No	Sulfa drugs	○ Yes ● No
Aspirin ○ Yes ● No	Other	○ Yes ● No

3. Have you ever had:

Extractions (Oral surgery)	○ Yes ● No
Root canals (Endodontics)	○ Yes ● No
Fillings (Operative)	● Yes ○ No
Missing teeth replaced (Prosthodontics)	○ Yes ● No
Teeth straightened (Orthodontics)	○ Yes ● No
Gum surgery (Periodontics)	○ Yes ● No

4. Have you been examined by your physician within the last year? ● Yes ○ No
5. Are you now being treated for any condition by a physician? ○ Yes ● No
6. Have you been taking any medications within the past year? ○ Yes ● No
7. Has there been any change in your general health during the last year? ○ Yes ● No
8. Have you lost or gained weight in recent months? ○ Yes ● No
9. Have you ever been seriously ill? ● Yes ○ No
10. Have you ever been hospitalized? ● Yes ○ No
11. Have you ever had surgery (an operation)? ● Yes ○ No
12. Have you ever had a blood transfusion? ○ Yes ● No
13. Have you ever been treated for a growth or tumor in any part of your body? ○ Yes ● No
14. Are you frequently ill? ○ Yes ● No
15. Do you often feel exhausted or fatigued? ○ Yes ● No
16. As a child, did you have growing pains? ○ Yes ● No
17. Have you ever had painful or swollen joints? ○ Yes ● No
18. Have you ever been told by a physician you have a heart murmur? ○ Yes ● No
19. Have you ever had any heart trouble? ○ Yes ● No
20. Do you have high blood pressure? ○ Yes ● No
21. Do you bleed for a long time when you cut yourself? ○ Yes ● No
22. Do you bruise easily? ○ Yes ● No
23. Do you have a blood disorder? ○ Yes ● No
24. Do you have any chest pain on exertion? ○ Yes ● No
25. Are you ever short of breath on mild exertion? ○ Yes ● No
26. Do your ankles ever swell? ○ Yes ● No
27. Do you have a pacemaker? ○ Yes ● No
28. Do you wear contact lenses? ○ Yes ● No

Continued.

HEALTH QUESTIONNAIRE—cont'd

29. Do you have a persistent cough?   ○ Yes   ● No
30. Do you ever have asthma?   ○ Yes   ● No
31. Do you ever have hay fever?   ● Yes   ○ No
32. Do you have any allergies (to drugs, food, animal fur, dust, etc.)?   ○ Yes   ● No
33. Do you ever have hives or skin rash?   ○ Yes   ● No
34. Have you ever experienced an unusual reaction to a dental anesthetic (e.g., Novocaine injection)?   ○ Yes   ● No
35. Do you smoke regularly?   ○ Yes   ● No
36. Do you regularly drink coffee or tea?   ○ Yes   ● No
37. Do you often have to get up at night to urinate?   ○ Yes   ● No
38. During the day, do you usually have to urinate frequently?   ○ Yes   ● No
39. Are you thirsty most of the time?   ○ Yes   ● No
40. Have you had kidney or bladder disease or infection?   ● Yes   ○ No
41. Has a doctor ever said you had a liver disease?   ○ Yes   ● No
42. Do you have any numbness or tingling in any part of your body?   ○ Yes   ● No
43. Has any part of your body ever been paralyzed?   ○ Yes   ● No
44. Do you ever have seizures or convulsions?   ○ Yes   ● No
45. Do you ever faint?   ○ Yes   ● No
46. Do you have frequent, severe headaches?   ○ Yes   ● No
47. Do you consider yourself to be a nervous person?   ○ Yes   ● No
48. Do you often feel unhappy and depressed?   ○ Yes   ● No
49. Do you often cry?   ○ Yes   ● No
50. Are you easily upset or irritated?   ○ Yes   ● No
51. Have there been any major diseases or deformities in your family?   ○ Yes   ● No
52. Do you have difficulty in chewing your food?   ○ Yes   ● No
53. Do you have sensitive teeth?   ○ Yes   ● No
54. Do you have bleeding gums?   ○ Yes   ● No
55. Have you noticed any loosening of your teeth recently?   ○ Yes   ● No
56. Have you ever had slow-healing sores in the mouth or on the lips?   ○ Yes   ● No
57. Do you have difficulty in opening your mouth wide?   ○ Yes   ● No
58. Do your jaws "pop" or "click" when opening wide?   ○ Yes   ● No
59. Have you ever had sinus trouble?   ○ Yes   ● No
60. Have you ever had any injury to your face, jaws, or teeth?   ○ Yes   ● No
61. Do you clench or grind your teeth while awake or asleep?   ○ Yes   ● No
62. Do you bite your lips or cheeks regularly?   ○ Yes   ● No
63. Do you bite objects with your teeth (pencils, pins, pipe, nails, etc.)?   ○ Yes   ● No
64. Do you breathe through your mouth while awake or asleep?   ○ Yes   ● No
65. Women—Are you pregnant at the present time?   ○ Yes   ○ No
66. Women—Are you menstruating regularly?   ○ Yes   ○ No
67. Women—Have you had a hysterectomy (uterus removed) or ovariectomy (ovary removed)?   ○ Yes   ○ No
68. How do you describe your general health?   *Very good.*

Form 2, cont'd

HEALTH QUESTIONNAIRE—cont'd

1. Why did you seek dental care at this office? If you were referred by another dentist, please give the dentist's name and address.

   I am new in town and this office was mentioned by another student.

2. Explain the symptoms or complaints which cause you to seek dental health care.

   Painful tooth and need general check-up for sports.

3. Please list all medications (drugs) which you have taken in the last 6 months.

   None

James Jones   9-26-77
PATIENT SIGNATURE   DATE

Patient resumé (to be completed by dentist)

James is a 19-year-old Caucasian male college student with a negative social-family history and a positive health history for seasonal hay fever and venereal disease (1½ years ago). His chief complaint is a painful tooth and in addition he desires a general dental examination.

Hospitalizations
    Meningitis, age 2 (1961), no complications.
    Bladder infection, age 4 (1963), no complications.
Surgeries
    Hand surgery, age 10 (1967), no bleeding, anesthesia, or drug complications.
Present medications
    None
Allergies
    None
Medical alert
    Venereal disease

Malcom E. Boone D.D.S.   10-5-77
DENTIST'S SIGNATURE   DATE

Form 2, cont'd

340   Records

   c. Mumps? *Yes*
   d. Venereal disease? *Yes*
 5. Chief complaint: *Has a painful tooth and needs a general check-up for sports.*
 6. Present medications: *None*

Patient interview

 After review of the information obtained in the health questionnaire, the dentist should interview the patient with special emphasis placed upon the positive responses obtained. Upon interviewing the patient, the dentist will hopefully discover that the patient experienced severe meningitis at age 2 for which he was hospitalized and successfully treated. Recovery was uneventful without any complications. James underwent successful hand surgery at age 10 and at present has no residual problems with his hand. He has had the childhood diseases. A past history of venereal disease was marked "yes" on the questionnaire. Further questioning revealed that he was treated for primary syphilis at age 17. James has suffered from previous bladder infections, which were treated with pencillin, and has seasonal bouts with hay fever.

 This information is quite complete; the problem is that most dentists fail to record these historical facts, attempting to keep them in their heads. As a result, problems develop because they find it hard to recall the important historical facts when needed.

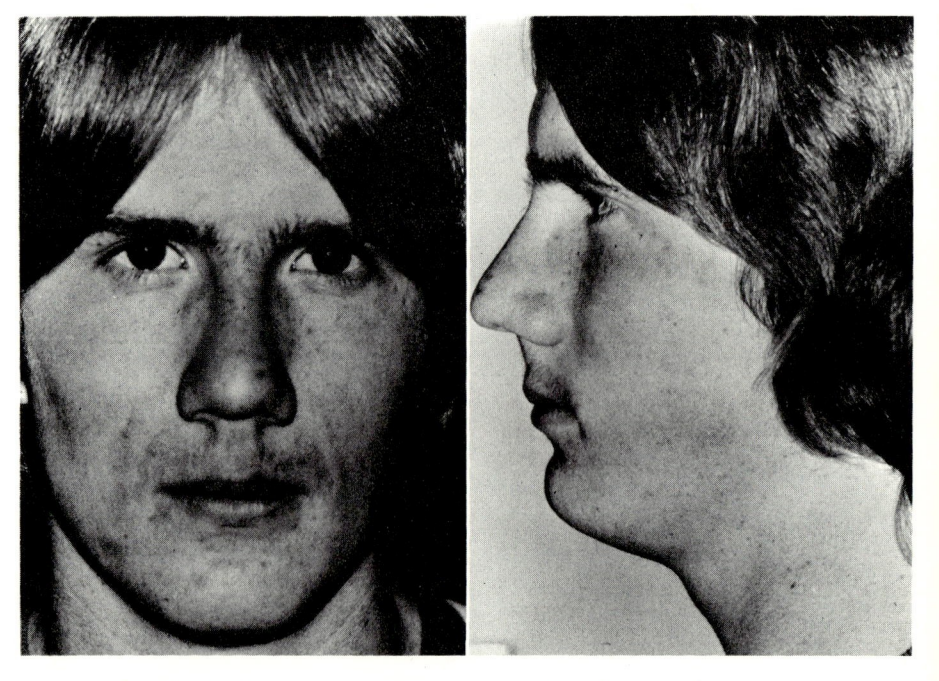

Fig. 20-1. Patient is a 19-year-old male college student.

Patient resumé

The *patient resumé* is the dentist's assimilation and translation of the data illicited from the patient via this objective-subjective interview. As well as serving as a reference summary for the dentist, it serves as a communications baseline when discussing this patient with other professions. The patient resumé for James was written as follows:

> James is a 19-year-old Caucasian male college student with a negative social-family history and a positive health history for seasonal hay fever and venereal disease (1½ years ago). His chief complaint is a painful tooth and in addition he desires a general dental examination.
>
> 1. Hospitalizations: meningitis, age 2 (1961), no complications. Bladder infection, age 4 (1963), no complications.
> 2. Surgeries: Hand surgery, age 10 (1969), no bleeding, anesthetic, or drug complications.
> 3. Present medications: None
> 4. Allergies: None
> 5. Medical alert: Venereal disease

With the increasing number of legal problems associated with the practice of dentistry, it is advisable to have a simple consent form that has been discussed with your legal counsel (see Form 3).

A full-mouth roentgenographic survey was accomplished using normal precautions to prevent exposure to unnecessary radiation (Figs. 20-2 to 20-4).

PATIENT CONSENT

I give permission for diagnosis and/or treatment in this dental office for myself or for the minor patient named below. In consideration of acceptance for diagnosis and/or treatment, I hereby release and forever discharge the dentists, agents, and employees of and from any claims of liability of any kind and nature arising out of dental services performed, or in any way connected with service or advice at this dental office. In regard to any and all claims by or on behalf of the minor patient named below, or by third parties arising out of diagnosis and/or treatment of the minor patient named below, I agree to release the above parties from all liability.

September 26, 1977
DATE

James Jones
PATIENT SIGNATURE

_____
SIGNATURE OF PATIENT'S AGENT

_____
RELATION TO PATIENT

_____
WITNESS

Form 3

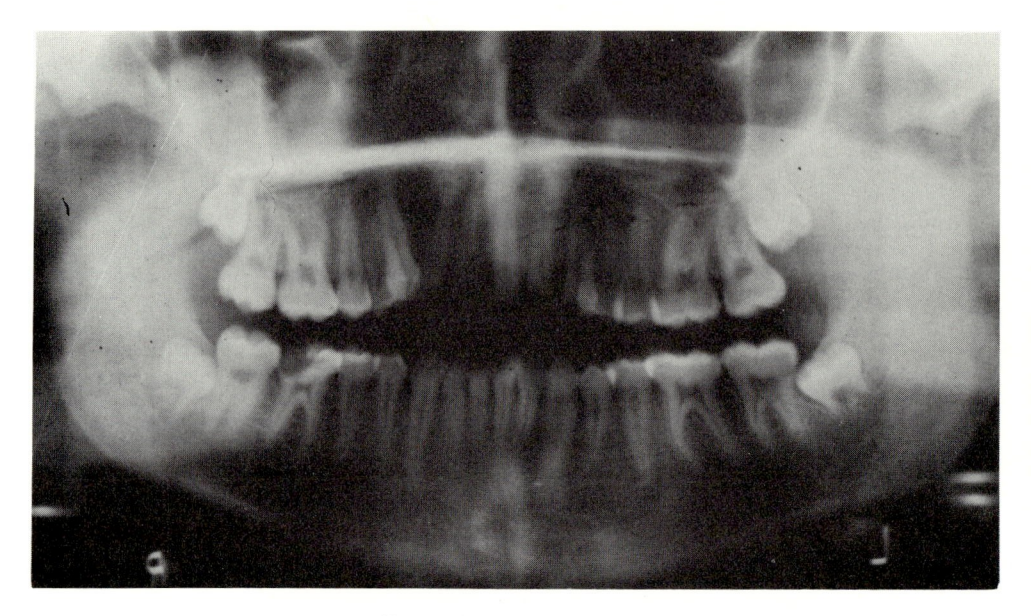

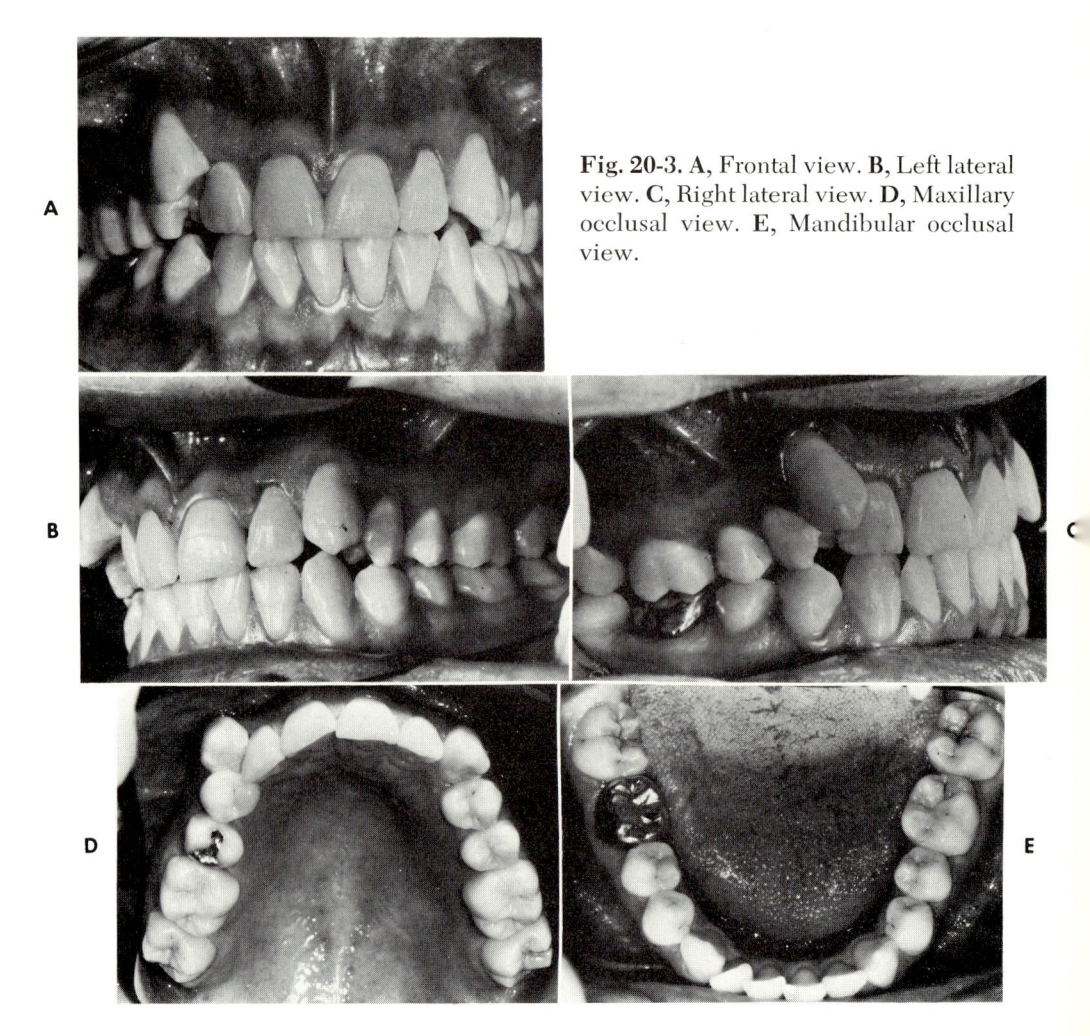

Fig. 20-2. Full-mouth panographic roentgenogram.

Fig. 20-3. A, Frontal view. **B,** Left lateral view. **C,** Right lateral view. **D,** Maxillary occlusal view. **E,** Mandibular occlusal view.

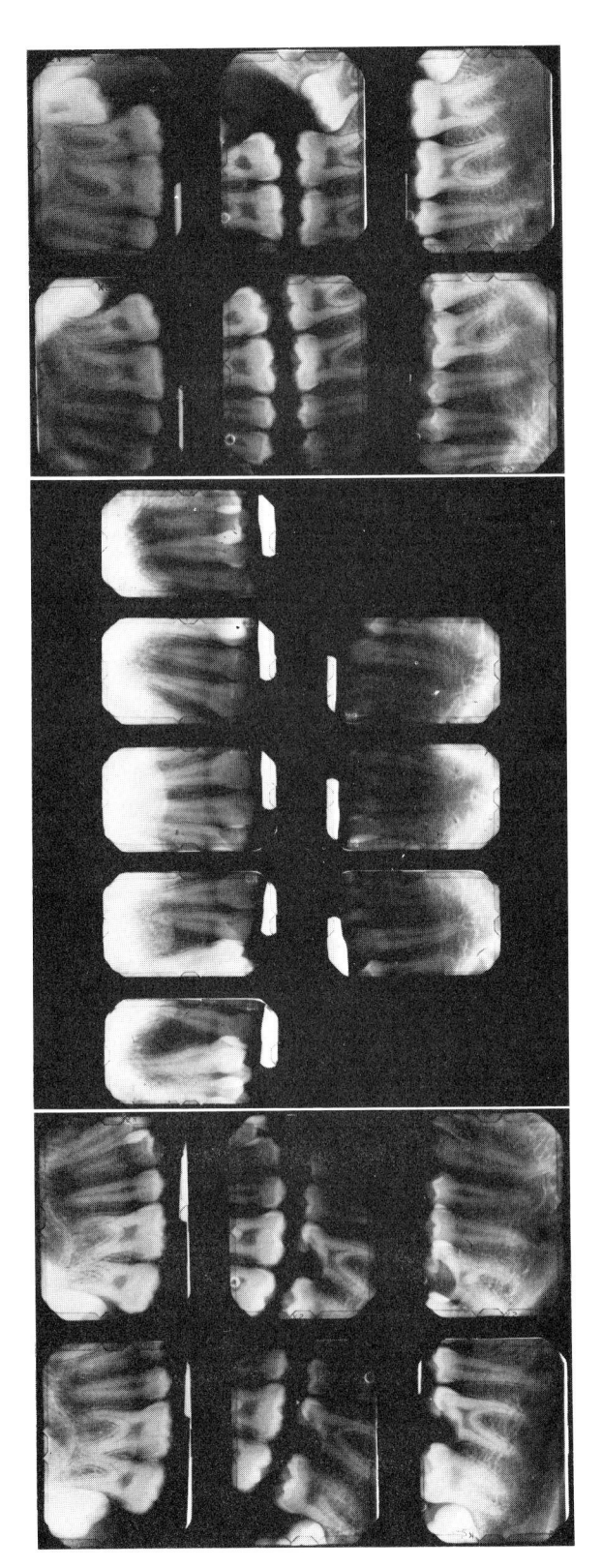

Fig. 20-4. Full-mouth roentgenograms.

Physical examination data base

The administration of the physical examination is done in the same manner as is described in current textbooks in the field of oral diagnosis and oral medicine, using the techniques of visualization, palpation, percussion, probing, and so on. An examination form is used that acts as a guide to help ensure that the dentist does not overlook any areas in the examination, and also so that a logical and systematic method of patient examination will occur (see Form 4).

All areas are examined, noting either no problem or possible problem. Space is provided for writing or drawing if any pathology is noted. The dental charting (Fig. 20-5) is done on one standard sheet that incorporates the dental examination, periodontal examination, and occlusal examination findings. Above and below, the teeth are designated for pockets, present restorations, defective restorations, carious lesions, and the planned restoration, with an area for comments. Standard symbols are used in these spaces, that is, red for

Text continued on p. 350.

PATIENT PHYSICAL-PHYSIOLOGIC-LABORATORY DATA BASE

	No problem	Possible problem		No problem	Possible problem
1. Review of systems					
Systems review	●	○			
2. Physical examination-laboratory tests					
General			*Eyes*		
Physical status ____	●	○	Position	●	○
_____			Pupils	●	○
B.P. _120/80_	●	○	Sclera	●	○
Pulse _80_	●	○	Cornea	●	○
Resp. _20_	●	○	Lids	●	○
Temp. _98.6_	●	○	Conjunctiva	●	○
RBC _____	○	○	Musculature	●	○
CBC _____	○	○	Vision	●	○
Glucose _____	○	○	Orbital margins	●	○
Serology _VDRL_	●	○	*Nose*		
Hematocrit _____	○	○	Nasal bridge	●	○
Skin			Size, shape	●	○
Quality, texture, moisture	●	○	Septal deviation	●	○
			Discharge	●	○
Color, pigmentation	●	○	Turbinates, capacity	●	○
Eruptions, lesions	●	○	*Ears*		
Swellings	●	○	Position	●	○
Scalp, hair			Morphology	●	○
Distribution, amount, texture	●	○	Developmental abnormalities	●	○
Nails			Hearing	●	○
Morphology	●	○			
Color	●	○			

Form 4

	No problem	Possible problem		No problem	Possible problem
2. Physical examination—cont'd.			*Lips*		
Head, facies			Position (at rest)	●	○
Irregularities, asymmetry	●	○	Position (in function)	●	○
			Moisture, texture, color	●	○
Skeletal	●	○	Lesions, swellings	●	○
Musculature	●	○	Developmental abnormalities	●	○
Neck					
Nodes	●	○	Mentalis area	●	○
Swellings, masses	●	○	Habits	●	○
Developmental abnormalities	●	○	Tonicity	●	○
			Thickness	●	○

Limitation, deviation, or discomfort in mandibular excursions:

Opening ○   Left ○   Protrusive ○
Closure ○   Right ○   Retrusive ○

Muscle pain   Right ○   Left ○   (circle muscles)
Muscle tenderness Right ○   Left ○   (circle muscles)
 R/L Masseter   R/L Digastric   R/L Temporalis
 R/L Med. Pterygoid R/L Trapezius
 R/L Lat. Pterygoid R/L S.C.M.   ● ○
TMJ pain   Right ○   Static ○   Excursions ○   ● ○
           Left ○   Static ○   Excursions ○   ● ○
TMJ sounds   Right ○   Left ○   ● ○

3. Roentgenographic examination

	No problem	Possible problem		No problem	Possible problem
Maxillary sinuses	●	○	Dentition		
Mandibular rami	●	○	Tooth number	●	○
TMJ	●	○	Ankyloses/impacted	●	○
Bone pattern	●	○	Tooth morphology	●	○
Radiolucencies	●	○	Crown:root ratio	●	○
Alveolar bone height	●	○	Pulpal therapy	○	●
			Pulpal morphology	●	○
PDL width	●	○	Pulpal abnormalities	●	○
Furcation involvement	●	○	Defective restorations	●	○
			Carious/hypoplasia	○	●
Radiopacities	●	○	Dental eruption	○	●

4. Intraoral examination

	No problem	Possible problem		No problem	Possible problem
Breath	●	○	Buccal mucosa		
Swallow, deglutition	●	○	Color, pigmentation	●	○
Tongue			Eruptions, lesions	●	○
Position (at rest)	●	○	Palate		
Position (swallow)	●	○	Morphology	●	○
Morphology, developmental abnorm.	●	○	Developmental abnormalities	●	○
			Color, pigmentation	●	○
Eruptions, lesions	●	○	Eruptions, lesions	●	○
Color, pigmentation	●	○	Functions	●	○
Floor of mouth			Pharyngeal area		
Color, pigmentation	●	○	Color, pigmentation	●	○
			Eruptions, lesions	●	○
Eruptions, lesions	●	○	Functions	●	○
			Tonsillar morphology	●	○
Frenums, muscle attachments	●	○	Gag reflex	●	○
			Salivary glands and function	●	○
			Saliva consistency	●	○

Form 4, cont'd

Continued.

PATIENT PHYSICAL-PHYSIOLOGIC-LABORATORY DATA BASE—cont'd

	No problem	Possible problem		No problem	Possible problem
Vestibules					
Color, pigmentation	●	○			
Eruptions, lesions	●	○			
Frenums	●	○			

5. Periodontal examination (Record on dental chart)

Pocket depth	●	○	Characterize the gingival unit:		
Mobility	●	○	Form, color, tone, texture is:		
Gingival recession	●	○	Physiologic _____	●	○
Furcations	●	○	Pathologic _____	●	○
Frenum attachments affecting gingival margins	●	○	Quantity of plaque: Hy ○ Md ● Lt ○	○	○
			Quantity of calculus: Hy ○ Md ○ Lt ●	○	○
Lack of attached gingiva	●	○	Bleeding on probing	○	●
			Fibrosis	●	○

6. Dental examination (Record on dental chart)

Missing/extra teeth	●	○	Diastemas, rotations contacts, etc.	○	●
Caries, hypoplasia	○	●			
Defective restorations	●	○	Tooth discoloration	●	○

7. Pulpal status (Date as recorded)

Tooth no.	History	Cold	Heat	EPT	Percussion	Palpation		
	+ −	N AB NR	N AB NR	NO NR	+ −	+ −		
	○ ○	○ ○ ○	○ ○ ○	○	○ ○	○ ○	○	○
	○ ○	○ ○ ○	○ ○ ○	○	○ ○	○ ○	○	○
	○ ○	○ ○ ○	○ ○ ○	○	○ ○	○ ○	○	○
	○ ○	○ ○ ○	○ ○ ○	○	○ ○	○ ○	○	○
	○ ○	○ ○ ○	○ ○ ○	○	○ ○	○ ○	○	○
	○ ○	○ ○ ○	○ ○ ○	○	○ ○	○ ○	○	○

8. Pathology status

In the diagrams on the opposite page, outline all existing pathosis in red with attention to the extent of possible lesions.

Findings: _____

_____

_____

Impressions: _____

_____

Form 4, cont'd

Right   Left

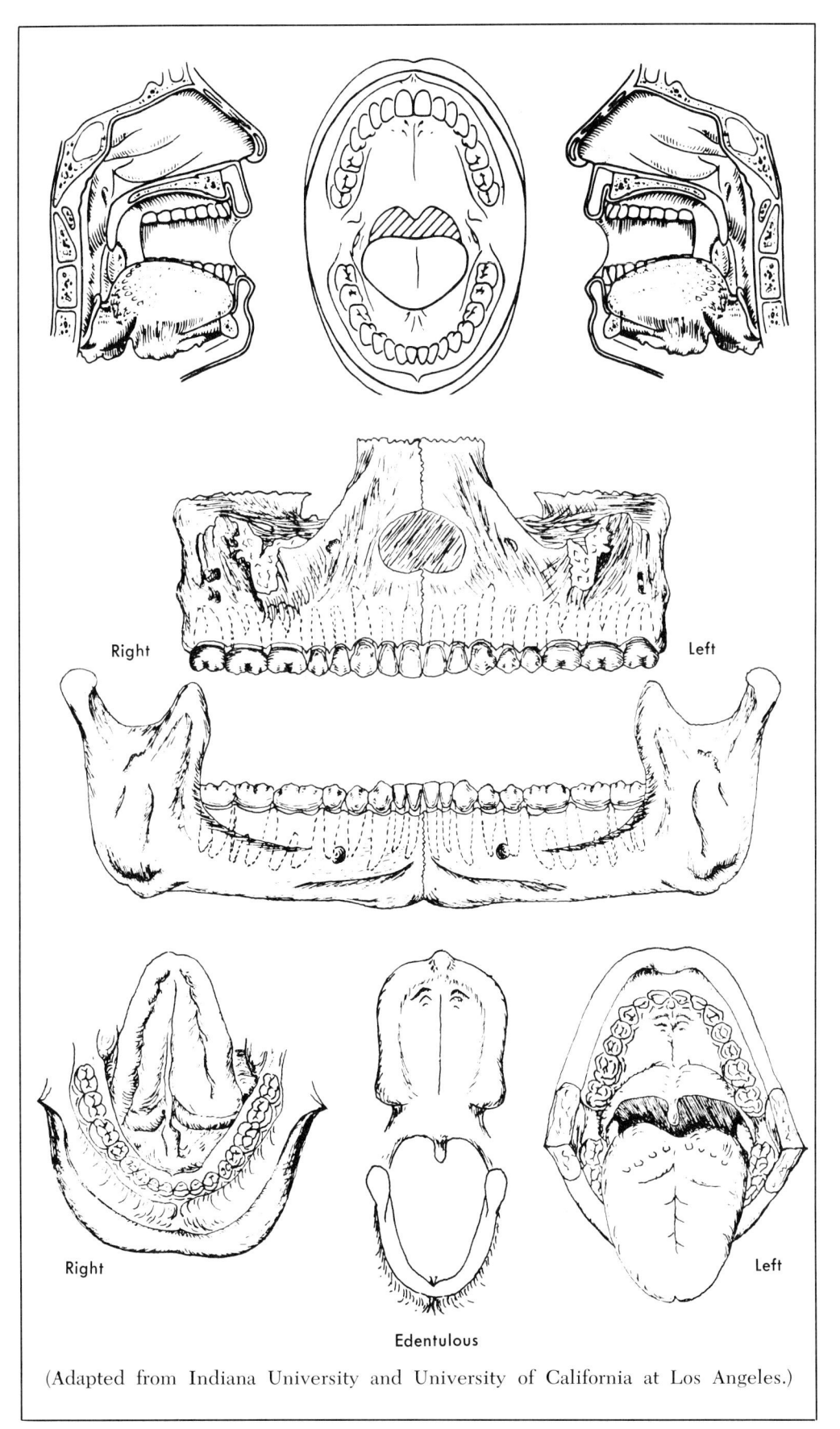

Right   Left

Edentulous

(Adapted from Indiana University and University of California at Los Angeles.)

PATIENT PHYSICAL-PHYSIOLOGIC-LABORATORY DATA BASE—cont'd

	No problem	Possible problem		No problem	Possible problem
9. Occlusal examination			*Malocclusion assessment*		
(Record on dental chart)			Molar class ○ 1 ● 2 ○ 3	●	○
			Overbite (or 1 + 2 mm)	●	○
Wear	●	○	Overjet (or 1 + 2 mm)	●	○
Mobility	●	○	Arch length	○	●
Fremitis	●	○	(2mm crowding)		
Centric relation discrepancy	●	○			
10. If patient is edentulous or requires prosthetic therapy:					
Ridge relationship ○ 1 ○ 2 ○ 3					
Throat form (soft palate) ○ 1 ○ 2 ○ 3					
Lateral throat form ○ 1 ○ 2 ○ 3					
Ridge form ○ Round ○ Thin ○ Flat				○	○
Tuberosities ○ Unsuitable ○ Suitable ○ Needs surgery				○	○
Vault form ○ Square ○ Flat ○ Arched ○ Tapering				○	○
Interarch distance				○	○
Tissue condition				○	○
Mental attitude				○	○
Previous denture history					
Subjective					
More than three dentures in last 2 years				○	○
More than 3 years since last dentures made				○	○
Dentures last relined more than 3 years ago				○	○
No dentures ever worn				○	○
Existing dentures					
Appearance				○	○
Speech				○	○
Masticatory ability				○	○
Vertical dimension				○	○
Broken dentures				○	○
Comfort of soft tissue				○	○
Comfort of abutments (partial dentures only)				○	○
Objective					
Existing dentures					
Aesthetics				○	○
Phonetics				○	○
Vertical dimension				○	○
Centric occlusion				○	○
Retention				○	○
Stability				○	○
Excursive occlusion				○	○
Tissue adaptation				○	○
Border extension				○	○

Form 4, cont'd

Problem-oriented record system—case example

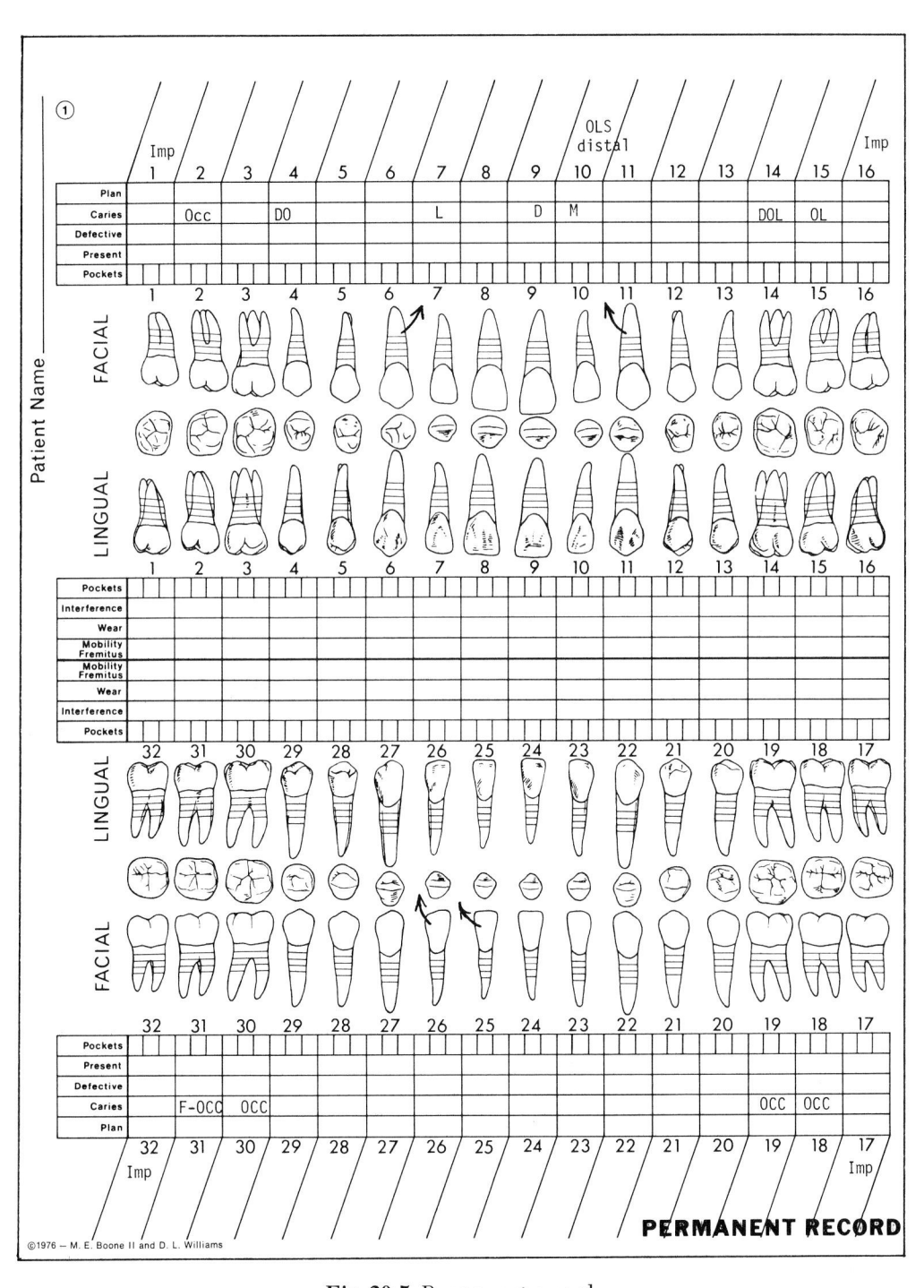

Fig. 20-5. Permanent record.

caries, blue for present restorations, blue line to bone level, red line to gingival level, and so on.

PROBLEM IDENTIFICATION

After all physical examination data has been collected, the next logical step is to assimilate all of the patient's problems (caries, pain, rheumatic fever, and so on) and organize these problems into a list of complete problems (Form 5),

COMPLETE PROBLEM LIST

Patient *James Jones*

Synthesize the *data base* into a complete list of numbered and titled problems. Judgment must be exercised, since each numbered and titled problem will require a correspondingly numbered and titled *plan* for its resolution. Ideal formulation of this list will synthesize the greatest number of possible problems from the *data base* into a minimum number of titled problems. Inactive or resolved problems must be signed and dated by the dentists. To reactivate a problem, simply make a new entry on this list, using the previous numbered title, but include a current date. New problems should reflect changes in the data base and must be assigned a number and title as they occur.

Problem no.	Active problem	Date entered/sig.	Problem resolved	Date resolved/sig.
1	Medical–venereal disease	10-26-77		
2	Periodontal plaque, gingival bleeding	10-26-77		
3	Pulpal pain – #30	10-26-77		
4	Dental caries	10-26-77		
5	Occ/Ortho – teeth 6 and 11 rotation	10-26-77		
6	Surg – impacted teeth 1, 16, 17, 32	10-26-77		

Form 5

not recognizing that a patient has 20 or 30 problems, but rather identifying problems related to a system, that is, medical, dental, pulpal, and so on. If all the patient's problems are listed, the result is a list of treatment to be rendered, not a list of the problems. Therefore we have derived a systems approach to problem identification, as illustrated below. All problems must be listed by systems as follows: After each problem is resolved, an arrow is drawn

Problem	Active problem	Date entered	Resolved	Date
1	Perio	9-26-76	→	10-10-76

to indicate the resolution and it is dated. Each time a new problem is discovered, it is added to the complete problem list. This procedure allows the dentist to note that problems have not been solved if they keep recurring on the problem list.

DIAGNOSTIC AND THERAPEUTIC PLANS (FORM 6)

After the data collection and problem identification has been accomplished, it is imperative that each of the identified problems from the *complete problem list* have a numbered and titled plan. Each plan should include (1) the *goal* of treatment, that is, elimination of plaque and gingival bleeding, (2) *diagnosis* (Dx) of gingivitis, (3) *therapy*—prophylaxis, and (4) *patient education plan* (Pt. ed. plan), that is, oral hygiene instruction.

DIAGNOSTIC AND THERAPEUTIC PLANS

Each plan will refer to a numbered and titled problem. Each plan will consist of *goals of treatment*. *Diagnostic* criteria logically sequences what is necessary to complete a differential diagnosis. *Therapeutic* plans, with means to achieve them, must be clearly stated. *Patient education plan* includes instructions, limitation of treatment, and prognosis for this problem.

Patient name _____

Problem no.	Title	Seq.	Plan	Additional data
1	Medical	1	Goal: Determine nature of positive history of venereal disease	VDRL
			Dx: —	
			Tx: As indicated by test results and medical consultation	
			Pt. ed. plan: Advise of reasons for VDRL and medical consult	

Form 6

Continued.

DIAGNOSTIC AND THERAPEUTIC PLANS—cont'd

Problem no.	Title	Seq.	Plan	Additional data
2	Perio	3	Goal: Elimination of plaque and gingival bleeding	
			Dx: Gingivitis	
			Tx: Prophylaxis	
			Pt. ed. plan: Oral hygiene instruction	
3	Pulpal	2	Goal: Eliminate pain #30	
			Dx: Pulpitis	
			Tx: Root canal therapy #30	
			Pt. ed. plan: Success, failure rates, and prognosis of tooth	
4	Dental	6	Goal: Remove disease from teeth (caries)	
			Dx: Caries	
			Tx: Restore as indicated	
			Pt. ed. plan:	
5	Occ/ortho	4	Goal: Eliminate rotation of #6 and #11 and accomplish an adequate occlusal relationship	
			Dx: Pending orthodontic evaluation	Referral
			Tx: Pending orthodontic evaluation	
			Pt. ed. plan: Need for orthodontic evaluation	
6	Surg	5	Goal: Evaluation of #1, 16, 17, 32 as to prognosis	
			Dx:	
			Tx:	
			Pt. ed. plan: Need for evaluation by oral surgeon	

Form 6

MASTER TREATMENT PLAN

Format:
1. List in sequence of planned treatment
2. List each procedure separately
3. Start and completion dates *must be* inserted and agree with treatment progress notes

Date ___/___/___   Total estimated fee _____   Name _James Jones_

Line no.	Prob. no.	Div.	Proced. no.	Tooth no.	Procedure (Use ink or type)	Fee	Start date	Comp. date
1	1				VDRL medical consult			
2					Full-mouth roentgenograms			
3					Panorex			
4					Examination			
5	5				Diagnostic study models			
6	5				Cephalometric survey			
7	3	Endo		30	Start endodontic therapy			
8	2	Perio			Prophylaxis			
9	5	Ortho			Orthodontic consult (Tx as needed)			
10	6				Surgery consult (Tx as needed)			
11								
12	3	Endo		30	Complete endodontic therapy			
13	4	Oper	7011	2	Occ amalgam			
14	4	Oper	7025	4	DO inlay			
15	4	Oper	7011	7	L amalgam			
16	4	Oper	7021	9	D composite			
17	4	Oper	7021	10	M composite			
18	4	Oper	7015	14	D-O-L amalgam			
19	4	Oper	7011	15	Occ—Ling amalgam			
20	4	Oper	7011	18	Occ amalgam			
21	4	Oper	7011	19	Occ amalgam			
22	4	Oper	7051	30	7/8 gold crown			
23	4	Oper	7011	31	F—Occ amalgam			

I give permission for diagnosis and/or treatment in this dental office for myself or for the minor patient named below. In consideration of acceptance for diagnosis and/or treatment, I hereby release and forever discharge the dentists, agents, or employees of and from any claims of liability of any kind and nature arising out of dental services performed, or in any way connected with service or advice at this dental office. In regard to any and all claims by or on behalf of the minor patient named below, or by third parties arising out of diagnosis and/or treatment of the minor patient named below, I agree to release the above parties from all liability.

_____   _____   _____
DATE   PATIENT SIGNATURE   SIGNATURE OF PATIENT'S AGENT

                    _____   _____
                    RELATION TO PATIENT WITNESS

Form 7

After establishment of a plan for each of the identified problems, a discussion of the problems and plans with your patient is desired. The actual treatment plan (Form 7) for the patient may be arrived at after discussion of the suggested plans or after urgent care has been accomplished.

TREATMENT PROGRESS NOTES

Each person has his or her own way of making entries in progress notes (Form 8). This is an acceptable procedure in your own private practice as long

TREATMENT PROGRESS NOTES

Include in procedure box areas and/or surfaces, restorative material, anesthetic, and other pertinent information, using the SOAP format. Each entry must be complete and have signature of dentist

Patient _James Jones_

Date	TP Line no.	Prob. no.	Area	Proced. no.	Tooth no.	Procedure	Dentist	Fee	Pay.	Bal.
2/16/75	—	—	Rad			4 BW's, pano, screening	Boone	$5	$5	$0
5/10/76	—	—	Diag			PBDB, PEDB	Boone	$9	$9	$0
6/8/76	—	—	Diag			Pt failed	Boone	—	—	—

Form 8

as you never leave the office or anyone else must read your record. That should not be the case for the problem-oriented record system concept. We must use a standard format that anyone could interpret. Therefore a suggested format is as follows:

The treatment progress notes are the legal entry for every patient contact. Entries will include the date, treatment plan line number, problem number, area, procedure number, tooth number, procedure (using the SOAP* format where possible), dentist signature, and fee. The payment and balance columns will be recorded by the payment clerk.

The following abbreviations are suggested:

Prep = Preparation	R = Right
Ins = Inserted	L = Left
Anes = Anesthetic	Con = Consultation
V = Varnish	Pt = Patient
Dy = Dycal	DDx = Differential diagnosis
Imp = Impression	Dx = Diagnosis
Zoe = Zinc oxide and eugenol	Fx = Fracture
$\bar{c}$ = with	Rem = Remove
c = cement	RCT = Root canal therapy
SSC = Stainless-steel crown	FC = Formocreasol
Rx = Prescription	

SUMMARY

The simple case has been presented using the problem-oriented dental record as an alternative to the more traditional treatment-oriented dental record.

In the future, with increasing consumer awareness, peer review, and quality assessment implications, the use of the problem-oriented record system can be of enormous value. Within the problem-oriented record system one can derive a wealth of statistical data. Some uses of this data might be:

1. Descriptions of practice profiles
2. Incidence of problems seen in patients
3. Profile of problems and plans related to long-term prognosis

Implementation of a problem-oriented record system in your practice, clinic, or dental school can only enhance the health care delivery system.

---

*S = subjective reactions or feelings of the patient toward the situation or treatment; O = objective statement of procedures attempted; A = assessment as to changes in diagnosis; P = plan for future treatment.

Index

A

Abortion, spontaneous, 59-60
Abutment designs, 259
Acetaminophen, 51, 62
Achlorhydria, 107
Acidosis
   lactic, 65
   respiratory, 97
   role in renal failure, 45, 47
Acids, role in dental caries, 156-157, 159
Acidulated phosphate fluoride (APF), 155, 156
Acrylics, 79, 162
ACTH, 53, 54
Acute necrotizing ulcerative gingivitis, 113, 121
Addison's disease, 52, 54, 55, 58
Adrenal glands
   disorders of, 52
   hyperfunction of, 83
   insufficiency of, secondary to chronic steroid administration, 52-59, 71
      dental treatment planning considerations, 57-59
      etiology, 52
      incidence and prevalence, 52-53
      medical management, 56-57
      pathophysiology, 53-55
      signs and symptoms, 55-56
Adult diabetes, 65, 66
Aerobic bacteria, role in dental caries, 156
Aesthetic appearance of dentition
   as consideration in fixed bridge work, 30, 31
   as consideration in full dentures, 33
   management of problems of, 183, 189
   normal, rehabilitation for, 184
   patient perceptions regarding, 147
   temporary management of, 187
   treatment to improve, case example, 250-256
Aged, treatment planning for, 175-176, 316
Agranulocytosis, 111
Air pollution, 94
Alcohol, 101, 153, 163
Aldosterone, 53-59
Alexidine mouthwash, 160
Alkaline phosphatase, 103

Alkylating agents, 110
Allergic rhinitis, 95
Allergies, role in periodontal disease, 163
Alopecia, 98
Aluminum hydroxide, 99
Amalgam restorations of teeth, 41
ϵ-Aminocaproic acid, 116
Aminophenazone, 111
Aminophylline, 84, 96, 97
Ammonia intoxication, 103
Amputations of roots, 40, 41, 274-276, 277, 278
   contraindications, 274, 276
   indications, 274
Anaerobic bacteria, role in dental caries, 156
Analgesics, 62, 66, 84, 85
Anaphylaxis, 185
Andrews bridges, 263, 279, 280
   contraindications, 279
   indications, 279
Androgens, 56
Anemia, 104-110, 113, 118, 121, 186
   of decreased erythrocyte production, 105, 107-108
   dental treatment planning considerations, 108-110
   hemolytic, 104-105
   related to loss of blood, 104
   role in renal failure, 45, 46, 47
Anesthetics, 62
Angina pectoris, 83-86, 185
   dental treatment planning considerations, 84-86
   medical management, 84
Angiotensin, 53
Anorexia, 55
Antacids, 98, 99
Antibiotics, 50, 62, 66, 91
Anticholinergics, 99, 100, 122
Antigen, Australia, 67
Antihistamines, 96
Antihypertensives, 82
Antilymphocyte globulin, use in suppression of kidney graft rejection, 49
Antimetabolites, 111, 118, 274

356

Antineoplastics, 111
Antiplatelet IgG, 113
Antistreptolysin O, 90
Aorta, coarctation of, 83, 93
APF gel, 126, 155, 156
Aplastic anemias, 107-108, 109-110
Arteriosclerosis, 45, 63
Arteriovenous shunt for hemodialysis, 48
　　dental treatment planning considerations for patients with, 50
Arthritis, 70-74
　　rheumatoid, 70-72
　　　　medical management, 71-72
Arthrocentesis, 116
Ascorbic acid, 158
Ascoxal, 158
Ascutal T, 158
Aspirin, 51, 62, 71, 73, 99, 115
Asthma, 52
　　hay fever and, 95-98
　　　　dental treatment planning considerations, 96-98
　　　　medical management, 96
Atmospheric irritants, role in periodontal disease, 163
Atrophic testes, 98
Atropine, 84, 97, 122
Australia antigen, 67
Autoimmune diseases, 53
Autoimmunogenic drugs, 113
Autonomic nervous system, effect of xerostomia on, 122-123
A-V shunt for hemodialysis, 48
　　dental treatment planning considerations for patients with, 50
Azathioprine, use in suppression of kidney graft rejection, 49
Azotemia, role in renal failure, 44, 45, 46, 47

B

Baby bottle syndrome, 158
Bacteremia, A-V shunt infection resulting from, 50
Bacteria
　　role in dental caries, 154, 156
　　role in gingivitis, 159-160
Bacterial activity in plaque, 156-158, 159-160
Bacterial endocarditis and rheumatic heart disease, 89-93
　　dental treatment planning considerations, 91-93
　　medical management, 91
Baker bar, 259
Banthine, 97
Bar bridges, 263, 279, 280
　　contraindications, 279
　　indications, 279
Barbiturates, 62, 84
Behavioral considerations in dental treatment planning, 131-150
　　dental interview, 132-140
　　developing treatment plan, 140-149
Benadryl, 109

Beta blocking agents, 84
Beta-thalassemia, 105, 106
Biliary cirrhosis, 101
Bilirubin, 68
Bilirubin cholelithiasis, 105
Blade implant, 270, 271, 272, 273
Bleeding following hemodialysis, 51
Bleeding disorders, 113-115
　　dental treatment planning considerations, 114-115
　　platelet deficits, 113, 114
　　thrombocytosis and functional disorders of platelets, 114-115
Blindness, 63
Blood, anemia related to loss of, 104
Blood creatinine test for renal function, 47, 49
Blood dyscrasias, role in periodontal disease, 163
Blood urea nitrogen (BUN) test for renal function, 47, 49
Bone and joint diseases, 70-75
　　arthritis, 70-74
　　joint prostheses, 72, 74-75
Bone marrow
　　effect of renal failure on, 45, 46
　　role in anemias, 104-108
Bony pathology, 19-20
Bony radiolucencies, 186
Bridges for tooth replacement; *see specific entries*
Bronchitis, chronic, 95
Bruxism, 21, 26, 35, 41, 188
"Buffalo hump," 56
BUN test for renal function, 47, 49

C

Calcium, 45, 47, 159
Calcium carbonate, 99
Calcium hydroxide, 162, 166
Calculus, 160, 163
Cancer; *see* Carcinoma
Candida albicans, 112
Candidiasis, 46, 50, 112, 120, 121, 128
Carbocaine, 62
Carbohydrate, role in dental caries, 155, 156, 157, 158-159
Carbon tetrachloride, 101
Carcinoma
　　oral, prevention of, 153
　　squamous cell, of oral cavity, 20
Cardiac decompensation, 86-89
Cardiac murmurs, 90, 91
Cardiac tamponade, 85
Cardiovalvular disease, 84
Cardiovascular disease, 267
　　oral hypoglycemics associated with, 65
Cardiovascular shunts in cyanotic and acyanotic anomalies, 93
Cardiovascular system, diseases of, 81-94
　　congenital heart disease, 93
　　congestive heart failure, 86-89
　　hypertension, 81-83
　　intracardiac prosthesis, 93-94

Cardiovascular system, diseases of—cont'd
  ischemic heart disease, 83-86
  rheumatic heart disease and bacterial endocarditis, 89-93
Caries, dental; *see* Dental caries
Carious lesions, 23
Case presentation in dental treatment planning, 3, 6, 282-295
Catecholamines, 82
Cavity liners, 162
Central nervous system, 123
Chemical irritants, role in periodontal disease, 163
Chemoprophylactic regimens for dental procedures involving upper respiratory tract, 92-93
Chemotherapy, use in suppression of kidney graft rejection, 49
Children
  chemoprophylactic regimen for dental procedures involving upper respiratory tract in, 92-93
  hematologic neoplasms in, 118-122
  preventive dental hygiene in, 157
Chlorambucil, 110
Chlorhexidine gluconate, 157
Chlorpromazine, 101
Chordae tendineae, 90
Christmas disease, 115, 116
Chronic bronchitis, 95
Cirrhosis of liver, 101-103
  biliary, 101
  dental treatment planning considerations, 103
  Laennec's, 101
  postnecrotic, 101
Classic hemophilia, 115-116
Cleft palate, nonrepaired, 24
Closed-ended questions as verbal communication, 136
Clubbing, digital, 101, 102
Coagulation disorders, 115-117
  acquired, 117
  dental treatment planning considerations, 117
  hemophilia A, 115-116
  hemophilia B, 116
  medical management, 116
  von Willebrand's disease, 116
Codeine, 51, 62
Collagen diseases, 53
Coma, diabetic, 185
Communal fluoridation, 155
Communication
  in case presentation, 290-294
  in dental interview, 136-140
Composite resin restorative materials, 41-42, 162
Condensing osteitis, 38, 39
Confrontation as verbal communication, 138-139
Congenital heart disease, 93
Congestive heart failure, 86-89, 193
  dental treatment planning considerations, 88-89
  medical management, 87-88
  role in renal failure, 47

Consent form, 341
Convulsion as late symptom of uremia, 46
Cooley's anemia, 105, 106
Coombs positive anemia, 104
Copalite, 162
Copper sulphate, 158
Cor pulmonale, 87, 95
Coronary artery atherosclerosis, 83
Coronary artery bypass surgery, 84
Corticosteroids, 69, 109, 113, 126
  chronic administration of, adrenal insufficiency secondary to, 52-59, 71
  in treatment of patients with
    duodenal ulcers, 99-100
    hepatitis, 103
    rheumatoid arthritis, 71
Cortisol, 53-59
Cortisone, 58, 193
Cortisone glucose tolerance test, 65
Cotton rolls, 161
Coumarin drugs, 117
Creatinine level in blood, test for renal function, 47, 49
Crowns
  porcelain-bonded-to-metal, 30, 41, 42
  porcelain-jacket, 41, 42
  telescoped, 167
Cushing's disease, 56, 57
Cyanocobalamin, 105, 107
Cyclic neutropenia, 112
Cytotoxins, 118
  use in suppression of kidney graft rejection, 49

D

Data, use in dental treatment planning
  analysis and synthesis, 3, 5
  collection, 3, 4-5
Data base, 328, 331-332, 334, 335, 336, 344-348
Debilitating diseases, role in periodontal disease, 163
Degenerative joint disease, 72-74
  characteristics, 72
  dental treatment planning considerations, 72-74
  medical management, 72
Demerol, 51
Dental care
  primary, 183, 185-187
  secondary, 183, 187-189
Dental caries
  gross, case example, 242-246
  prevention of
    primary level, 153-159
    secondary level, 161-162
Dental cases
  difficult, 215-234
    alternative treatment plans, 216-217
    dentist-patient relationship, 215-216
    examples, 218-234
    factors in, 216
    flexibility, 217
    interdisciplinary tooth replacement case, 200-214

Dental cases—cont'd
  interdisciplinary tooth replacement case—cont'd
    examples, 201-214
  simple, 192-199
    clinical findings, 192-193
    example, 193-199
    medical considerations, 193
    psychological considerations, 193
Dental floss, role in removal of plaque, 157, 160
Dental history of family, 149
Dental interview, 132-140
  nonverbal communication, 139-140
  process, 136
  purpose and goals, 132-134
  setting the stage, 136
  site, 134-136
    furniture arrangement, 135-136
    verbal communication, 136-139
Dental treatment planning; *see* Treatment planning
Dentiforms, use in case presentations, 295
Dentifrices and rinses, fluoride, 156
Dentist, general
  as coordinator of the team, 12-15
  dental laboratory and specialist availability for, 172-174
  experience and competence of, 171-172
  organization of, 292-293
  personal appearance and mannerisms of, 293-294
  professional attitude of, 293
  relationship with patient, 215-216
  time availability of, 172
Dentistry
  operative, preventive and prognostic aspects, 166
  restorative, 300-303
Denture wearers, irradiation in, 127
Dentures
  full, 33-34, 79
  overlay, 280-281
  partial
    case example, 205-210
    precision- or semiprecision-attachment, 276, 278, 279
    removable, 31-33, 79
      evaluations, 302-303
Depression as symptom of uremia, 46
Dermatitis, pruritic, 72
Dermatoses, 53
Desiccation, 162
Dexamethasone, 58
Dextranase, 158
Dextrans, 156, 158
Dextrostix, 65
Diabetes, 21, 186, 193, 267, 274
Diabetes insipidus, 122
Diabetes mellitus, 63-66, 122
  adult, 65
  dental treatment planning considerations, 66
  juvenile, 63, 65
  laboratory findings, 65
  medical management, 65-66

Diabetic coma, 185
Diabetic nephropathy, 63
Diagnosis, establishing of, in dental treatment planning, 3, 5
Diagnostic and therapeutic plans, 329-330, 332, 351-354
Diagrams, use in case presentation, 295
Dialysis
  hemodialysis, 48
  kidney; *see* Renal failure
  peritoneal, 48
Diaphragmatic hernia, 98-99
  dental treatment planning considerations, 98-99
  medical management, 98
Diazepam, 51, 62, 76
Diencephalic syndrome, 83
Diet, nondetergent, role in periodontal disease, 163
Difficult dental case, 215-234
  alternative treatment plans, 216-217
  dentist-patient relationship, 215-216
  examples, 218-234
  factors in, 216
  flexibility, 217
Digitalis, 87
Digits, clubbing of, 101, 102
Dilantin, 77
Diphenhydramine hydrochloride, 109
Diphenylhydantoin, 77
Disaccharides, 158
Disclosing solution, 157
Diuretic agents, 82
Dolder bar, 259
Dopamine, 87
Drug nephropathy, 44
Drug-induced hepatitis, 67
Drugs
  administration during pregnancy, 62
  anticholinergic, 122
  autoimmunogenic, 113
  myelosuppressive, 113
  parasympathomimetic, 122, 125
  psychotropic, 123
  reactions to, role in periodontal disease, 163
Ducts, Wharton's and Stensen's, 125
Duodenal ulcers, 99-100
Dysfunctional tooth contacts, 25

E

Eclampsia, 83
Economics of patient as consideration in dental treatment planning, 149, 317
Edema, pitting, role in renal failure, 46, 47
Edentulous ridges, conditions of, as consideration in dental treatment planning, 19, 24-25
Elderly patient, dental treatment planning for, 175-176, 316
Electric toothbrush, 162
Electrolytes, disturbances of, in renal failure, 45
Emergency dental care, 183, 185-186
Emphysema, 94-95

Encephalopathy, role in renal failure, 47
Endoarteritis, 50
Endocarditis, bacterial; see Bacterial endocarditis and rheumatic heart disease
Endocrine diseases, 52-59
Endocrine dysfunction, role in periodontal disease, 163
Endodontics, 37-39, 300-301
Endosseous implants, 270-274
    contraindications, 274
    indications, 270, 274
Endotoxins, 160
Epidemic hepatitis, 67-70
Epilepsy, 75, 174-175
Epileptic seizure, 185
Epinephrine, 86, 87, 96, 97
Erythema multiforme, 52
Erythremia, 110
Erythroblastosis fetalis, 105
Erythrocytes
    decrease in, as cause of anemia, 104, 105, 107-108
    increase in, as cause of polycythemia, 110-111
Erythrocytosis, 110
Erythromycin, 51, 62
    in treatment of patients with
        congenital heart disease, 93
            rheumatic heart disease and bacterial endocarditis, 91-93
Erythropoietin, role in renal failure, 45
Esophagitis, 98
Ethacrynic acid, 87
Eugenol, 162
Exostoses, 164
Extracorpuscular defects of erythrocytes, 104

F

Factor V, 116
Factor VIII, 116
    deficiency, 103, 115-116
Factor VIII protein, 46
Factor IX, 116
    deficiency, 115, 116
Factor X, 116
    deficiency, 103
Factor XI, 116
Fallot, tetralogy of, 93
Family dental history, 149
Fanconi's syndrome, 108
Fasting blood glucose test, 65
Fat-soluble vitamins, 101
Feedback as verbal communication, 137-138
Fetal injury as consideration in dental treatment planning, 59-62
Fibrinogen deficiency, 103
Financial resources of patient as consideration in dental treatment planning, 149, 317
Fissure and pit sealants, 156, 188
Fixed abutment tooth design for fixed bridge construction, 30
Fixed bridge construction for tooth replacement, 28-30, 31
    advantages, 30
    case example, 201-204

Fixed bridge construction for tooth replacement—cont'd
    causes of failure, 28-30
    disadvantages, 30
    evaluation, 301-302
Fixed partial prosthesis, preventive and prognostic aspects, 166-167
Floss, dental, 157, 160
Floss threaders, 157, 160
Fluoridation, communal, 155
Fluoride, 188, 259
    role in prevention of dental caries, 155-156
Fluoride dentifrices and rinses, 156
Fluoride tablets, 155
Focal seizure, 76-77
Folic acid, 105, 107, 111
Food impaction, role in periodontal disease, 163
Fructose, 158
Full dentures for tooth replacement, 33-34
    case example, 210-214
Furniture arrangements for dental interview, 135-136
Furosemide, 87
Fusospirochetal necrotizing gingivitis, 112

G

Gamma globulin, pooled, for prevention of hepatitis, 69
Gangrene, 63, 64
Gastric ulcers, 100
Gastroesophageal reflux, 98
Gastrointestinal diseases, 98-103
    cirrhosis of the liver, 101-103
    hepatitis, 100-101
    hiatal hernia, 98-99
    peptic ulcer, 99-100
Gelfoam, 115
Geriatric patient, treatment planning for, 175-176, 316
Gingival tissue, recession or loss of, 165
Gingivectomy, 164
Gingivitis, 159
    acute necrotizing ulcerative, 113, 121
    fusospirochetal necrotizing, 112
    prevention of, 162
Gingivoplasty, 164
Glomerular tuft, role in renal failure, 44, 45
Glomerulonephritis, 44
Glossitis in anemia, 107
Glucocorticoids, 56, 57
Glucose, 66, 158
Glucose tolerance test, 65
Glycoprotein, 156
Gold casting restorations, 41
Gold foil restorations, 41, 42
Gold salts, 71, 72
Gout, 70, 71
Graft rejection in kidney transplantation, 49
Gram-negative streptococci, 159
Grand mal seizure, 76, 77, 78-79
    status epilepticus, 76, 78
Group A beta hemolytic streptococci, 44, 89
Guanethidine, 82
Gynecomastia, 98, 101

H

Halothane, 101
Hard tissue, condition of, patient perceptions regarding, 146
Hay fever and asthma, 95-98
    dental treatment planning considerations, 96-98
    medical management, 96
HBsAg, 67, 68, 69, 70
Health questionnaire, 334, 337-340
Health-threatening systemic conditions, management of, 183, 186
Heart attacks, 63
Heart disease
    congenital, 93
    ischemic, 83-86
    rheumatic, and bacterial endocarditis, 89-93
Heart failure
    congestive, 86-89
    left-sided, 85, 86, 87
    right-sided, 86, 87
Heart murmurs, 90, 91
Heart valves, prosthetic, 92
Heartburn, 98
Heberden's node, 73
Hemarthrosis, 115
Hematocrit, 103, 104
Hematologic diseases, 103-122
    anemia, 104-110
    bleeding disorders, 113-115
    coagulation disorders, 115-117
    neoplasms, 118-122
    neutropenia, 111-113
    polycythemia, 110-111
Hematologic neoplasms, 118-122
    leukemia, 118-121
    lymphoma, 121-122
Hematuria, 45
Hemisections, 40, 274-276
    contraindications, 274, 276
    indications, 274
Hemodialysis, 48, 50-51
Hemoglobin
    decrease in, as cause of anemia, 104, 105, 107-108
    increase in, as cause of polycythemia, 110-111
Hemolytic anemias, 104-105, 108-109
Hemophilia
    A, 115-116
    B, 116
Hemosiderosis, 108
Heparin
    anticoagulant effect of, 51
    use during hemodialysis, 48
Hepatitis, 100-101, 110, 186
    A, 67-70
    B, 67-70, 153
    dental treatment planning considerations, 69-70
    medical management, 68-69, 101
    prevention, 69
Hepatomegaly, 101
Hepatosplenomegaly, 101, 105, 108, 121
Hernia

Hernia—cont'd
    diaphragmatic, 98-99
    hiatal, 98-99
Hiatal hernia, 98-99
    dental treatment planning considerations, 98-99
    medical management, 98
Hip replacement, total, 74
Histiocytes, 121
History taking, pitfalls in, 306-310
Hydralazine, 82
Hydrocortisone, 54, 58, 59
Hyperadrenalism, 56
Hyperglycemia, 65
Hyperinsulinism, 65
Hyperkalemia, 45, 47
Hyperparathyroidism, role in renal disease, 45
Hyperpigmentation of skin as symptom of uremia, 46
Hyperplasias, 83
Hyperpyrexia, 56
Hypertension, 81-83, 186
    essential, 81
        dental treatment planning considerations, 82-83
        medical management, 82
    secondary, 83
Hypertension, 216
    role in renal failure, 44, 46, 47
Hyperthyroidism, 84
Hypnotics, 62
    in treatment of symptoms of chronic renal failure, 47
Hypoalbuminemia, 98
Hypoglycemia, 65, 66
Hypoglycemics, oral, 63, 65, 66
Hypoplasia of teeth, 23
Hypoplastic anemias, 107-108, 109-110
Hypoprothrombinemia, 101, 103
Hypotension, 55, 56
    orthostatic, 82-83
Hypothalamus, 53
Hypothyroidism, 186
Hypoxia in pregnant dental patient, 62

I

Icterus, 68
Idealistic versus pragmatic dental treatment planning, 9-11
Idiopathic thrombocytopenic purpura (ITP), 113
IgG, antiplatelet, 113
Implants
    blade, 270, 271, 272, 273
    endosseous, 270-274
    pterygoid extension, 270
    ramus, 270
    subperiosteal, 268-270
Indomethacin, 71, 73
Infection
    deep, around joint prosthesis, 74-75
    orofacial, in diabetic patient, 64, 66
Infectious disease, 67-70
Infectious hepatitis, 67-70
Inhalants, steroid, 96

Insulin, 63, 65, 66
Interdisciplinary tooth replacement case, examples, 200-214
  fixed bridges, 201-204
  full dentures, 210-214
  partial dentures, 205-210
Intracardiac prosthesis, 93-94
Intracorpuscular defects of erythrocytes, 104
Intracranial pressure, elevated, 83
Intrinsic factor in vitamin B_{12} absorption, 107
Ionizing radiation, 111, 113, 126-128
Iron deficiency, induced, 110
Iron-deficiency anemia, 104, 105, 107-108, 122
Irradiated patients, 126-128
Irradiation, 159
  damage to fetus, 61
Ischemic heart disease, 83-86
  angina pectoris, 83-85
  myocardial infarction, 85-86
Isoproterenol, 87, 96, 97
ITP, 113

J

Jacksonian motor seizure, 77
Janeway lesions, 91
Jaundice, 68, 101
Jaws and oral mucous membranes, prevention of disease of, 153
Joint
  destruction of, 115
  diseases of, and bone diseases, 70-75
    arthritis, 70-74
    degenerative, 72-74
    prostheses, 72, 74-75
Jones criteria, modified, 91
Juvenile diabetes, 63, 65, 66
Juvenile periodontitis, 21

K

Kaopectate, 109
Ketoacidosis, 65
Ketone bodies, 66
Kidney
  disease of; *see* Renal failure
  polycystic, 44
Knee
  destruction of, 115
  replacement, total, 74

L

Lactic acidosis, 65
Lactobacilli, 159
Lactose, 158
Laennec's cirrhosis, 101, 102
Lead apron as safety precaution during radiation exposure, 61
Left-sided heart failure, 85, 86, 87
Lente insulin, 66
Leukemia, 118-121
  dental treatment planning considerations, 119, 121
  medical management, 118-119
Leukocytes, neutrophilic, depression of, as cause of neutropenia, 111

Leukopenia, 111, 113
Lichen planus, 52
Lidocaine, 51, 62, 74
Life-threatening dental care, 183, 185
Liver, disease of, 67-70, 101-103
Lymphocytes, 121
Lymphoma, 121-122
  dental treatment planning considerations, 122
  medical management, 122

M

Magnesium oxide, 99
Maintenance
  medical examination, 296-304
    periodontal evaluation, 299-300
    soft tissue examination, 298
    temporomandibular joint evaluation, 298-299
  monitoring and, 181, 183-184, 189-190
    in complex cases, 241-242
    in gross caries case, 244
    in interdisciplinary tooth replacement case, 210, 214
    in simple dental case, 199
  restorative dentistry, 300-303
  roentgenology, 303-304
Malaria, 104
Malignant hypertension, 81
Mandible, fracture of, 186
Mannitol, 158
Manual dexterity of patient as consideration in dental treatment planning, 174-175
Mastication
  muscles of, and temporomandibular joint, 19, 25-26
  role in periodontal disease, 163
  role in plaque accumulation, 160
  temporary management of conditions preventing, 187
Mechanical irritants, role in periodontal disease, 163
Megakaryocytes, 113
Menorrhagia, 104
Mental handicaps as pitfall in dental treatment planning, 316-317
Mental retardation, 174-175
Mental slowness as symptom of uremia, 46
Meperidine, 51
Mercurials, 87
Metallic poisoning, role in periodontal disease, 163
Methaneline, 97
Methotrexate, 107
Methyldopa, 82
Methylprednisolone, 58
Microangiopathy, 63
Microorganisms
  role in dental caries, 154, 156
  role in gingivitis, 159-160
Milk bottle syndrome, 159
Milontin, 77
Mineralocorticoid, 56
Models, use in case presentation, 295
Monamine-oxidase inhibitors, 82

Monitoring, 3, 7
  maintenance and, 181, 183-184
    in complex cases, 241-242
    in gross caries case, 244
    in interdisciplinary tooth replacement case, 210, 214
    in simple dental case, 199
Mononucleosis, 67
Monosaccharides, 158
Morphine, 85
Mouth breathing, 163
Mouth odor, patient perceptions regarding, 147
Mouthrinses and dentifrices, fluoride, 156
Mucogingival surgery, 164
Mucolytic agents, 158
Mucous membranes, oral, prevention of disease of, 153
Muscles of mastication and temporomandibular joint, 19, 25-26
Muscular disorders, 174-175
Muscular hyperactivity as symptom of uremia, 46
Mycostatin, 121, 128
Myelitis, ascending, 83
Myelomas, 118
Myelosuppressive drugs, 113
Myocardial infarction, 85-86, 185, 193
  dental treatment planning considerations, 85-86
  medical management, 85
Myofascial pain syndrome, 25-26, 35
Mysoline, 77

N

Neoplasms, 186
  hematologic, 118-122
    leukemia, 118-121
    lymphoma, 121-122
Neostigmine, 122
Nephritis, 44
Nephropathy
  diabetic, 63
  drug, 44
Nephrosclerosis, 45
Nervous system
  autonomic, 122
  central, 123
  sympathetic, 122
Neuritis, peripheral, 83
Neurologic diseases, 75-79
Neutropenia, 109, 111-113
  dental treatment planning considerations, 112-113
  medical management, 112
Neutrophils, 111-113
Newborn, hemolytic anemia of, 105
Nitrites, 84
Nitrogen compounds, role in renal failure, 45, 47
Nitroglycerin, 83, 84, 85
Nitrous oxide, 62
Nondetergent diet, role in periodontal disease, 163
Nonocclusion, role in periodontal disease, 163
Nonthreatening oral disease, management of, 183, 188-189
Nonverbal communication
  in case presentation, 292-294
  in dental interview, 139-140
NPH Iletin, 66
Nutrition, 188
  role in dental caries production, 158
  role in periodontal disease, 163
Nystatin, 50, 121, 128

O

Obstructive uropathy, 44
Occlusal considerations in dental treatment planning, 19, 25
Odontoblasts, 162
Odontotomy, prophylactic, 161
Odor of mouth, patient perceptions regarding, 147
Open heart surgery, 193
Open-ended questions, 137
Operative dentistry, preventive and prognostic aspects, 166
Oral conditions, threatening, management of, 183, 186-187
Oral contraceptives, 101
Oral disease, nonthreatening, management of, 183, 188-189
Oral emergencies, 183, 185-186
Oral findings as consideration in dental treatment planning, 19-42
  case classification for individual teeth, 27-35
    difficult case, 34-35
    simple case, 27
    tooth replacement case, 27-34
    transitional case, 35
  extraction, 35-36, 37
  major categories, 19-26
    edentulous ridges, conditions of, 19, 24-25
    occlusal considerations, 19, 25
    patient hygiene, 19, 20-21
    periodontium, pathology of, 19, 21-23
    salivary abnormalities, 19, 20
    soft tissue and bony pathology, 19-20
    teeth, pathology of, 19, 23-24
    temporomandibular joint and muscles of mastication, 19, 25-26
  questionable or borderline, 36
  retention, 36-42
    periodontal considerations, 39-40
    restorations, 41-42
    root canal treatment, 37-39
  treatment planning for individual teeth, 35-42
Oral hygiene, 20-21
  following periodontal surgery, 39
Oral hypoglycemics, 63, 65, 66
Oral mucous membranes and jaws, prevention of disease of, 153
Oral surgery, 264-267
  contraindications, 267
  indications, 266-267
Orofacial infection in diabetic patient, 64, 66
Orthodontia, 33, 34, 162
  improper, role in periodontal disease, 163

Index

Orthodontia—cont'd
  surgical, 264-267
    contraindications, 267
    indications, 266-267
Orthostatic hypotension, 82-83
Osler nodes, 91
Ostectomy, 164
Osteitis, condensing and rarefying, 38, 39
Osteoarthritis, 26, 72-74
  characteristics, 72
  dental treatment planning considerations, 72-74
  medical management, 72
Osteodystrophy, renal, role in renal failure, 45, 47
Osteomalacia, 101
  role in renal disease, 45
Osteomyelitis, 126
Osteoplasty, 164
Osteoradionecrosis, 126, 127
Overdentures, 256-259
  abutment designs, 259
  advantages, 257
  contraindications and maintenance, 259
  indications, 257-259
Overlay dentures, 280-281
  contraindications, 281
  indications, 281
Oxazolidinediones, 77

P

Pancreas, 63
Pancytopenia, 108
Panoramic roentgenograms, 303
Papaverine, 84
Paradione, 77
Paralysis as consideration in dental treatment planning, 174-175
Paramethadione, 77
Parasympathomimetic agents, 84, 122, 125
Parathormone, role in renal disease, 45
Parathyroid glands, role in renal disease, 45
Parkinson's disease, 160
Parotitis as symptom of uremia, 46
Partial dentures
  case example, 205-210
  fixed, 166-167
    precision- or semiprecision-attachment, 276, 278, 279
  removable, 31-33, 168, 302-303
Patent ductus arteriosus, 93
Patient
  attitudes toward dental treatment, 148-149
  background data base, 334, 335, 336
  case presentation to, 6
  consent form for, 341
  elderly, 175-176, 316
  examination of, 3, 4-5
  initial classification of, 3-4
  expectations of, 141-143
  financial resources, 149, 317
  hygiene of, 19, 20-21
  interview with, case example, 340

Patient—cont'd
  management of, pitfalls in, 305-319
    consultations with specialists, 313
    diagnosis, 314-315
    examination, 310-312
    history taking, 306-310
    prognosis, 318-319
    reception by dentist, 306
    special investigations, 312-313
    treatment plan, 315-318
  manual dexterity of, 174-175
  past experiences of, 143-146
  perceptions of, regarding oral condition, 146-147
    aesthetic appearance, 147
    hard tissue, condition of, 146
    mouth odor, 147
    soft tissue, condition of, 146-147
  physical examination data base, case example, 344-348
  problem identification, case example, 350-351
  resumé of, 341
  time availability of, 172
Penicillin, 51, 62
  in treatment of patients with
    congenital heart disease, 93
    rheumatic heart disease and bacterial endocarditis, 91-93
  use in prevention of dental caries, 158
Penicillin G, 92, 99
Penicillin V, 92, 99
Peptic ulcers, 99-100
  duodenal, 99-100
  gastric, 100
Percarbonate, 158
Periarteritis nodosa, 83
Pericarditis, 47
Periodontal disease, 21
  prevention of
    primary level, 153-154, 159-160
    secondary level, 162-164
    therapy in tertiary level, 164-165
Periodontal evaluation, 299-300
Periodontal therapy for retained teeth, 39-40
Periodontitis, 21, 159, 162-164, 274
  advanced, treatment of, 164-165
  hopeless, with tooth replacement, case example, 247-250
  moderate to severe, in patient with limited finances, case example, 247
Periodontium, pathology of, 19, 21-23
  etiologies, 21
  treatment, 21-23
Peripheral neuritis, 83
Peritoneal dialysis, 48
Pernicious anemia, 105, 109, 122
Petit mal seizure, 76, 77
Pharyngoesophageal ulcerations, 105
Phenacetin, 109
Phenergan, Syrup of, 50, 74
Phenformins, 65
Phenobarbital, 77
Phenothiazine tranquilizers, 111, 123

Phensuximide, 77
Phenylbutazone, 71, 72
Pheochromocytomas, 83
Phlebotomy, 110
Phosphatase, alkaline, 103
Phosphate, 45, 160
Photographs, use in case presentation, 295
Pilocarpine, 122, 125
Pin-retained bases and castings, 41
Pit and fissure sealants, 156, 188
Pitting edema, role in renal failure, 46, 47
Pituitary gland
  disorders of, 52, 53
  tumors of, 83
Pituitary-adrenal axis and feedback system, 53
Plaque, role in dental caries and periodontal disease, 154, 156, 159-160
  bacterial activity in, 156-158, 159-160
Plasma cells, 121
Platelet deficits, 113, 114
Plummer-Vinson syndrome, 105, 109
Polycystic kidney, 44
Polycythemia, 83, 95, 110-111
  dental treatment planning considerations, 111
  medical management, 110
Polycythemia vera, 110
Polypropylene, 83
Polysaccharides, 156, 158
Porcelain, 79
Porcelain-bonded-to-metal crowns, 30, 41, 42
Porcelain-jacket crowns, 41, 42
Postnecrotic cirrhosis, 101
Postprandial blood glucose test, 65
Potassium balance, 53
Pragmatic versus idealistic dental treatment planning, 9-11
Precision-attachment partial dentures, 276, 278, 279
  contraindications, 279
  indications, 279
Prednisolone, 58
Prednisone, 58, 59, 98
  use in suppression of kidney graft rejection, 49
Pregnancy, 59-62
  dental roentgenograms, 61
  drug administration, 62
  role in periodontal disease, 163
  treatment timing, 60-61
Prevention
  current measures evident at initial patient visit, 151-152
  home care improvement, evaluation of, 152
  primary level
    dental caries, 153-159
    oral mucous membranes and jaws, diseases of, 153
    periodontal disease, 153-154, 159-160
    systemic disease, 153
  in secondary dental care, 183, 187-188
  secondary level, 160-164
    dental caries, 161-162
  tertiary level, 164-165

Preventive and prognostic considerations in dental treatment planning, 151-170; see also Prevention
  fixed partial prosthesis, 166-167
  importance, 168
  operative dentistry, 166
  removable partial prosthesis, 168
Primary dental care, 183, 185-187
  emergency, 183, 185-186
  urgent, 183, 186-187
Primidone, 77
Pro-Banthine, 122
Problem list, 328-329, 332, 350-351
Problem-oriented dental record system, 323-333
  case example, 334-355
  components, 327-330
    data base, 328, 331-332, 334, 335, 336, 344-348
    diagnostic and therapeutic plans, 329-330, 332, 351-354
    problem list, 328-329, 332, 350-351
    progress notes, 330, 332-333, 354-355
  model, 330-333
Procaine penicillin G, 92
Progress notes, 330, 332-333, 354-355
Promethazine, 74
Propantheline bromide, 122
Propoxyphene, 51
Propranolol, 82, 84
Prosthesis
  fixed partial, 166-167
  heart valve, 92
  intracardiac, 93-94
  joint, 72, 74-75
  removable partial, 168, 302-303
Prosthodontics, removable, evaluations of, 302-303
Protamine sulfate, 51
Proteinuria, 45
Prothrombin deficiency, 103
Pruritic dermatitis, 72
Pruritus as symptom of uremia, 46
Pseudohemophilia, 116
Pseudoneutropenia, 111
Psychiatry in treatment of symptoms of chronic renal failure, 47
Psychomotor seizure, 76, 77
Psychosis as symptom of uremia, 46
Psychosocial considerations in dental treatment planning, 132-133
Psychosomatic factors in periodontal disease, 163
Psychotropic drugs, 123
Pteroylglutamic acid, 107
Pterygoid extension implant, 270
Pulmonary edema, 85, 86, 90
Pulpal disease, 38-39
Pulpitis, acute and chronic, 38
Pulpoperiapical lesions, 38
Purpura, 101
  intraoral, 117
Pyelonephritis, 44
Pyrosis, 98

Q

Questions, open- and closed-ended, in dental interview, 136, 137

R

Radiation
  ionizing, 111, 113, 126-128
  role in periodontal disease, 163
Radiation therapy, use in suppression of kidney graft rejection, 49
Ramus implant, 270
Rarefying osteitis, 38, 39
Rauwolfia alkaloids, 82
Record keeping in dental treatment planning, 3, 7-8
Records, 321-355
  problem-oriented dental record system, 323-333
    case example, 334-355
    components, 327-330
      data base, 328, 331-332, 334, 335, 336, 344-348
      diagnostic and therapeutic plans, 329-330, 332, 351-354
      problem list, 328-329, 332, 350-351
      progress notes, 330, 332-333, 354-355
    model, 330-333
Reflection as verbal communication, 138
Rehabilitation, 181, 183, 184, 190-191
  in interdisciplinary tooth replacement, 210, 214
  in simple dental case, 199
Removable partial denture for tooth replacement, 28, 31-33
  advantages, 32
  disadvantages, 32
  indications for, 31-32
  preventive and prognostic aspects, 168
Removable prosthodontics evaluations, 302-303
Renal disease, unilateral, 83
Renal failure, 44-52
  dental treatment planning considerations, 49-52
    chronic renal failure, 49-50
    dialysis, 50-51
    renal transplant, 51-52
  dialysis, 48
  etiology, 44
  medical management, 47
  pathophysiology, 44-45
  signs and symptoms, 45-47
  transplantation, 49
Renal osteodystrophy, role in renal failure, 45, 47
Renal tubules, role in renal failure, 44, 45
Renal vascular disease, 44
Renal vasculature, role in renal failure, 44, 45
Respiratory acidosis, 97
Respiratory diseases, 94-98
  chronic bronchitis, 95
  emphysema, 94-95
  hay fever and asthma, 95-98
Restorative dentistry, 300-303
  endodontics, 300-301

Restorative dentistry—cont'd
  fixed and operative evaluations, 301-302
  removable prosthodontics, 302-303
Rh incompatibility, 104, 105
Rheumatic carditis, 90
Rheumatic heart disease and bacterial endocarditis, 50, 89-93
  dental treatment planning considerations, 91-93
  medical management, 91
Rheumatic valvulitis, 90
Rheumatoid arthritis, 52, 70-72
  characteristics, 72
  medical management, 71-72
Rhinitis, allergic, 95
Ridge extensions, 267-268
  contraindications, 267-268
  indications, 267
Right-sided heart failure, 86, 87
Rinses and dentifrices, fluoride, 156
Roentgenology, 303-304
Root amputations, 40, 41, 274-276, 277, 278
  contraindications, 274, 276
  indications, 274
Root canal treatment, 37-39, 166
Root caries, 165
Root sensitivity, 165
Rubber dams, 97, 161
Rubella, 93

S

Salicylates, 71, 72
Saliva
  artificial, 128
  role in dental caries, 159
Salivary abnormalities, 19, 20
Salivary gland
  infection of, 186
  xerostomia and, 122-128
Scleroderma, 34, 174
Sealants, pit and fissure, 156, 188
Secondary dental care, 183, 187-189
  interim evaluation of therapy and nonthreatening conditions, 183, 189
  nonthreatening oral disease, management of, 183, 188-189
  prevention, 183, 187-188
  provisional aesthetic and functional management, 183, 189
Secondary hypertension, 83
Sedatives, 47, 62
Seizure disorders, 75-79
  dental treatment planning considerations, 77-79
  etiology, 75
  medical management, 77
  types, 76-77
    focal seizure, 76-77
    grand mal seizure, 76, 77, 78-79
      status epilepticus, 76
    petit mal seizure, 76
    psychomotor seizure, 76

Semiprecision-attachment partial dentures, 276, 278, 279
　contraindications, 279
　indications, 279
Sequencing and flexibility of treatment planning, 179-191
　categories, 183-191
　criteria, 182-183
Serum glutamic-oxaloacetic transaminase (SGOT), 68, 103
Serum hepatitis, 67-70
Shunts, cardiovascular, in cyanotic and acyanotic anomalies, 93
Sickle cell disease, 104, 105, 108-109
Sideropenic dysphagia, 105
Silence as verbal communication, 137-138
Silicates, 162
Simple dental case, 192-199
Sinusitis, 95
Sjögren's syndrome, 122, 123, 124, 159
Skin, hyperpigmentation of, as symptom of uremia, 46
Smoking, 21, 94, 95, 96, 99, 188
Snyder test, 158-159
SOAP format, 330, 355
Sodium
　depletion of, role in renal failure, 45, 47
　imbalance of, 53
Sodium bicarbonate, 73, 97
Sodium fluoride, 155
Sodium monofluorophosphate dentifrice, 156
Soft tissue
　bony pathology and, 19-20
　condition of, patient perceptions regarding, 146-147
　examination, 298
Solucortef; see Hydrocortisone
Sorbitol, 158
Speech, temporary management of conditions preventing, 187
Spherocytosis, hereditary, 104
Spironolactones, 87
Spleen, 113
Splenectomy, 108, 112, 113
Splenomegaly, 91
Spontaneous abortion, 59-60
Sprue, 107
Squamous cell carcinoma of oral cavity, 20
Stabilization, 181, 183, 184, 185-189
　in complex cases, 241-242
　in gross caries case, 244
　in interdisciplinary tooth replacement case, 210, 214
　in simple dental case, 198-199
Staining of teeth, 23
Stannous fluoride gel, 126, 155, 156
Starch, 158
Status epilepticus, 76, 78
Steatorrhea, 101
Stem cell leukemia, 118
Stem cells, 121
Stensen's ducts, 125
Steroid inhalants, 96
Steroids, 109, 118, 267, 268, 274

Steroids—cont'd
　chronic administration of, adrenal insufficiency secondary to, 52-59, 71
　use in suppression of kidney graft rejection, 49
　in treatment of dental patients with asthma, 98
Stomatitis, 73, 105, 112
　chronic, 186
　as symptom of uremia, 46
　treatment of, in dental patients with chronic renal failure, 50
　ulcerative, 72
Streptococci
　gram-negative, 159
　group A beta hemolytic, 44
　viridans, 91
Streptococcus mutans, 156
Streptococcus organisms, 91
Streptomycin, 62, 92
Stress from dental procedures precipitating asthmatic attacks, 97
Strokes, 63, 160
Subacute bacterial endocarditis, 50
Subperiosteal implants, 268-270
　contraindications, 270
　indications, 270
Sucrose, 156
　role in dental caries, 158-159
Sugar, role in dental caries, 158-159
Sulfadiazine, 91
Sulfonylureas, 65
Sulfur dioxide, 94
Support as verbal communication, 138
Supracontacts, 25
Sympathetic nervous system, 122
Sympathomimetic amines, 87
Syncope in supine pregnant dental patient, 60-61
Syphilis, 67, 153
Syrup of Phenergan, 50, 74
Systemic conditions, health-threatening, management of, 183, 186
Systemic disease, prevention of, 153
Systemic lupus erythematosus, 53, 113

T
Telescoped crown, 167
Temporomandibular joint, 188
　evaluation, 298-299
　muscles of mastication and, 19, 25-26, 35
Testes, atrophic, 98
Tetracycline, 51, 62, 99
Tetralogy of Fallot, 93
Thalassemia, 104, 105, 106, 109
Thalidomide, 93
Thiazides, 82, 87
Thrombocytopenia, 109, 113, 114-115, 118
Thrombocytosis, 114-115
Thyroid storm, 185
Thyrotoxicosis, 83
Tobacco, 153
Tomes' fibers, 162
Tooth (teeth)
　as aspect in periodontal therapy, 39-40, 165

Tooth (teeth)—cont'd
  individual
    case classification for, 27-35
    treatment planning for, 35-42
      extraction, 35-36, 37
      questionable or borderline teeth, 36
      retention, 35, 36-42
  interdisciplinary replacement case, examples, 200-214
  pathology of, 19, 23-24
  restorations of, 41-42
  role in plaque accumulation, 160
  root canal treatment, 37-39, 166
  susceptibility to dental caries, 155-156
Toothbrush
  electric, 162
  use in removing plaque, 157, 160
Toothbrushing, improper, role in periodontal disease, 163
Total hip replacement, 74
Total knee replacement, 74
Toxic hepatitis, 67
Tranquilizers, 84, 85
  phenothiazine, 111, 123
Transitional dental case, 235-259
  case presentation, 238-239
  case reevaluation and monitoring, 239
  early identification, 237
  examples
    complex case with severe medical problems, 239-241
    complex cases that have failed in stabilization or monitoring stages, 241-242
    gross caries, 242-246
    hopeless periodontitis with tooth replacement, 247-250
    moderate to severe periodontitis in patient with limited finances, 247
    overdentures, 256-259
    treatment to improve aesthetics only, 250-256
  general approach, 237
  patient attitudes, 237-238
Transplantation, kidney; see Renal failure
Treatment-oriented dental record system, 323-324, 326, 327
Treatment planning
  behavioral considerations in, 131-150
  case presentation, 3, 6, 282-295
    communication skills, 290-295
      nonverbal, 292-294
      verbal, 290-292
      visual aids, 294-295
    considerations to increase effectiveness, 287-290
      treatment-plan summary letter, 287-290
    format, 283-287
      areas of concern, 284
      conclusions, 286-287
      consequence of neglecting treatment, 284
      establishing mutual goals of therapy, 285-286
      introduction, 283-284
      policies, 286

Treatment planning—cont'd
  case presentation—cont'd
    format—cont'd
      treatment plan proposal, 284-285
  dental laboratory and specialist availability, 172-174
  development of plan, 140-149
    attitudes, 148-149
    economics, 149, 317
    family dental history, 149
    past experiences, 143-146
    patient expectations, 141-143
    perceptions regarding oral condition, 146-147
  difficult case, 215-234
  for elderly patient, 175-176, 316
  innovative approaches in, 263-281
  interdisciplinary tooth replacement case, 200-214
  manual dexterity of patient, 174-175
  medical considerations, 43-130; see also specific entries
  operator experience and competence, 171-172
  operator and patient time availability, 172
  oral findings as consideration in, 19-42
  patient management and, pitfalls in, 305-319
  pragmatic versus idealistic, 9-11
  records, 321-355; see also Records
  role of general dentist in, 12-15
  sequence and flexibility, 179-191
  simple case, 192-199
  steps in, 3-8
    analysis and synthesis of data, 3, 5
    case presentation and adoption of plan, 3, 6
    data collection, 3, 4-5
    development of plan, 3, 6
    implementation of plan, 3, 7
    initial classification of patient, 3-4
    monitoring, 3, 7
    record keeping, 3, 7-8
  transitional case, 235-259
Tridione, 77
Trimethadione, 77
Tuberculosis, 52, 67
Tylenol, 62

U

Ulcerations, pharyngoesophageal, 105
Ulcerative stomatitis, 72
Ulcers
  duodenal, 99-100
  gastric, 100
  peptic, 99-100
Ultralente insulin, 66
Upper respiratory tract
  chemoprophylactic regimens for dental procedures involving, 92-93
  infection of, 44
Uremia, 44, 45
Uremic frost as symptom of uremia, 46
Urgent dental care, 183, 186-187
Urinary glucose and acetone test, 65
Uropathy, obstructive, 44

V

Valium, 51, 62, 76
Valves, heart, prosthetic, 92
Valvular disease, 91
Vancomycin, 92
VA-Oralube, 128
Varnish, 162
Vascular disease, renal, 44
Venereal disease, 186
Ventricular fibrillation, 85
Verbal communication
  in case presentation, 290-292
  in dental interview, 136-139
Viral hepatitis, 67-70
Viridans streptococci, 91
Visual aids in case presentation, 294-295
Vitamin(s)
  A, 101
  B_{12}, 105, 107, 111
  C, 117
  D, 47, 101
  fat-soluble, 101
  K, 101, 103, 116, 117

Von Willebrand's disease, 116

W

Water, use in restorative dentistry, 161
Weight loss, 55
Wharton's ducts, 125
White, S. S., cavity liners, 162

X

Xerostomia, 122-128
  dental treatment planning considerations, 125-126
  irradiated patients and, 126-128
  oral findings, 123, 125
Xylitol, 158
Xylocaine, 74
Xylose, 158

Z

Zinc oxide eugenol, 166